"The book is fantastic and very comprehensive! I really enjoyed reading it. It is much more in depth and informative than anything available. The format is great as well— very easy to follow, and the standard format between chapters makes it easy to use it as a reference guide after an initial read-through. I learned about several items that I had been afraid to try, too! "

—Laurie R., living in Singapore
with allergies to corn, dairy, eggs, gluten, nuts, and soy

"This book is amazing! It's packed full of so much information if I just want to eat down the street or going on vacation in the states. I'll also bring it with me when I travel to Europe for the first time. I think it's terrific that you are filling a need that no one else has been addressing. Great job!!"

—Dawn W., living in Chicago, IL with allergies to corn, soy and wheat

"I can't tell you how excited I am by your book. I have a severe allergy to soy that I developed in my late 20's. Since then I too have figured out how to eat out (out of necessity!) in the US. I'm still struggling when I travel overseas. In fact, I'm going to Germany, France and the UK next month and am panicked about what to do with eating. Just today, I had my allergist prescribe 4 EPI pens for me just in case."

(After her trip)…" Your information was very helpful and gave me the confidence that I would likely have no issues eating out overseas and I did not. Again, I can't tell you how excited I am by what you are doing and thank you."

—Debbie P., living in New York, NY with an allergy to soy

"I have read your book and it is excellent. It is true that us Brits eat a lot of Indian food especially living so close to Birmingham, where we are told Chicken Tikki Masala originated. I think you got the recipes spot on, especially when you use proper English words like coriander instead of cilantro!!!"

—Margaret W., living in Shustoke, UK with an allergy to wheat

Family members supporting loved ones living with food allergies and specialized diets say:

"My oldest daughter has celiac and I am glad to know that you are improving the lifestyle for someone like my daughter—I appreciate it and I am sure when she eventually comes of age (a little to hard to comprehend at 3 years old), she will also appreciate the path that you are plowing for her!"

—John A., a father, living in San Francisco, CA
with a daughter diagnosed with celiac/coeliac disease

"I just want to say that I am greatly inspired by your book. I truly believe you are doing something that may even save people's lives, not to mention return to them a quality of life they are surely longing for."

—Janie G., a daughter, living in Chicago, IL with a father allergic to wheat

Culinary professionals serving guests with food allergies and specialized diets say:

"A well researched and interesting book allowing the reader to get good background knowledge about the cuisines, the different cultures and the ingredients used. The breakdown of each dish gives the reader the opportunity to see where any hidden allergy foods may be or what questions they need to ask in the restaurant to ensure that their meals are safe to eat."

—Tariq Z., restaurant owner in Birmingham, England

"Your new book is fascinating. It will help to change the social conscience of our population and significantly impact lives. A young woman once commented that waiters often rolled their eyes because of her diet constraints. She said she'd rather not bother dining out. This is absurd considering over three million Americans suffer from celiac/coeliac disease."

—Matthew M., restaurant industry veteran in Chicago, IL

Let's Eat Out!
Your Passport to
Living Gluten and Allergy Free

Kim Koeller & Robert La France

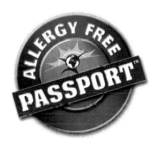

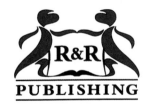

PUBLISHING

LCCN 2005929744

Front Cover photos (left to right):
PhotoDisc/Getty Images; Masterfile; Stockbyte/Getty Images.

Interior photos provided by:
Brand X Pictures™, Creatas Images, Digital Vision, Getty Images®, Ingram, Istockphoto™, MedioImages™, Photodisc®, Shutterstock™, and Thinkstock™ Images.

Book design: Emily Brackett/Visible Logic, Chicago, IL

Published by:
R & R Publishing, LLC
446 N. Wells, Ste. 254
Chicago, IL 60610
info@rnrpublishing.com
http://www.rnrpublishing.com

ISBN 0-9764845-0-1

Dedication

This book is dedicated to our parents:

Vivi	Norma
&	&
Ed	Roland

Thank you for your love, confidence and continuous encouragement.
You've helped us follow and realize our dreams all of our lives.

— For our angels Robbie and Robert —

Acknowledgements

Let's Eat Out! has been made possible by the collaborative efforts of our team, advisors, family and friends. You have inspired us to deliver this pioneering book and helped to achieve our vision. We are forever grateful for your gifts of time, great ideas and never-ending support.

We would like to thank our team for their energy, enthusiasm and expertise in helping to make this book and business foundation a reality including: Richard La France, Katie Koeller, Christopher Bodenner, Emily Brackett, Ellen Senrich, Janie Gabbett, John Myers, Maureen Zabloudil, Gene Jacobs, Bart Lazar, Bob Sell, Bennett Berg, Paula Carlin, Diane MacWilliams, Cal Thixton, Malka Greene, John Uppgren and John Park.

Thank you to our Board of Directors—Faris Aoun, Michael McEachran, and Brad Rugger for challenging our thinking. We are especially grateful to our allergy and health advisors for their insights, recommendations and commitment including: Michelle Melin-Rogovin, Shelley Case, Barbara Griffin, Dr. Christy Furey, Laurie Rosini, Dawn Warner, Margaret Williams, Nijie Relaeh and Margaret Phillip. Special thanks to our culinary advisors who confirmed the cuisine content including: Crystal Crawley, Arber Murici, Lumi Devine, Freddy Sanchez, Billy Wilcoxen, Sueson Vess, Lisa Artz, Tim Gannon, Laura Cherry, domenica catelli, Tariq Zaman, Samir Majmudar, Pam Panyasiri, Nicolas Bergerault, Stephane Tremolani, Alfredo Rosiv and Jeff Dattilo.

We appreciate the continued guidance and encouragement that we have received from our business advisors including: Peter Guidew, Beth Miles-Barry, Laura Roberts, Consuelo Martinez, Dr. Salvador Antonio Martinez-Matiella, Kim Olson, Lisa Carney, Jan Sabelstrom, Pat Veverica, Paula Carney, Vivi & Ed Koeller, Norma & Roland La France Sr., Scott Boone, Mark Jacobson, Ryan LaSalle, Julia Reiter, Jon Karp, Andrea Au, Deb Miller, Colleen Koeller, Dennis Sakurai, Zack Klein, Paul Nevarez, Nick Sanzo, Tim Pritchard, Lawrence Anderson, Jay Tindall, Eva Mangas, Jeff Field, Catherine Caldwell, Nicolas Guenat, Patty Frost and Marianna Dumont.

From Kim, a special thanks to the health professionals who helped "put me back together" throughout the years including: Dr. Mildred Geiger, Dr. Margaret Hannon, Dan Cubacub, Dr. John Hefferon, Dr. Preston Wolin, David Buchanan, Dr. Rocky Yapp, Suzanne Shaw, Jan Hamlin, Todd Nelson, Eriks Jekabsons, Dr. Kenneth Schiffman, Karen Granato, Beverly Holcomb, Dr. Lorene Wu, Dr. Dean Politis, Josette Pritchett, Dane Baptiste, Leslie Stevenson, Carol Kats and Alan Wolf.

Happy and healthy travels wherever your journeys may lead you—be it around the corner or around the world.

—Kim and Robert

Intention of This Book

This book—*Let's Eat Out! Your Passport to Living Gluten and Allergy Free,* is intended to provide information useful to people living with food allergies and specialized diets. AllergyFree Passport™, LLC as the authors, R & R Publishing, LLC as the publisher, the contributors and reviewers of this book (collectively "we") have made reasonable efforts to make sure that the information provided is accurate and complete. We believe that factual information contained in this book was correct to the best of our knowledge at the time of publication. However, we do not warrant or guarantee that any of the information is accurate or complete. It is not possible for us to have gathered all the information available or independently analyzed or tested the information.

We assume no responsibility for errors, inaccuracies, omissions or typographical errors contained in this book. We expressly disclaim responsibility for any adverse effects arising from the use or application of the information contained herein, as well as responsibility for any liability, injury, loss or damage, whether it be actual, special, consequential, personal or otherwise, which is incurred or allegedly incurred as a direct or indirect consequence of the use and application of any of the contents of this book or for references made within it.

The information contained in this book should not be viewed as medical advice. Questions regarding specific food allergies, specialized diets, drug and food interactions and anything related to a specific individual should be addressed to a doctor or other medical practitioner.

We are not responsible for any goods and/or services referred to in this book. By providing this information, we do not endorse any business or advocate the use of any products or services referred to in this book, and the owners or operators of the businesses referred to in this book do not endorse AllergyFree Passport™, LLC or R & R Publishing, LLC. We expressly disclaim any liability relating to the use of any goods and/or services referred to in this book.

Although the authors and the publishers of this book are appreciative of the support and information received, AllergyFree Passport™, LLC and R & R Publishing, LLC are not affiliated with (and have not received any compensation from or related to) any of the individuals, products, organizations, associations, airlines, restaurants or businesses identified in this book.

Contents

French Cuisine

Indian Cuisine

Italian Cuisine

Mexican Cuisine

Thai Cuisine

Chapter Overview

Breakfast Meal and Side Dish Overview

Sample Breakfast Menu

Breakfast Quick Reference Guide

Chapter Overview

Allergy Awareness in Beverages

Non-Alcoholic Beverage Suggestions

Non-Alcoholic Beverage Quick Reference Guide

Alcoholic Beverage Suggestions

Alcoholic Beverage Quick Reference Guide

Chapter Overview

Snack and Light Meal Overview

No Preparation Suggestions: Sample Shopping Checklist

Hot Water Preparation Suggestions: Sample Shopping Checklist

Cooler Required Suggestions: Sample Shopping Checklist

Snack and Light Meal Quick Reference Guide

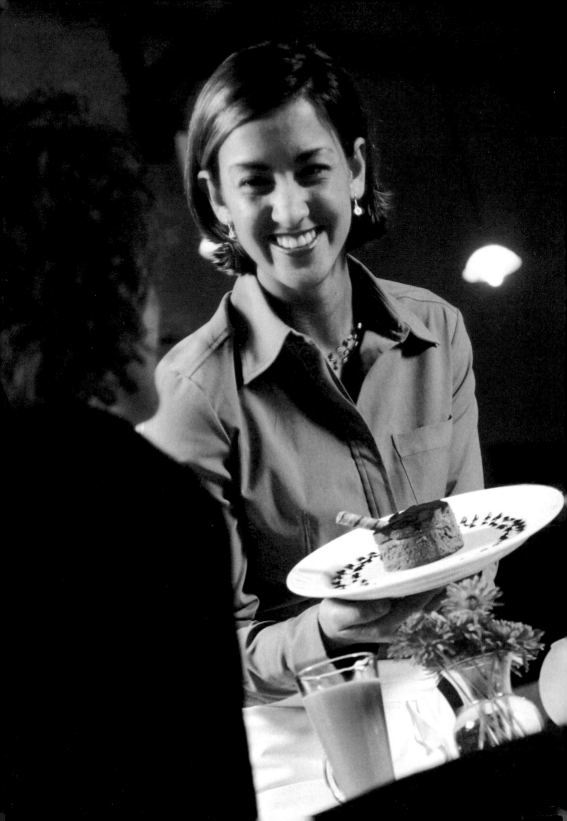

*"If I have helped just one person in exploring
a new location, be it in the city or country side,
within their own country and/or on foreign lands,
I will feel as though I have succeeded."*
—Ralph Waldo Emerson

Introduction

Overview

Let's Eat Out! Your Passport to Living Gluten and Allergy Free is the first book dedicated to eating outside the home by cuisine while managing 10 common food allergens including: corn, dairy, eggs, fish, gluten, peanuts, shellfish, soy, tree nuts and wheat. This pioneering effort focuses on what you can eat by providing allergy considerations for 175-plus sample menu items from seven international cuisines. The book is designed to facilitate a safe eating experience whether you are traveling around the corner from your home or around the world.

This book was written to help those impacted by specialized diets from seven varying perspectives. It is intended to assist each of you who:

1. Have food allergies, intolerances and sensitivities

2. Have celiac/coeliac disease

3. Have auto-immune related diseases that may benefit from a specialized diet

4. Choose to follow special diets based upon lifestyle preferences

5. Support or have the desire to help individuals with special dietary needs such as family, friends, and business colleagues

6. Serve individuals requiring specialized diets such as restaurant staff and management as well as educate professionals in culinary institutions

7. Treat individuals impacted by dietary considerations, such as health professionals including physicians, gastro-enterologists, nutritionists, naturopaths and dieticians

This book can be used as a daily resource, a reference guide, an educational tool or a training manual depending upon your perspective. We hope it meets your diverse needs and empowers you with the knowledge to achieve your desired gluten and allergy-free objectives.

This introduction addresses background information on the:

• Book approach

• Birth of our idea

• Book design and methodology

Book Approach

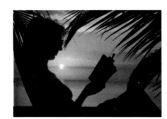

The book is organized in a manner that allows you to use the information in a number of different ways. One of our key guiding principles was to develop an easy-to-use guide that is succinct and flexible to meet an individual's needs. 50% of the content details seven international cuisines and specific menu items. The remainder is devoted to practical eating and travel guidelines concerning snacks, beverages, airlines, and multi-lingual phrases, as well as references for stores, associations, web sites and reading materials.

As with any book, it can be read cover to cover as a reference guide, or if you prefer, by chapter or appendix depending upon what topics you are most interested in learning about. It is also written in a format that allows you to skip around and focus on one or more specific chapters without reading the entire book. Each chapter stands on its own. It's all about your needs, preferences and areas of concern during that particular moment of the day.

For example, if you're planning to go to an Italian restaurant, you may want to learn about Italian cuisine, potential menu items, associated guidelines and how to navigate through the restaurant menu. If you're going to purchase gluten and allergy-free products that day and need a shopping checklist, you can flip to the snack and light meal chapter to review applicable suggestions or view the appendix for potential stores. If you're going to meet friends for breakfast, you can review the breakfast chapter to investigate potential allergy-free menu options. If you're going to a restaurant and just need to re-familiarize yourself on possible choices or want a "cheat sheet" to bring with you to help guide your choices, you can view the Quick Reference Guides. If you are booking airline tickets and want to request an allergy-free meal, you could reference the airline chapter for special meal availability and contact information. The list goes on and on.

Birth of Our Idea
After years of misdiagnosis, Kim learned that she had allergies and intolerances to dairy, fish, seafood, pork, chemicals and preservatives. She was also told that she had an autoimmune disease spelled celiac disease in North America or coeliac throughout other parts of the world. This is a permanent intolerance to gluten (the protein found in wheat, rye and barley) which can only be controlled by strictly adhering to a gluten-free diet. When she first received this comprehensive diagnosis, she felt relief that her team of specialists finally figured it out and had names for "it".

From her perspective, she relates the following: "I just sat there dumbfounded thinking, "Wow! How do you even spell these words? What in the world do they mean? What exactly is my diagnosis? What do I do? What is gluten? What are hidden allergens? More importantly, what can I eat when I'm away from home either in Chicago, traveling in the States or overseas? How do I eat in airports and hotels?"

Intro

Typically after diagnosis, many people think just the opposite, "What meals can be prepared at home? What cookbooks can be purchased? How can my favorite recipes be modified? How do I ensure that my home is gluten and allergy-free? What items and brands can I purchase?" Eating outside the home and travel may or may not be on many people's priority list.

For Kim, learning to eat anywhere and traveling with all of her allergies was priority number one. Global travel was an integral part of her personality and career. She had already flown over a million miles by this time, eating 80% of her meals away from home, and was not willing to give up what she loved to do, both from a personal and professional standpoint. In order to continue with her lifestyle, she needed to figure out how to eat gluten and allergy-free food anywhere in the world, regardless of her location or destination.

As a result, she conducted extensive research to determine how to eat outside the home and travel safely. She scoured over 100 web sites, subscribed to allergy-related publications and joined 20-plus international allergy and celiac/coeliac associations. She also read over 40 books, numerous publications and hundreds of articles on allergies, auto-immune diseases and celiac/coeliac disease.

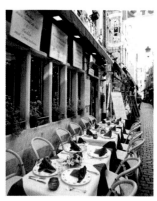

The focus of this literature was either on gluten and allergy-free cooking in the home or background information about coping with allergies. A very small percentage of these books discussed eating in restaurants and traveling with gluten and other food allergies. She was very surprised to realize that books devoted to these topics had not been written. She then contacted 100-plus global associations for information, researched various cities and traveled to numerous destinations. She explored many restaurants and stores first hand, and sampled local cuisines and available snacks. Realizing how valuable this research could be for other individuals living with food allergies and specialized diets, friends and family encouraged her to write a book that could help people on a global basis.

Based upon Kim's dining experiences with Robert and his extensive background in the restaurant industry, they began to experiment with restaurants and menu items. From Kim and Robert's standpoint, "We went through extensive trial and error determining what foods to eat in restaurants, what are the safest menu items, and what has the highest probability of having hidden allergens. We started to develop our own list of what questions to ask and what areas of food preparation may pose the biggest concerns. We began to identify what could make things easier on the restaurant staff and what could simplify the ordering process for both the guest and the server while still ensuring a safe dining experience. Then, we decided to team up to share this knowledge, coupled with more extensive research to empower individuals with food allergies and specialized diets to eat outside the home, travel and explore the world." Voilá! The idea for the book that you are reading was born!

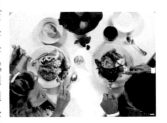

Design and Methodology

The contents of this book are based on years of personal experience, extensive research, proven results and the collaborative efforts of many individuals and organizations around the world. We have organized the book's contents into the following six areas to give you a better understanding of how each was researched, designed, tested and confirmed:

- Eating outside the home approach

- Ingredient and preparation technique guidelines

- International cuisines

- Quick reference guides

- Eating and travel suggestions

- Our personal perspectives

- Resource and reference materials

Eating Outside the Home Approach— Chapter 1

This chapter focuses on eating outside the home while managing food allergies and specialized diets. In addition to our personal experience, we consulted many individuals impacted by food allergies to get a better understanding of what personal factors influence them on a daily basis and alter their approach to eating outside the home. We also consulted with numerous restaurant and culinary professionals to identify key areas of considerations in handling special dietary requests. Based upon these factors, we have developed suggestions and recommended approaches to eating out from both the guest and restaurant perspectives.

Ingredient and Preparation Technique Guidelines—Chapter 2

Key ingredients and food preparation techniques that you need to understand to successfully navigate through a restaurant menu are outlined, based upon your dietary requirements. Basic areas of food preparation where common allergens may exist are discussed, as well as common food allergy myths and product labeling regulations. This information has been confirmed by culinary experts from all over the world.

Questions and requests are also provided to facilitate mutual understanding between you and the restaurant staff as to your specific needs. These were derived through personal experience, consultation with individuals impacted by food allergies and restaurant professionals. In many cases, these questions and requests may give you a sense of comfort, knowing that the restaurant staff understands your special dietary requirements. They may also educate your server about the areas of food preparation where common allergens may be hidden. This collaborative effort helps improve the level of awareness in the restaurant industry, as well as increase your personal comfort level when dining out.

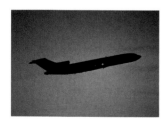

International Cuisines— Chapters 3 through 9

We have researched seven of the most common international cuisines you can find around the world, regardless of location or destination. These cuisines include American Steak and Seafood, Chinese, French, Indian, Italian, Mexican and Thai. The chapter format is standardized across the cuisines, allowing the reader to easily recognize each section of information. This content and structure are the result of years of development, consultation with individuals and extensive testing in North America and Europe. Through trial and error, this format has proven to be effective in disseminating the necessary information for each cuisine.

Each chapter begins with an overview, detailing background information on the history, culture, standard ingredients and traditional preparation techniques that are indicative of the cuisine. Since the culinary world is a constantly changing discipline, this information gives you a better understanding of the factors involved in the evolution of the cuisine and the development of traditional practices.

Gluten Awareness details the areas of food preparation you must consider in order to effectively adhere to a gluten-free diet. These areas of food preparation are explained in detail and a series of requests are presented to help simplify the ordering process. Many of these considerations are identical from chapter to chapter, while others may vary slightly based upon cuisine.

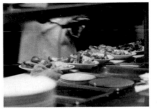

Other Allergy Considerations identify the potential sources of hidden food allergens that may be present in a cuisine based upon both traditional and non-traditional culinary practices. Through our research, we noticed a common theme across all cuisines: practicality. There are many reasons why a restaurant may incorporate non-traditional culinary practices into their cuisine. Lack of availability, associated costs of importing special ingredients and regular customers' preferences can influence an establishment's approach to cooking.

Dining Considerations outline relevant service styles for each cuisine. We describe what to expect from a dining experience based on meal schedules and cultural customs. Regardless of your location or destination, we have also included information on how menus may be presented.

Sample Cuisine Menus identify the name of each dish in its native language with the English equivalent. In the case of cuisines from countries that do not use the Latin alphabet, such as India and Thailand, we have provided the names of each dish phonetically. In our global research, we discovered that international cuisines often present each menu item in the language of the country you are in, as well as the native language. Whether you are enjoying an Italian restaurant in Amsterdam or eating Thai food in Brussels, this information can help you navigate the menu and make informed choices based upon your special dietary needs.

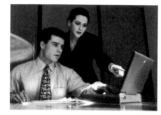

We researched cuisine menus and recipes from all over the world to determine which items are most commonly found in each cuisine. Once established, we reviewed each menu item to determine which dishes had the highest likelihood of being gluten/wheat-free. We further narrowed the selection by determining which menu items had the highest likelihood of not including the eight other common food allergens discussed in this book.

Cuisine Menu Item Descriptions summarize each dish's ingredients and the culinary preparation techniques involved in its creation. We determined what areas of food preparation had to be confirmed with the restaurant to ensure each dish was gluten/wheat-free, what other common food allergens could be potentially included and the areas of food preparation that must be questioned to ensure an allergy-free dining experience. After each description, we outline the following concerns:

Gluten-Free Decision Factors:
- "Ensure" an ingredient is not present as part of the food preparation

- "Request" an item is not included or inquire about a substitution

Food Allergen Preparation Considerations:
- "Contains" an allergen from an ingredient in alphabetical order

- "May contain" an allergen from an ingredient in alphabetical order

This information has been further confirmed by culinary experts and tested by various individuals impacted by specialized diets on a global basis.

Cuisine Quick Reference Guides— Chapter 10

The *Cuisine Quick Reference Guides* are designed to give the reader easy access to information previously discussed in each cuisine chapter. Each of the ten common food allergens discussed in this book have been color coded for easy reference in the following manner:

- Brown for corn and soy
- Yellow for dairy and gluten/wheat
- Blue for fish and shellfish
- Green for peanuts and tree nuts
- Pink for eggs

Color Key for the Quick Reference Guides

Corn–dark brown
Soy–light brown
Dairy–light yellow
Gluten/wheat–dark yellow
Fish–dark blue
Shellfish–light blue
Peanuts–dark green
Tree Nuts–light green
Eggs–pink

The Quick Reference Guides provide an overview of each item in the respective cuisine sample menus and indicate whether a dish "typically contains" or "may contain" an allergen. These guides highlight what you need to be aware of to order specific menu items, avoid specific allergens and adhere to your specialized diet at a glance.

Eating and Travel Suggestions— Chapters 11 through 15

These helpful suggestions are designed to assist you while eating outside the home and traveling across the globe. Breakfast, beverages, snacks and light meals, airlines and essential multilingual phrases are discussed individually in these chapters. Each chapter begins with a standardized overview outlining the structure of what is included. We analyzed what information was useful in our previous travels and noted what information was lacking that could have enhanced these experiences. We leveraged personal experience, surveyed other individuals, conducted significant research and compiled our results.

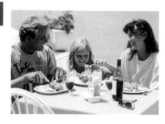

Breakfast Meal Suggestions guide you through breakfast options while away from home, whether on the road, in your hotel room or at a breakfast buffet. These suggestions were developed from personal experience and consulting culinary professionals. We have provided a sample menu of common breakfast items found in the Western world and created a quick reference guide similar to the cuisine specific guides that help you determine the safest breakfast choices.

Allergy-Free Beverage Suggestions focus on both non-alcoholic and alcoholic beverage options. Each category is further subdivided into different beverage types for easy reference. We have outlined a list of common ingredients found in non-alcoholic beverages and what potential food allergens these ingredients may be derived from.

In the case of alcoholic beverages, international law does not require manufacturers to list ingredients on their product labels. As a result, we were unable to confirm ingredients contained in these beverages. Through our research of alcoholic beverages, we outline some important considerations in the manufacturing process that may help you to determine which products might be safe for you to consume. We received input from bartenders and beverage distributors in conjunction with our personal research to develop this information. We have also created quick reference guides for non-alcoholic and alcoholic beverages.

On the Go Snack and Light Meal Suggestions are divided into three category types: no preparation, hot water preparation and cooler required. *The Quick Reference Guide* gives an overview of each snack and light meal type and whether they "typically contain" or "may contain" the ten common food allergens addressed in this book. Next are sample shopping checklists organized by snack and light meal type to assist you while purchasing products.

Airline Meal Suggestions were created based upon our research of global air carriers. We have provided a list of 25-plus standard meal types with descriptions that are available on 50-plus global airlines based upon medically prescribed lifestyles, recommended lifestyles, age considerations, religious considerations and health preferences. In addition to identifying which air carriers offer each specific meal, we have also provided detailed contact information for each airline and the necessary requirements for ordering your meal in advance. All telephone numbers provided are the contacts for customer service in the English language for the respective airlines as of June 2005. We have provided both local and in country numbers to assist you with your travel concerns.

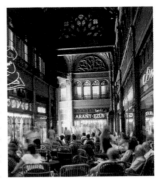

Communicating Essential Multi-lingual Phrases provides over 300 phrases integral to international travel while managing food allergies. These phrases were developed based upon our research and global travel experience. Each phrase has been translated into French, German, Italian and Spanish by a professional technical translation service. We conducted quality assurance testing with native speakers of each language to ensure phrase accuracy and applicability based upon contemporary cultural idioms. These phrases include a variety of concerns you may need to communicate including dining and health phrases. Even if you do not know how to pronounce these words, the format is designed so that you may refer to these phrases when scanning a menu or point directly to the guide to express your request while in a foreign language speaking country.

Our Personal Perspectives—Chapter 16

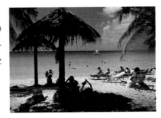

This chapter reflects the authors' personal insights into living with food allergies, supporting friends and family, the restaurant perspective, dining outside the home and global travel.

Resource and Reference Materials— Appendices I, II, III and IV

These appendices represent extensive research conducted to define helpful resources available in your search for information and knowledge. *Appendix I—Contributors to Let's Eat Out!* acknowledges the chefs, restaurants, culinary institutions and health professionals involved in reviewing the book contents, as well as country-specific product reference materials. *Appendix II—Global Association and Organization Listing* details

180-plus global organizations specializing in food allergy, celiac/coeliac disease and autoimmune disease. *Appendix III—Additional Global Resource and Reference Listings* are a comprehensive listing of 170-plus helpful web sites and reading materials concerning food allergies, celiac/coeliac disease and autoimmune disease. Also listed are 100-plus stores and manufacturers including brick and mortar operations as well as online facilities that provide allergy-free products around the world. *Appendix IV—About the Authors and Additional Products* outlines background details and convenient pocket-size passports.

Closing Remarks

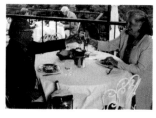

Knowledge is power. Our mission from the outset was to empower individuals with food allergies and specialized diets to safely dine outside the home regardless of location or destination. From our own experiences, we realize that knowledge alone, however, is not enough to avoid encountering food allergens while eating out and traveling. This requires due diligence, persistently asking the right questions of restaurant professionals, educating yourself and reading labels to ensure a safer dining experience. Mistakes may happen even after reading this book. Since we go through this process ourselves, we feel confident that posing the right questions, combined with a basic understanding of the cuisines and suggestions, helps to alleviate some of the stress experienced when living with food allergies and specialized diets.

And remember,

**"Life loves to be
taken by the lapel and told,
'I am with you kid. Let's go!'"**

—Maya Angelou

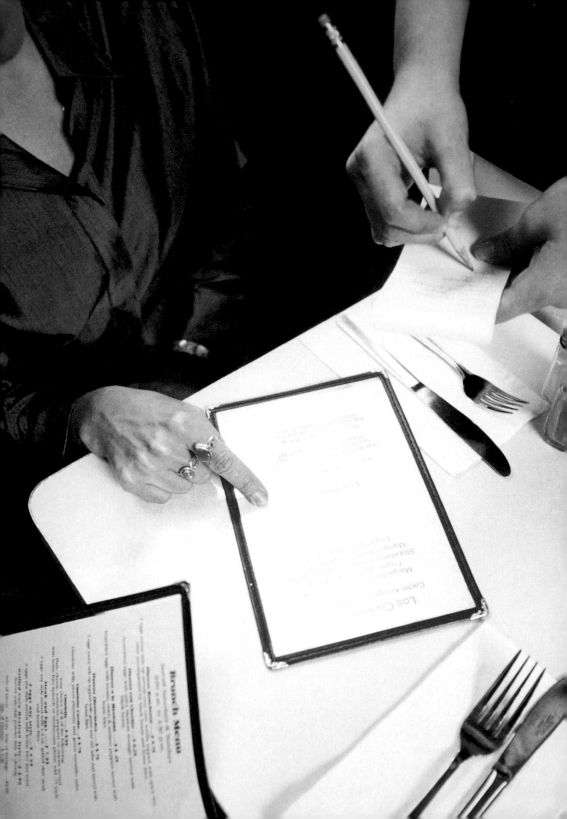

Confidence, like art, never comes
from having all the answers; it comes
from being open to all the questions.
—Earl Grey Stevens

Chapter 1
Eating Outside the Home Approach

Chapter Overview

Dining in restaurants, around the corner or anywhere around the world, is truly one of life's pleasures. Food has tremendous power in our lives. It gives us physical nourishment and provides us with the opportunity to socialize with friends and family. The collaborative effort between guests and eating establishments has been a tradition for hundreds of years, dating back to the 18th century when Mathurin Roze de Chantoiseau opened the first restaurant in Paris which claimed to serve "only those foods that either maintain or re-establish health[1]." Little did he know that the slogan for the world's first documented restaurant would mean so much to the estimated 300-plus million people in the Western world potentially requiring specialized diets.

Following a specialized diet increases the level of complexity involved in eating outside the home, particularly in restaurants. It requires a higher level of education and understanding compared to the general public, who can easily eat whatever they want, wherever they want. Knowing what foods are safe and control-

[1] Sprang, Rebecca L.
"The Invention of the Restaurant,"
Harvard University Press, 2000.

1

ling what you eat is of the utmost importance. Without knowledge, eating outside the home while managing a specialized diet is a lot like surfing on a lake...you're extremely limited in how far you can travel.

The suggestions outlined in this chapter may help give you a greater sense of comfort when you venture beyond your front door. Regardless of your location and destination, key factors involved in managing specialized diets covered in this chapter include:

- Learning Curve Associated with Specialized Diets

- Collaborative Process of Dining Out

- Approach to Eating Outside the Home—the Guest's Perspective

- Approach to Handling Special Dietary Requests —the Restaurant's Perspective

Learning Curve Associated with Specialized Diets

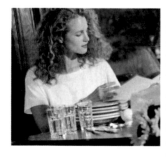

There are stages involved in understanding specialized diets, both from an individual and a restaurant professional perspective. The two paths taken in this learning process are similar in many ways, the most important of which is awareness. For the individual, the first step in understanding exactly what you are allergic to or what specialized diet you are required to follow is educating yourself. You may be asking, "What have I been diagnosed with and where do I begin my research? What resources are available to me and what do I do?" These are all common questions associated with learning about your new way of life. On the other side of the table, restaurant professionals go through a similar experience. "What type of specialized diets may be required by our guests? What do we need to learn to better understand their needs? What resources are available to help us?"

The next step in the learning curve is information. As an individual, you must learn what you can and cannot eat on a fundamental level. Once this is understood, it is important to investigate where problematic foods can be hidden in cooking and what you need to do to adjust for this unexpected variable. Likewise, restaurant professionals follow a similar thought process. "What can this guest eat and what is not allowable?" "Where in our food preparation techniques could these concerns be an issue and how can we adjust to suit their requirements?" The parallel is undeniable.

Once this understanding is accomplished, the third step is knowledge. You need to apply what you have learned while eating at restaurants, as well as at home. Furthermore, you must learn to communicate your special requirements and devise an effective strategy for ordering meals. The restaurant has a different set of concerns to address, such as how to train the staff and how to accurately convey the information between all employees involved in the process. If they are truly organized in their training efforts, an establishment teaches their staff how to assist the guests by guiding them through the menu.

The final step of the learning curve is empowerment. You need to know where and what you can eat, as well as what modifications can be made to easily accommodate your dietary requirements. Once this is achieved, you can focus on enjoying your dining experiences, while remaining diligent about the food you eat. For the restaurant, the focus becomes how to simplify menu options to adjust for special dietary needs. This allows the restaurant to concentrate on providing safe and delicious meals for their guests, while ensuring a high standard of service.

Collaborative Process of Dining Out

The collaborative process between guests and restaurants is critical in successfully eating outside the home with special dietary requirements. As outlined in the chart on the next page, this process is comprised of two primary components—the planning effort and the continuous interaction throughout the dining experience between the two parties.

1

Collaborative Process Between Guests and Restaurants

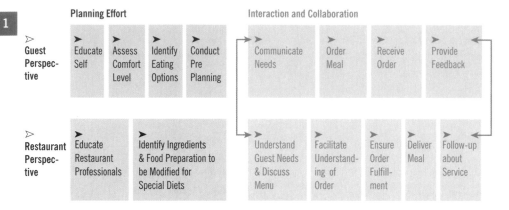

	Planning Effort				Interaction and Collaboration			
▷ **Guest Perspective**	➤ Educate Self	➤ Assess Comfort Level	➤ Identify Eating Options	➤ Conduct Pre Planning	➤ Communicate Needs	➤ Order Meal	➤ Receive Order	➤ Provide Feedback
▷ **Restaurant Perspective**	➤ Educate Restaurant Professionals	➤ Identify Ingredients & Food Preparation to be Modified for Special Diets			➤ Understand Guest Needs & Discuss Menu	➤ Facilitate Understanding of Order	➤ Ensure Order Fulfillment	➤ Deliver Meal / ➤ Follow-up about Service

The planning effort from both the guest and restaurant perspective focuses on education and is completed prior to any interaction between the two parties. Interaction and collaboration begins once contact is initiated by the guest with the restaurant. Each step associated with this process from the guest's and restaurant's perspectives are described in detail within the respective approach sections. We have provided guidelines for the steps as well as suggested questions to ask which are intended to stimulate ideas prior to and during the collaborative process of dining out.

Approach to Eating Outside the Home—The Guest's Perspective

Based upon experience and research, the following approach may help you have an enjoyable dining experience regardless of restaurant, cuisine or location. These suggestions include how to:

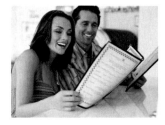

1. Educate yourself about eating outside the home with specialized diets

2. Assess your dining comfort level for the meal

3. Identify your eating options and preferences

4. Determine the level of pre-planning efforts desired

5. Communicate your special dietary needs with the restaurant

6. Order your meal

7. Receive order and appreciate your meal

8. Provide feedback on dining experience

Each of the suggestions detailed below can help you streamline your approach to eating outside the home. The questions to ask yourself may be helpful in assessing your level of preparedness along the way. If you are new to your diet, these ideas may give you some food for thought during the early stages of your learning curve. For those who have been following a specific diet for some time, you might find it interesting to reflect upon your previous experiences, correlate them to this recommended approach and, perhaps, learn something new in the process.

1. Educate yourself about eating outside the home with specialized diets

a. Read applicable materials:

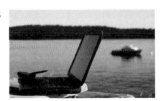

- Review books, publications, restaurant reviews and awareness programs

- Research the Internet and other reference materials

b. Talk with other individuals dealing with specialized diets:

- Become a member of applicable associations and organizations

- Participate in support groups and discussion forums

c. Attend educational sessions:

- Participate in associated conferences

- Participate in cooking classes to learn more about food preparation

- Hire a personal chef for consultation

1

Suggested Questions to Ask Yourself:

Do I have the information that I need to make informed choices and increase my comfort level in restaurants?

What additional research do I need to expand my knowledge?

2. Assess your dining comfort level for the meal

a. Identify your safety factors:

- Determine how you feel physically

- Assess how safe you need to feel

b. Based upon your previous needs and experience, evaluate what cuisines are low risk and high risk

c. Assess specific cuisines:

- Determine what type of cuisine satisfies your comfort level and tastes

- Identify your desired level of complexity in food preparation

Suggested Questions to Ask Yourself:

How comfortable do I feel eating out in restaurants today?

What foods appeal to me?

How safe do I need to feel today with the food that I will be eating based upon my current state of being?

Do I have an event tomorrow that may require me to be extremely cautious today?

3. Identify your eating options and preferences

a. Determine what type of establishment and atmosphere you prefer:

- Fine dining establishment

- Family-oriented restaurant
- Fast food/quick service establishment
- Carry out/take away

b. Assess what type of cuisine you prefer:

- New and different
- Familiar with menu items
- Understand preparation considerations

c. Determine if it is most important to go somewhere:

- New and different
- You have eaten before and know the safe items
- Gluten and allergy friendly
- Featuring a specific gluten and allergy-free menu
- Where people know who you are

d. Select your restaurant

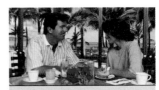

Partial List of Gluten-Free Restaurant Programs

UK /Europe–
Gluten-Free On The Go Program
Sponsored by: Coeliac UK
http://www.gluten-free-onthego.com

US – Gluten-Free Restaurant Awareness Program
Sponsored by: Gluten Intolerance Group
http://www.glutenfreerestaurants.org

Suggested Questions to Ask Yourself:

How much effort do I want to spend on deciding what to eat at this restaurant?

How comfortable do I feel with this restaurant, the cuisine and my menu options?

4. Determine the level of pre-planning effort desired

a. Conduct research as necessary on:

- Cuisine ingredients and preparation
- Restaurant menu options

b. Determine the best time for your reservation or meal:

- Decide to walk into a restaurant when convenient
- Reserve a time that is convenient
- Reserve a time that is typically not crowded

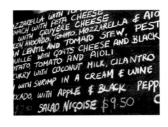

1

based on access to the people who can help you as well as your level of comfort

c. Determine the level of communication and interaction necessary with the restaurant prior to your meal:

- None required

- Review menu on the Internet

- Call ahead to discuss dietary requirements

Suggested Questions to Ask Yourself:

What level of planning and preparation do I want to do prior to going to the restaurant?

Do I need to conduct more research to increase my comfort level about this cuisine and restaurant?

Based on my needs, what areas of food preparation do I need to review?

What hidden allergens do I need to be aware of?

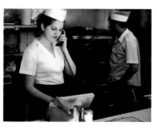

5. Communicate your special dietary needs with the restaurant

a. Determine your approach to explaining your dietary needs:

- Vulnerable to anaphylactic shock

- Following a medically prescribed diet

- Have severe food allergies

- On a specialized diet

b. Initiate your first contact with restaurant

- Go to restaurant without prior communication

- Prior to walking in the door, call ahead during non-peak times and discuss menu options with restaurant professionals

- Pre-order your meal based upon your comfort level

c. Discuss requirements with the restaurant staff and based upon their knowledge of specialized diets, potentially request a manager or the chef, as needed, to help ensure a safe experience

Suggested Questions to Ask Yourself:

How do I want to communicate the severity of my condition?

When and how do I want to explain my special dietary needs?

Are my needs understood or do I need to speak with someone else to feel safe and comfortable?

6. Order your meal:

a. Determine reference materials required to order meal:

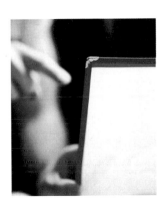

- Assess if a restaurant card or other materials outlining dietary requirements should be given to your server based upon your comfort level or language considerations

- Refer to your notes, books, cuisine passports, quick reference guides, translation cards and foreign language phrase books as needed

b. Discuss the menu with the restaurant professionals:

- Ask the appropriate questions to determine meal choices based upon cuisine, dishes and preferences

- Explain your concerns to the restaurant professionals

- Realize that if the restaurant is extremely busy it may be best to keep special requests to a minimum

c. Place your order:

- Request special food preparation

- Confirm your order with restaurant professionals

Suggested Questions to Ask Yourself:

How do I want to communicate my needs to the restaurant—ask questions, give them materials outlining requirements or provide materials and ask questions?

What areas of food preparation do I need to question?

What hidden allergens do I inquire about?

How comfortable do I feel that my order will be prepared as requested?

7. Receive order and appreciate your meal

    a. Confirm your order upon delivery:

- Reiterate your special order request
- Receive dish and assess preparation

    b. Enjoy your meal:

- Accept the dish
- Request dish be returned if special request is not met

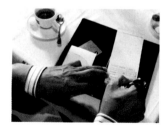

    c. Relax and appreciate the dining experience:

- Compliment the staff on attention to detail if your special requests are met
- Include a generous tip for good and conscientious service
- Frequent the restaurant again based on experience

Suggested Questions to Ask Yourself:

Is my meal what I ordered?

What needs to be modifed to correct the order?

Would I come back to this restaurant?

8. Provide feedback on your dining experience

   a. Provide constructive feedback to restaurant professionals on your dining experience

   b. Recommend the dining establishment to your friends and family

   c. Notify applicable restaurant awareness programs of your experience

Suggested Questions to Ask Yourself:

What do I want to communicate to the staff regarding their service?

Would I recommend this establishment to others?

Approach to Handling Special Dietary Requests—The Restaurant's Perspective

Based upon experience and discussions with culinary and restaurant professionals, the following suggestions are designed to help restaurants enable their staff to assist individuals with specialized diets. These include how to:

1. Educate staff about potential dietary requirements

2. Identify restaurant-specific ingredients and food preparation techniques to be potentially modified for specialized diets

3. Communicate with guests and understand their special dietary needs

4. Facilitate accurate understanding of the order and special requirements

5. Ensure fulfillment of special orders

6. Deliver meal

1

7. Follow-up with guests about service and ensure satisfactory dining experience

Each of the suggestions detailed below helps restaurants address the special dietary requirements of their guests. The questions to ask yourself, as the restaurant, may be helpful in assessing training effectiveness and the level of preparedness in handling special requests. These ideas are provided for restaurants that are concerned about assisting their guests, as well as for those individuals who are curious and want to understand the restaurant's perspective.

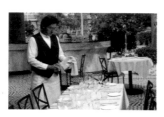

1. Educate staff about potential dietary requirements

a. Conduct training for management and staff on:

- Specialized diets and requirements
- Interacting with individuals who require specialized diets

b. Obtain certification from appropriate organizations and restaurant awareness programs

c. Talk with other restaurants dealing with specialized diets

d. Monitor training effectiveness and guest feedback

Suggested Questions for the Restaurant:

Is the staff knowledgeable about specialized diets?

Are there training programs we can implement to improve awareness and effectiveness with the staff?

What are other restaurants doing to satisfy their guests with special dietary requirements?

What type of certification process can we participate in to promote our efforts to guests?

How can we maintain the desired level of quality with our continued training efforts?

2. **Identify restaurant-specific ingredients and preparation techniques to be potentially modified for specialized diets**

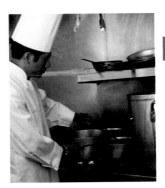

   a. Identify common food allergens and associated ingredients

   b. Assess what areas of food preparation specific to our kitchen contain common food allergens

   c. Identify which menu items are naturally free of specific allergens

   d. Explore potential modifications to menu items based upon specific allergens and ingredients

   e. Determine possible cross-contamination and potential changes required in our kitchen

   f. Identify what ingredients and areas of food preparation cannot be modified

Suggested Questions for the Restaurant:

What are the most common food allergens?

What are the common ingredients?

Where can these allergens be hidden in our methods of food preparation and menu items?

What do we offer on the menu that is safe for certain specialized diets?

Are there dishes we offer that can be easily altered for those with special dietary needs?

How do we want to communicate this information to our guests?

3. **Understand guest's special dietary needs and discuss menu**

   a. Discuss guest's dietary conditions:

   • Vulnerable to anaphylactic shock

   • Following a medically prescribed diet

   • Have severe food allergies

   • On a specialized diet

1

b. Discuss menu items and safety factors of dishes:

- Which menu items are safe based upon requirements

- Identify which items can be modified to be safe

c. Discuss which menu items must be avoided

d. Confirm menu items and preparation with chef based upon requirements

Suggested Questions for the Restaurant:

Are the special dietary needs of the guest clear?

Does the chef understand these special dietary needs?

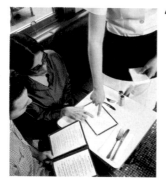

4. Facilitate accurate understanding of the order and special requirements

a. Determine if the special order is understood by the cooks under the chef's supervision

b. Assess and factor in language considerations with the kitchen staff

c. Determine the feasibility of executing special requests based upon how busy the kitchen is

d. Assess if order can be prepared as requested

e. Follow-up with guest if a change to the order is required

Suggested Questions for the Restaurant:

Do the cooks understand how to prepare specialized meals?

Is there a potential language barrier between waiters and kitchen staff that could result in miscommunication?

Is the kitchen staff capable of executing a special request based upon the restaurant's capacity at that time?

Does anything need to be changed from the original order based upon feedback from the kitchen?

5. Ensure fulfillment of special order

 a. Confirm with the chef if special request can be handled

 b. Monitor fulfillment of special request

 c. Re-confirm order with kitchen staff prior to delivery

Suggested Questions for the Restaurant:

Can the chef confirm that the special request was effectively addressed?

Has the special order been prepared as requested?

6. Deliver meal

 a. Deliver meal to guest

 b. Confirm their special dietary request when the meal is delivered

 c. Handle situation il meal does not meet the guest's expectations

Suggested Questions for the Restaurant:

Are we delivering the appropriate meal to the guest with special dietary requirements?

Have we confirmed with the guest that their special order is prepared as requested?

7. Follow-up with guests about service and ensure satisfactory dining experience

 a. Follow-up with guest to ensure meal is satisfactory

1

    b. Provide guest feedback to manager and chef as needed

Suggested Questions for the Restaurant:

Did we follow-up with the table to confirm that the meal meets the guest's expectations?

Are there any improvements we can implement to streamline our special order process?

Summary

There is no doubt that the level of awareness in the restaurant industry concerning specialized diets has been improving over the last decade. There is an increasing number of special menus and nutritional programs found in many restaurants. There is also an increase in the number of health conscious establishments thriving in many parts of the Western world. This trend can be directly tied to the relationship between restaurants and their guests. Due to a desire to provide quality service in a highly competitive market, restaurants typically have the best intentions when it comes to guest satisfaction. They want you to be happy with your experience, because they want you to come back often.

Most restaurants are flexible with special requests. In fact, a great number of restaurants these days prepare dishes that are made to order. There is a movement growing in the industry to make every effort to accommodate individuals with special dietary requirements. Omitting an obvious ingredient that an individual is allergic to is generally not a problem. Accommodating special requirements can sometimes be more difficult during exceptionally busy hours. However, for the most part, it is possible to eliminate certain ingredients from a menu item depending upon the dish.

The collaboration between guests and restaurants has contributed to advancements in special dietary awareness. We learn from each other, so it is important to take note of any new knowledge that results from each dining experience from both perspectives. Going forward, our collective efforts will continue to increase the understanding of specialized diets so that it becomes a universally supported way of living

Like some lessons in life, managing specialized diets has an educational process and tuition to be paid. We all learn one way or another. Hopefully, reading this book can help you along your learning curve and make the process easier. Eat out! Explore the world! Have Fun!

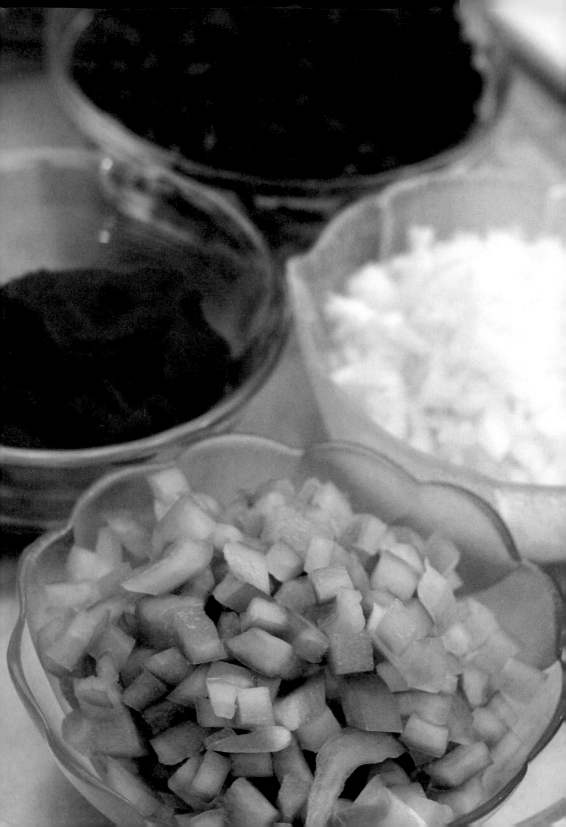

You don't have to cook fancy or complicated
masterpieces—just good food from fresh ingredients.
—Julia Child

2

Chapter 2
Ingredient and Preparation Technique Guidelines

Chapter Overview

When you dine at a restaurant there are almost no
labels, nor is there the handy nutritional analysis
that you find on most products manufactured and
sold in the western world. The best way to increase
your comfort level about eating outside the home is to
educate yourself on food ingredients, how food can be
prepared and what techniques require your attention.
Knowledge is power! With a little bit of effort and
courage, you can learn to navigate through any menu,
empowered by an understanding of common culinary
practices and the ability to ask the right questions to
ensure an allergy-free dining experience.

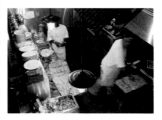

To accomplish this, you need to know a few things
about how restaurants prepare food, which include:

- Areas of considerations

- Worldwide product labeling regulations

- Common food allergy myths

- Quick Reference Guide

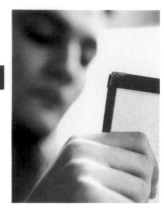

2

• Ingredient and preparation techniques by allergen

Believe it or not, the areas that require your attention are actually very manageable. When it comes to common food allergens, there are three major areas to consider:

• Allergens as ingredients

• Allergens hidden in food preparation techniques

• Cross-contamination

Allergens as ingredients are typically much easier to identify and manage while eating outside the home. Obviously, if you are allergic to shrimp, you can request no shrimp on your salad. If you are allergic to dairy, you can request no cheese on your beef carpaccio. If you are allergic to fish, don't order it. That's the easy part.

Allergens hidden in food preparation techniques require a bit more investigation on your part. Are the French fried potatoes fried in peanut oil? Is the chicken dusted with wheat flour prior to pan frying? Does the marinade for your pork chops contain soy sauce? As you can imagine, this can get complicated with unexpected surprises lurking around many corners. That being said, asking the right questions is extremely important.

Cross-contamination occurs in two primary instances and should be considered at any restaurant you choose to dine in. One may occur when your meal is prepared in the same frying oil as foods containing other possible allergens. The second may occur when microbes or food particles are transferred from one food to another by using the same knife, cutting board, pan, grill or other utensils without washing the surfaces or tools in between uses. To avoid cross-contamination, restaurants need to dedicate fryers for specific foods and wash all materials and cooking surfaces that may come in contact with food in hot, soapy water prior to preparing items for those with special dietary requirements. In the case of open flame grills, the intense heat typically turns most protein into carbon;

however, scraping the grill may be required as a safety precaution. It is important to ensure that restaurants follow these procedures to avoid cross-contamination between foods.

2

Worldwide Product Labeling Regulations

In recent years, various geographic regions have instituted product labeling regulations for manufacturers. Product labeling legislation in Australia, Europe, New Zealand and North America varies by terms, definitions, food allergens covered, compound ingredients, substitutions, exemptions, placement and legibility. There are hundreds of pages of regulations and requirements outlining the specific details of the various geographic labeling laws. These regulations encompass various combinations of food allergens such as celery, dairy and milk, eggs, fish, gluten, mustard, peanuts, sesame, shellfish, soy, sulphur dioxide, tree nuts and wheat. These allergens are responsible for over 90% of allergic reactions to food on a worldwide basis.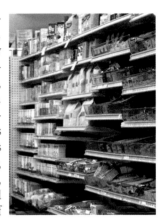

It is currently mandatory to label ingredients derived from defined food allergens in Australia, New Zealand and Europe. In 2002, Food Standards Australia New Zealand (FSANZ) required top food allergens to be named on ingredient lists under Standard 1.2.4. The European Union Directive (2003/89/EC) on product labeling requires manufacturers to identify 12 allergens and their derivatives by November 2005.

In 2004, the US Food Allergen Labeling and Protection Act (FALCPA) was signed for full implementation by January 2006. Canada is in the process of approving regulations on product labeling for various food allergens and their derivatives. It should be noted that labeling laws apply to the products manufactured in their country of origin. Frequently, imported products do not need to adhere to the export country's labeling regulations.

When traveling, it is advised that you review the labeling requirements and standards of each country

2

you plan to visit. To obtain country-specific ingredient and labeling information, it is recommended that you refer to Appendix II and III for potential websites and listings in your home country or travel destination location. You may elect to contact the respective associations and/or organizations for more details based upon your personal requirements and specific concerns.

Common Food Allergy Myths

Sources of ingredients, manufacturing processes and labeling regulations for products vary on a worldwide basis. Definitions of terms and acceptable levels of various food allergens also differ based on country and/or geographic region. Acknowledging these differences, through our global research we uncovered three myths regarding specific food ingredients which have triggered concerns within the food allergy and celiac/coeliac community. These myths have been perpetuated by the worldwide variances of food manufacturing practices, word of mouth, the Internet and outdated reference materials.

These discussions have revolved around three primary ingredients found in food manufacturing and preparation. Based upon significant research and discussions with health professionals, a summary of our findings are outlined for the following ingredients:

- Vinegar

- Colors or flavors

- Caramel color

Vinegar

According to *Gluten-Free Living,* "there are several types of vinegar, most of which do not begin with wheat. 'Gluten is not present in the starting material commonly used in the manufacture of vinegar. Apple, grape, corn and rice sugars are the most frequently used sources of alcohol that is fermented into vinegar,' according to The Vinegar Institute, an international trade association that represents the vast majority of vinegar manufacturers and bottlers in the United States, as well as producers in different countries around the world. In North America, most distilled white vinegars are made from corn. The Vinegar Institute says, 'Alcohol manufacturers and independent laboratories have tested alcohol produced from corn and been unable to detect the presence of any protein. While it is possible for white vinegars to be manufactured from grains other than corn, it is uncommon.' "

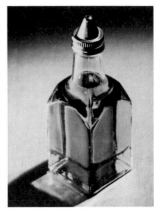

According to the Canadian Celiac Association, "...there is no detectable amount of gluten (prolamin) in distilled alcohol. There can therefore be no possibility of gluten in distilled white vinegar which contains acetic acid equivalent to about 4% alcohol. Celiacs/coeliacs should therefore have no cause for concern about distilled white vinegar or foods such as pickles and condiments which may contain it."

As stated in *Gluten-Free Living,* "it bears noting that wheat is used to make vinegar in Canada, and the Canadian Celiac Association has never warned celiacs/coeliacs to avoid vinegar. In fact, celiacs in every other country in the world have used vinegar without concern."

Distilled white vinegar is rendered corn and gluten-free through the distillation process. However, it may be possible for gluten-containing ingredients to be added after the distillation to some flavored vinegars which would be indicated on the product labels. Malt vinegar is not acceptable for those adhering to a gluten-free diet. Unlike distilled vinegar, malt vinegar is fermented and made from "an infusion of barley malt or cereals," according to the US Food and Drug Administration. Throughout this book, we have indicated the presence of malt with respect to corn and gluten as well as malt vinegar as a consideration for gluten. We have not identified those areas where flavored vinegars may be encountered.

Colors or Flavors

Global regulations differ in how they define the term colors or flavors. As stated in *The Gluten-Free Diet—A Comprehensive Resource Guide,* "according to flavor experts from industry and government in Canada and the USA, gluten-containing grains are not commonly used in flavorings. However, there are two exceptions:

1. Barley malt can be used as a flavoring agent and is usually (though not always) listed on the label. It might be listed as barley malt, barley malt extract or barley malt flavoring. Some companies may list it as 'flavor (contains barley protein)' or occasionally declare it only as 'flavor'.

2. Hydrolyzed wheat, corn and/or soy protein can be used as 'flavor' or 'flavor enhancers' in a variety of foods. However, in Canada and the USA, they must be declared as 'hydrolyzed proteins' and not hidden on the label as 'flavor' or 'natural flavor'[B.01.009 in Canada and Sec. 101.22 in the USA]"

In North America, flavors which may contain gluten/wheat may be found in cereals which use barley malt flavoring or extract, meat products, products containing meat, deli meats, beef jerky, imitation bacon bits and soy beverages. Additionally, flavor enhancers, fillers and thickening agents may be derived from barley extract, barley malt and Hydrolyzed Wheat Protein (HWP).

For purposes of this book, we have categorized "colors or flavors" as a term to encompass the possibility that manufactured or pre-fabricated products used in restaurants may contain common food allergens. With this in mind, our global research indicates that colors or flavors may contain corn, dairy, eggs, fish, gluten, soy or wheat, which are indentified as such throughout this book. The only way to be certain of the contents of the colors or flavors in manufactured or pre-fabricated food items is to refer to the product label and understand the labeling regulations of the country of origin for the respective product.

Caramel Color

Manufacturing processes and ingredients differ globally in the production of caramel color. As stated in *The Gluten-Free Diet—A Comprehensive Resource Guide,* "Caramel color is manufactured by heating carbohydrates, either alone, or in the presence of food-grade acids, alkalies and/or salts, and is produced from commercially available food-grade nutritive sweeteners consisting of fructose, dextrose (glucose), invert sugar, sucrose and/or starch hydrolysates and fractions thereof. Although gluten-containing ingredients [malt syrup (barley) and starch hydrolysates] can be used in the production of caramel color, they are not used according to food processors in North America. Corn is used most often, as it produces a longer shelf life and a much better product."

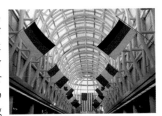

It should be noted that outside of North America, caramel color may contain gluten (from barley) or soy and therefore needs to be questioned at your restaurant of choice based upon the menu item ordered. The only way to be certain as to the contents of the caramel color in manufactured or pre-fabricated food items is to refer to the product label and understand the labeling regulations of the country of origin for the respective product. For purposes of this book, we have grouped caramel color within the colors or flavors and not as a separate item.

Ingredient and Preparation Techniques: Quick Reference Guide

Based upon the 175-plus menu items across seven international cuisines outlined in this book, the following represent the most common ingredients and preparation techniques that you may encounter while dining out anywhere in the world. It is acknowledged that this is not a complete list of every possible culinary practice. However, our research and discussions with many culinary professionals indicates that these are the most common culinary practices associated with each allergen.

These practices are mapped to the 10 allergens which are color-coded by allergen type for an easy-to-use format and include:

- Brown for corn and soy
- Yellow for dairy and gluten/wheat

- Blue for fish and shellfish

- Green for peanuts and tree nuts

- Pink for eggs

2

Color Key for the Quick Reference Guides

Corn–dark brown
Soy–light brown
Dairy–light yellow
Gluten/wheat–dark yellow
Fish–dark blue
Shellfish–light blue
Peanuts–dark green
Tree Nuts–light green
Eggs–pink

The 65-plus potential ingredients and techniques, listed in alphabetical order, identify where each allergen may be found. This is indicated by an ● for "typically contains allergen" or an ○ for "may contain allergen" recommending that you check with the restaurant professional to ensure the absence of your specific food allergen.

At first, the level of detail included may seem overwhelming. Keep in mind that every effort has been made to incorporate both traditional and non-traditional culinary techniques. For example, the possibility that you may find soy sauce in a Mexican restaurant, while remote, has nonetheless been proven by our research. The question must be asked when there is a possibility that a culinary practice may be used, although unusual to the cuisine, in order to ensure that the dish is safe for you to eat.

Ingredient and Preparation Techniques:
Quick Reference Guide
(Almonds – Custard)

	Corn	Dairy	Eggs	Fish	Gluten/Wheat	Peanuts	Shellfish	Soy	Tree Nuts
Almonds or Almond Extract	O								●
Anchovies				●					
Artificial Bacon Bits	O				O			O	
Artificial Mashed Potato Mix	O	O			O			O	
Batter	O		●		O				
Beans					O				
Bean Curd								●	
Bouillon	O				O			O	
Bread or Bread Crumbs	O	O	O		O	O		O	O
Breading	O	O	O		O			O	
Butter		●							
Cakes or Cookies		O	O		O	O			O
Calamari							●		
Cashew or Cashew Powder									●
Cheese or Blue Cheese	O	●			O			O	
Chocolate		O						O	
Colors or Flavors	O	O	O		O	O		O	O
Corn Flour or Corn Meal	●								
Corn Starch	●								
Corn Syrup	●								
Crab							●		
Cream, Sour Cream or Whipped Cream		●							
Croutons			O		O				
Custard			●						

Always ensure no cross-contamination in food preparation
● Typically contains allergen   O May contain allergen

Ingredient and Preparation Techniques:
Quick Reference Guide
(Dedicated Fryer – Salad Dressing)

	Corn	Dairy	Eggs	Fish	Gluten/Wheat	Peanuts	Shellfish	Soy	Tree Nuts
Dedicated Fryer					O				
Dumpling Skin			●		O				
Egg Sealer			●						
Egg Yolk			●						
Escargot							●		
Fish Sauce				●	O				
Flour Dusting	O				O				
Fluffing Agent					O				
Fresh Oil					O				
Garnish						O			O
Imitation Crabmeat or Seafood	O		O	●	O			O	
Ketchup								O	
Lobster							●		
Malt	O				O				
Malt Vinegar					●				
Marinade	O	O		O	O			O	
Masa	●							O	
Mayonnaise			●					O	
Milk or Buttermilk		●							
Mussels							●		
Noodles or Pasta			O		O				
Oysters							●		
Peanut Oil						●			
Pistachios									●
Salad Dressing	O	O	O	O	O			O	O

Always ensure no cross-contamination in food preparation

● Typically contains allergen   O May contain allergen

Ingredient and Preparation Techniques:
Quick Reference Guide
(Salmon – Yogurt)

	Corn	Dairy	Eggs	Fish	Gluten/Wheat	Peanuts	Shellfish	Soy	Tree Nuts
Salmon				●					
Sauce, Dipping Sauce or Salsa	O	O	O	O	O	O		O	O
Seasonings	O	O			O			O	
Shrimp							●		
Side Dishes or Accompaniments	O	O	O		O	O		O	O
Soy Sauce					O			●	
Stabilizers					O				
Stock or Broth				O			O		
Thickening Agent	O				O				
Tofu								●	
Tortillas or Tortilla Chips	O				O			O	
Tuna				●					
Vanilla Extract	O								
Vegetable Bisque						O			O
Vegetable Oil	O						O	O	
Walnuts									●
Wheat Flour					●				
Yogurt, Yogurt Curd or Yogurt Sauce		●			O			O	

Always ensure no cross-contamination in food preparation
● Typically contains allergen   O May contain allergen

2

Ingredient and Preparation Techniques by Allergen

The allergens detailed in this section include: corn, dairy, eggs, fish, gluten/wheat, peanuts, shellfish, soy and tree nuts. Each allergen description outlines:

- Basic information on the allergen

- List of ingredients and food preparation techniques specific to the allergen

- Specific ingredients and techniques on how to manage the consideration and a sample question to ask the restaurant professional to ensure its absence in dishes.

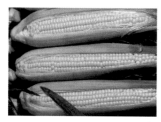

Corn

Corn, in its natural form, can obviously be detected as an ingredient in many dishes. In some parts of the world, it is referred to as maize. Additionally, hominy is another term for corn primarily found in North America.

The following potential ingredients and preparation techniques represent areas of concern while managing sensitivities to corn and its derivatives:

- Almond Extract
- Artificial Bacon Bits
- Artificial Mashed Potato Mix
- Batter
- Bouillon
- Bread or Bread Crumbs
- Breading
- Cheese
- Colors or Flavors
- Corn Flour or Corn Meal
- Corn Starch
- Corn Syrup

- Imitation Crabmeat or Seafood

- Malt

- Masa

- Salad Dressing

- Sauce, Dipping Sauce or Salsa

- Seasonings

- Side Dishes or Accompaniments

- Tortillas or Tortilla Chips

- Vanilla Extract

- Vegetable Oil

Almond Extract is used in many cuisines and found primarily in breads, desserts and pastries. Most almond extract typically contains corn and tree nuts.

- Ensure no almond extract is used in the preparation of breads, desserts and pastries.

- Sample question: *"Is there almond extract in the crème brulée?"*

Artificial Bacon Bits are used as substitutes for bacon primarily in North America and may contain corn, gluten/wheat and soy, as well as other ingredients. They are typically offered with baked potatoes and in salads.

- Ensure no artificial bacon bits that contain corn are used in the preparation of baked potatoes and salads.

- Sample question: *"Is the bacon included in this salad real or artificial?"*

Artificial Mashed Potato Mix is often used as a time saving and inexpensive solution for mashed potatoes in North America and may contain corn, dairy, gluten/wheat and soy.

- Ensure no artificial mashed potato mix that contains corn.

- Sample question: "Are the mashed potatoes included with this entree real or artificial?"

Batter typically contains corn or wheat flour combined with eggs and is used in many types of international cuisines.

- Ensure no corn flour, starch or oil in batter for appetizers, entrees and side dishes.

- Sample question: *"Is corn flour used to batter the chicken?"*

Bouillon is often used as a time saving and inexpensive solution for soup bases and sauces. It often contains corn, gluten/wheat and soy as well as other ingredients.

- Ensure no bouillon containing corn is used in the preparation of sauces and soups.

- Sample question: *"Is this soup made with fresh chicken stock?"*

Bread or Bread Crumbs may contain corn, dairy, eggs, gluten/wheat flour, peanuts, soy and tree nuts as well as other ingredients and are used in many types of international cuisines.

- Ensure no bread or bread crumbs containing corn.

- Sample question: *"Do you make your bread with corn oil?"*

Breading may contain corn, dairy, eggs, gluten/wheat flour and soy and is used in many international cuisines.

- Ensure no corn in breading.

- Sample question: *"Is the petti di pollo (Italian chicken breast) breaded with corn meal?"*

Cheese contains dairy and possibly gluten/wheat if blue or veined cheese. Pasteurized processed cheese may also contain corn or soy depending upon the manufacturer. It is used as an ingredient in sauces, salads, entrees, side dishes and desserts.

- Ensure no pasteurized processed cheese containing corn is used in any dish.

- Sample question: *"Is this salad topped with pasteurized processed cheese containing corn?"*

Colors or Flavors can be made from a variety of ingredients some of which contain corn, dairy, eggs, gluten/wheat, peanuts, soy and tree nuts. These may be included in prefabricated frozen desserts, beverages and food coloring.

- Ensure no colors or flavors containing corn are ingredients in any commercially made product.

- Sample question: *"Do you make your ice cream fresh in the restaurant or is it from a container that identifies corn or its derivatives as an ingredient on the label?"*

Corn Flour or Corn Meal may be used for battering, breading, flour dusting and tortillas in many international cuisines.

- Ensure no corn flour or corn meal is used in battering, breading and flour dusting.

- Sample question: *"Is there corn flour in these croquettes?"*

Corn Starch may be used to texture meats or fish and as a thickening agent for sauces and soups.

- Ensure no corn starch is used in flour dusting, sauces and soups.

- Sample question: *"Is the chicken dusted in corn starch prior to frying?"*

2

Corn Syrup is a common ingredient in commercially produced sauces and dressings, as well as a sweetener for beverages.

- Ensure no corn syrup in any commercially made products.

- Sample question: *"Do you make your cocktail sauce with ketchup containing corn syrup?"*

Imitation Crabmeat or Seafood is also known as surimi and is commonly used in Asian cuisines. It is made of fish paste and a number of additives, then molded into a shape, usually resembling crabmeat. In addition to fish, surimi may contain corn, eggs, gluten/wheat, and soy.

- Ensure no imitation crabmeat or seafood containing corn in any dish.

- Sample question: *"Do you use imitation crabmeat in your seafood bisque?"*

Malt is typically made from corn or barley, which contains gluten. It is commonly used in commercially produced beverages, confectionary products and frozen desserts.

- Ensure no malt containing corn in any commercially produced beverages, confectionary products and frozen desserts.

- Sample question: *"Does the ice cream container identify malt or corn as an ingredient on the label?"*

Masa is made from corn meal and lard or vegetable oil, which may be made with corn and soy. It is used primarily in Central and South American cuisine.

- Ensure no tamales and corn tortillas.

- Sample question: *"Are the tortillas made with flour or corn meal?"*

Salad Dressing that is commercially produced may contain ingredients derived from corn, dairy, eggs, fish, gluten/wheat and soy. Vinaigrettes made fresh in restaurants with vegetable oil may also include corn and soy. If used in a fresh vinaigrette, olive oil that does not state 100% on the container may be mixed with vegetable oil.

- Ensure no corn in any commercially made salad dressings or fresh vinaigrettes.

- Sample question: *"Is this vinaigrette made with 100% olive oil?"*

Sauce, Dipping Sauce or Salsa may contain corn as an ingredient and corn starch as a thickening agent, as well as dairy, eggs, fish, gluten/wheat, peanuts, soy and tree nuts. Commercially produced sauces may contain a number of different corn derivatives.

- Ensure no corn or its derivatives are ingredients in sauces.

- Sample question: *"Do you use corn starch to thicken the sauce?"*

Seasonings that are commercially produced sometimes contain ingredients derived from corn, dairy, gluten/wheat and soy.

- Ensure no corn in any commercially made seasonings.

- Sample question: *"What type of seasonings do you use to flavor the chicken?"*

Side Dishes or Accompaniments may contain corn, as well as other ingredients such as dairy, eggs, gluten/wheat, peanuts, soy and tree nuts.

- Ensure no corn as an ingredient in any side dish or accompaniment.

- Sample question: *"Are the refried beans made with corn oil?"*

Tortillas or Tortilla Chips may contain corn, gluten/wheat or soy and are common in Central and South American cuisines. They can be made from either corn or wheat flour and lard or vegetable oil.

- Ensure no corn tortillas or tortillas chips.

- Sample question: *"What type of tortilla is the taco salad bowl made from?"*

Vanilla Extract may contain a corn derivative as an ingredient and is primarily used in desserts.

- Ensure no vanilla extract containing corn is used in desserts.

- Sample question: *"Do you use fresh vanilla beans in your rice pudding?"*

Vegetable Oil can be a blend of corn, peanuts, soy and other types of oils.

- Ensure no corn oil in vegetable oil blends.

- Sample question: *"Can I have the asparagus sautéed in butter rather than vegetable oil?"*

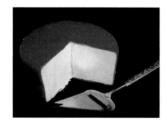

Dairy

Dairy products are commonly used in many international cuisines and have many forms. In the case of product labels, dairy products can be represented using alternative names such as casein, caseinates, hydrolysates, lactalbumin, lactoglobulin, lactose and whey.

The following potential ingredients and preparation techniques represent areas of concern while managing sensitivities to dairy and its derivatives:

- Artificial Mashed Potato Mix

- Bread or Bread Crumbs

- Breading

- Butter

- Cakes or Cookies

- Cheese or Blue Cheese

- Chocolate

- Colors or Flavors

- Cream, Sour Cream or Whipped Cream

- Milk or Buttermilk

- Salad Dressing

- Sauce or Dipping Sauce

- Seasonings

- Side Dishes or Accompaniments

- Yogurt, Yogurt Curd or Yogurt Sauce

Artificial Mashed Potato Mix is often used as a time saving and inexpensive solution for mashed potatoes in North America and may contain dairy, corn, gluten/wheat and soy.

- Ensure no artificial mashed potato mix that contains dairy.

- Sample question: *"Are the mashed potatoes included with this entree real or artificial?"*

Bread or Bread Crumbs may contain dairy, corn, eggs, gluten/wheat flour, peanuts, soy and tree nuts, as well as other ingredients and are used in many types of international cuisines.

- Ensure no bread or bread crumbs containing dairy.

- Sample question: *"Are your dosas (South Indian bread) made with butter?"*

Breading may contain dairy, corn, eggs, gluten/wheat flour and soy and is used in many international cuisines.

- Ensure no dairy in breading.

- Sample question: *"Does the breading for the chicken breast contain butter?"*

Butter is often used as an ingredient and to sauté foods.

- Ensure no butter is used in any dish.

- Sample question: *"Can you sauté the haricots verts (French green beans) in vegetable oil?"*

Cakes or Cookies can contain dairy, eggs, gluten/wheat flour, peanuts and tree nuts. They are included as ingredients or accompaniments to desserts in many international cuisines.

- Ensure no dairy in cakes and cookies.

- Sample question: *"Is there any butter in the wafer?"*

Cheese or Blue Cheese contains dairy and possibly gluten/wheat if blue or veined cheese. Pasteurized processed cheese may also contain corn or soy depending upon the manufacturer. It is used as an ingredient in sauces, salads, entrees, side dishes and desserts.

- Ensure no cheese or blue cheese is used in any dish.

- Sample question: *"Is this salad topped with cheese?"*

Chocolate contains dairy if it is identified as milk chocolate or listed on label. It may also contain soy if made in the United States. It is used as an ingredient in desserts and some sauces.

- Ensure no chocolate containing dairy as ingredient is used in desserts and sauces.

- Sample question: *"Is this dessert prepared with milk chocolate or dark chocolate?"*

Colors or Flavors can be made from a variety of ingredients some of which contain dairy, corn, eggs, gluten/wheat, peanuts, soy and tree nuts. These may be included in prefabricated frozen desserts, beverages and food coloring.

- Ensure no colors or flavors containing dairy are ingredients in any commercially made product.

- Sample question: *"Do you make your sherbet fresh in the restaurant or is it from a container that identifies dairy or its derivatives as an ingredient on the label?"*

Cream, Sour Cream or Whipped Cream can be used in many different areas of food preparation. Cream and sour cream are often used in sauces, while whipped cream is typically used for desserts.

- Ensure no cream, sour cream or whipped cream is used in any dish.

- Sample question: *"Do you top your fresh berries with whipped cream?"*

Milk or Buttermilk is often used as an ingredient in sauces, soups, entrees and desserts.

- Ensure no milk or buttermilk is used in any dish.

- Sample question: *"Is there milk in your green chile sauce?"*

Salad Dressing that is commercially produced may contain ingredients derived from dairy, corn, eggs, fish, gluten/wheat and soy.

- Ensure no dairy in any commercially made salad dressings.

- Sample question: *"Does this salad dressing identify dairy or its derivatives as an ingredient on the label?"*

Sauce or Dipping Sauce may contain dairy as an ingredient, as well as corn, eggs, fish, gluten/wheat, peanuts, soy and tree nuts. Commercially produced sauces may contain a number of different dairy derivatives.

- Ensure no dairy or its derivatives are ingredients in sauces.

- Sample question: *"Is there parmesan cheese in your marinara sauce?"*

Seasonings that are commercially produced sometimes contain ingredients derived from dairy, corn, gluten/wheat and soy.

- Ensure no dairy in any commercially made seasonings.

- Sample question: *"What type of seasonings do you use to flavor the chicken?"*

2

Side Dishes or Accompaniments may contain any number of dairy products including butter, cheese or cream, as well as other ingredients such as corn, eggs, gluten/wheat, peanuts, soy and tree nuts.

- Ensure no dairy or its derivatives are ingredients in any side dish or accompaniment.

- Sample question: *"Are the refried beans topped with cheese?"*

Yogurt, Yogurt Curd or Yogurt Sauce typically contains dairy as an ingredient and is commonly used in Mediterranean, Middle Eastern and Indian cuisines. Commercially produced yogurt may also contain gluten/wheat and soy.

- Ensure no yogurt is used in any dish.

- Sample question: *"Is there yogurt in this curry?"*

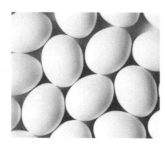

Eggs

Eggs are used in most international cuisines and are commonly found in commercially made food products. In the case of product labels, products derived from eggs can be represented using alternative names such as albumin (albumen), conalbumin, globulin, lecithin (from egg), livetin, lysozyme, ovalbumin, ovamucin, ovomucoid, ovotransferrin, ovovitellin and vitellin.

The following potential ingredients and preparation techniques represent areas of concern while managing sensitivities to eggs and its derivatives:

- Batter

- Bread or Bread Crumbs

- Breading

- Cakes or Cookies

- Colors or Flavors

- Croutons

- Custard

- Dumpling Skin

- Egg Sealer

- Egg Yolk

- Imitation Crabmeat or Seafood

- Mayonnaise

- Noodles or Pasta

- Salad Dressing

- Sauce or Dipping Sauce

- Side Dishes or Accompaniments

Batter typically contains eggs combined with either corn or wheat flour and is used in many types of international cuisines.

- Ensure no eggs in batter for entrees and side dishes.

- Sample question: *"Is the veal in this dish battered?"*

Bread or Bread Crumbs may contain eggs, corn, dairy, gluten/wheat flour, peanuts, soy and tree nuts, as well as other ingredients and are used in many types of international cuisines.

- Ensure no bread or bread crumbs containing eggs.

- Sample question: *"Are the cozze al vapor (Italian steamed mussels) topped with bread crumbs?"*

Breading may contain eggs, corn, dairy, gluten/wheat flour and soy and is used in many international cuisines.

- Ensure no eggs in breading.

- Sample question: "Does the breading with the beef Wellington contain eggs?"

Cakes or Cookies can contain eggs, dairy, gluten/wheat flour, peanuts and tree nuts. They are included as ingredients or accompaniments to desserts in many international cuisines.

- Ensure no eggs in cakes and cookies.

- Sample question: *"Are there any eggs in the almond cookie?"*

Colors or Flavors can be made from a variety of ingredients some of which contain eggs, corn, dairy, gluten/wheat, peanuts, soy and tree nuts. These may be included in prefabricated frozen desserts and beverages.

- Ensure no colors or flavors containing eggs are ingredients in any commercially made desserts and beverages.

- Sample question: *"Do you make your gelato fresh in the restaurant or is it from a container that identifies egg as an ingredient on the label?"*

Croutons typically contain eggs and gluten/wheat flour, as well as other ingredients and are used in salads and soups in many types of international cuisines.

- Ensure no croutons containing eggs.

- Sample question: *"Is the salad topped with croutons?"*

Custard always contains eggs as an ingredient.

- Ensure no custard in desserts.

- Sample question: *"Is the fruiti di stagione (Italian fresh fruit in season) served with zabaglione (Italian custard)?"*

Dumpling Skins are common in Asian cuisines, typically contain eggs and may contain gluten/wheat.

- Ensure no eggs in dumpling skins.

- Sample question: *"Does the dumpling skin for the kanom jeeb (Thai shrimp dumplings) have eggs in it?"*

Egg Sealer is a term used for the process of sealing dumplings and parchment bags used for cooking.

- Ensure no eggs are used to seal dumplings and parchment paper.

- Sample question: *"Is egg used to seal the parchment paper bag in the saumon en papillote (French baked salmon)?"*

Egg Yolks are often used as an ingredient in sauces, entrees and desserts.

- Ensure no egg yolks are used in any dish.

- Sample question: *"Does this sauce contain egg yolks?"*

Imitation Crabmeat or Seafood is also known as surimi and is commonly used in Asian cuisines. It is made of fish paste and a number of additives, then molded into a shape, usually resembling crabmeat. In addition to fish, surimi may contain eggs, corn, gluten/wheat and soy.

- Ensure no imitation crabmeat or seafood containing eggs in any dish.

- Sample question: *"Do you use imitation crabmeat in your seafood bisque?"*

Mayonnaise contains eggs and is used as an ingredient in sauces, as well as a condiment. In commercially produced mayonnaise, soy may also be included.

- Ensure no mayonnaise as a condiment or in sauces.

- Sample question: *"Can I have my hamburger without mayonnaise?"*

Noodles or Pasta may contain eggs and gluten/wheat flour as ingredients.

- Ensure no noodles or pasta containing eggs.

- Sample question: *"Do the rice noodles contain eggs?"*

Salad Dressing that is commercially produced may contain ingredients derived from eggs, corn, dairy, fish, gluten/wheat and soy. Fresh Caesar dressing is typically made with eggs and some fresh French vinaigrettes may contain hard boiled eggs.

- Ensure no eggs in any commercially made or fresh salad dressings.

- Sample question: *"Does the dressing in the asperge à la vinaigrette (French asparagus salad) contain eggs?"*

Sauce or Dipping Sauce may contain eggs as an ingredient, as well as corn, dairy, fish, gluten/wheat, peanuts, soy and tree nuts.

- Ensure no eggs are included as ingredients in sauces.

- Sample question: *"Can I have my filet mignon without béarnaise sauce?"*

Side Dishes or Accompaniments may contain eggs, as well as other ingredients such as corn, dairy, gluten/wheat, peanuts, soy and tree nuts.

- Ensure no eggs as an ingredient in any side dish or accompaniment.

- Sample question: *"Is the pasta in the side salad made with eggs?"*

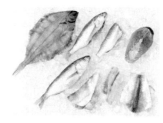

Fish

Fish is an easier allergy to manage, since it is used primarily as a main ingredient in most dishes. There are some commercially produced sauces that contain fish.

The following potential ingredients and preparation techniques represent areas of concern while managing sensitivities to fish:

- Anchovies

- Fish Sauce

- Imitation Crabmeat or Seafood

- Salad Dressing

- Salmon

- Stocks and Broths

- Tuna

Anchovies are a common ingredient in European style salads and some commercially produced sauces.

- Ensure no anchovies are included as ingredients in salads and sauces.

- Sample question: *"Does your salade niçoise contain anchovies?"*

Fish Sauce is a common sauce in Southeast Asian cuisine and may also contain gluten/wheat based upon manufacturing processes outside of Thailand.

- Ensure no fish sauce is used in any Southeast Asian dish.

- Sample question: *"Is there fish sauce in your thom kha gai (Thai chicken and coconut soup)?"*

Imitation Crabmeat or Seafood is also known as surimi and is commonly used in Asian cuisines. It is made of fish paste and a number of additives, then molded into a shape, usually resembling crabmeat. In addition to fish, surimi may contain corn, eggs, gluten/wheat and soy.

- Ensure no imitation crabmeat or seafood in any dish.

- Sample question: *"Do you use imitation crabmeat in your seafood bisque?"*

Salad Dressing that is commercially produced may contain ingredients derived from fish, corn, dairy, eggs, gluten/wheat and soy. Fresh Caesar salad dressing typically contains anchovies.

- Ensure no fish in any commercially made or fresh Caesar salad dressings.

- Sample question: *"Does the Caesar salad dressing contain anchovies?"*

Salmon, like most fish, may be found in appetizers and entrees in many international cuisines.

- Ensure no salmon is included in any dish.

2

- Sample question: *"Do you grill your steaks on the same side of the grill as your salmon and other fish?"*

Stocks and Broths may contain fish and shellfish if they are used in the preparation of seafood dishes.

- Ensure no stocks or broths made from fish are used in any dish.

- Sample question: *"Is your risotto special made with fish stock?"*

Tuna, like most fish, may be found in appetizers and entrees in many international cuisines.

- Ensure no tuna is included in any dish.

- Sample question: *"Does this salad contain tuna?"*

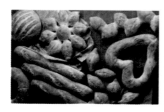

Gluten/Wheat

Gluten is the protein found in wheat, rye and barley. Although oats do not contain the gluten protein, the milling process in most manufacturing facilities may involve cross-contamination with other grains. It should be noted that an individual can have allergies, intolerances or sensitivities to wheat without having the dietary concerns for other grains that contain gluten.

The following potential ingredients and preparation techniques represent areas of concern while managing sensitivities to gluten/wheat and their derivatives:

- Artificial Bacon Bits

- Artificial Mashed Potato Mix

- Batter

- Beans

- Bouillon

- Bread or Bread Crumbs

- Breading

- Cakes or Cookies

2

- Cheese or Blue Cheese
- Colors or Flavors
- Croutons
- Dedicated Fryer
- Dumpling Skins
- Fish Sauce
- Flour Dusting
- Fluffing Agent
- Fresh Oil
- Imitation Crabmeat or Seafood
- Malt
- Malt Vinegar
- Marinade
- Noodles or Pasta
- Salad Dressing
- Sauce, Dipping Sauce or Salsa
- Seasonings
- Side Dishes or Accompaniments
- Soy Sauce
- Stabilizers
- Thickening Agent
- Tortillas or Tortilla Chips
- Wheat Flour
- Yogurt, Yogurt Curd or Yogurt Sauce

Artificial Bacon Bits are used as substitutes for bacon primarily in North America and may contain gluten/ wheat, corn and soy, as well as other ingredients. They are typically offered with baked potatoes and in salads.

2

- Ensure no artificial bacon bits that contain gluten/wheat are used in the preparation of baked potatoes and salads.

- Sample question: *"Is the bacon included in the baked potato real or artificial?"*

Artificial Mashed Potato Mix is often used as a time saving and inexpensive solution for mashed potatoes in North America and may contain gluten/wheat, corn, dairy and soy.

- Ensure no artificial mashed potato mix that contains gluten/wheat.

- Sample question: *"Are the mashed potatoes included with this entree real or artificial?"*

Batter typically contains wheat or corn flour combined with eggs and is used in many types of international cuisines.

- Ensure no wheat flour in batter of entrees and side dishes.

- Sample question: *"Is the chicken in the panang curry (Thai peanut curry) battered?"*

Beans may include wheat flour as an ingredient in many international cuisines.

- Ensure no beans containing wheat flour.

- Sample question: *"Do the fava beans contain wheat flour?"*

Bouillon is often used as a time saving and inexpensive solution for soup bases and sauces. It often contains gluten/wheat, corn and soy, as well as other ingredients.

- Ensure no bouillon containing gluten/wheat is used in the preparation of sauces and soups.

- Sample question: *"Is this soup made with fresh vegetable broth?"*

Bread or Bread Crumbs may contain gluten/wheat flour, corn, dairy, eggs, peanuts, soy and tree nuts, as well as other ingredients and are used in many types of international cuisines.

- Ensure no bread or bread crumbs containing wheat flour.

- Sample question: *"Are the escargots topped with bread crumbs?"*

Breading may contain gluten/wheat flour, corn, dairy, eggs and soy and is used in many international cuisines.

- Ensure no wheat flour in breading.

- Sample question: *"Is the petti di pollo (Italian chicken breast) breaded?"*

Cakes or Cookies can contain gluten/wheat flour, dairy, eggs, peanuts and tree nuts. They are included as ingredients or accompaniments to desserts in many international cuisines.

- Ensure no wheat flour in cakes and cookies.

- Sample question: *"Is there any wheat flour in the flourless chocolate torte?"*

Cheese or Blue Cheese contains dairy and possibly gluten/ wheat if blue or veined cheese. Pasteurized processed cheese may also contain corn or soy depending upon the manufacturer. It is used as an ingredient in sauces, salads, entrees, side dishes and desserts.

- Ensure no blue or veined cheese is used in any dish.

- Sample question: *"Is this salad topped with Roquefort?"*

Colors or Flavors can be made from a variety of ingredients some of which contain gluten/wheat, corn, dairy, eggs, peanuts, soy and tree nuts. These may be included in prefabricated frozen desserts, beverages, food coloring and meat products.

2

- Ensure no colors or flavors containing gluten/ wheat are ingredients in any commercially made product.

- Sample question: *"Is the smoked sausage made in the restaurant or do you use pre-packaged sausage that identifies gluten or wheat on the label?"*

Croutons typically contain gluten/wheat flour and eggs, as well as other ingredients and are used in salads and soups in many types of international cuisines.

- Ensure no croutons containing wheat flour.

- Sample question: *"Is the salad topped with croutons?"*

Dedicated Fryer is a term used for a fryer that only fries one particular food type (e.g. battered items only or French fries). Dedicated fryers eliminate the possibility of gluten/wheat cross-contamination from frying battered, breaded or wheat flour dusted foods with non-gluten containing foods.

- Ensure no cross-contamination with deep fried foods containing gluten/wheat.

- Sample question: *"Are your French fries fried in the same fryer as your beer battered onion rings?"*

Dumpling Skins are common in Asian cuisines; they typically contain eggs and may contain gluten/wheat.

- Ensure no gluten/wheat flour in dumpling skins.

- Sample question: *"Do you use wheat flour for the dumpling skins in the kanom jeeb (Thai shrimp dumplings)?"*

Fish Sauce is a common sauce in Southeast Asian cuisine and may also contain gluten/wheat based upon manufacturing processes outside of Thailand.

- Ensure no fish sauce containing wheat is used in any Southeast Asian dish.

- Sample question: *"Is the brand of fish sauce you use in this dish processed in Hong Kong?"*

Fluffing Agent is a term used for adding an ingredient, such as gluten/wheat flour, to eggs to enhance their appearance and increase their volume.

- Ensure no gluten/wheat flour is used as a fluffing agent for egg dishes.

- Sample question: *"Do you add wheat flour to the egg mix for your omelets?"*

Flour Dusting is a term used for coating meat and fish with an ingredient, such as gluten/wheat flour, for texture prior to pan-frying.

- Ensure no gluten/wheat flour is used to dust meat and fish.

- Sample question: *"Do you dust the beef in wheat flour prior to pan frying?"*

Fresh Oil is a request that may be necessary to eliminate the possibility of cross-contamination from used cooking oil.

- Ensure fresh cooking oil to avoid cross-contamination.

- Sample question: *"Can you use fresh oil to fry my huevos Mexicanos (Mexican eggs)?"*

Imitation Crabmeat or Seafood is also known as surimi and is commonly used in Asian cuisines. It is made of fish paste and a number of additives, then molded into a shape, usually resembling crabmeat. In addition to fish, surimi may contain gluten/wheat, corn, eggs and soy.

- Ensure no imitation crabmeat or seafood containing gluten/wheat in any dish.

- Sample question: *"Do you use imitation crabmeat in your seafood bisque?"*

Malt is typically made from barley, which contains gluten, or corn. It is commonly used in commercially produced beverages, confectionary products and frozen desserts.

- Ensure no malt in any commercially produced beverages, confectionary products and frozen desserts.

- Sample question: *"Does the ice cream container identify malt or wheat as an ingredient on the label?"*

Malt Vinegar is made by fermenting barley, which contains gluten, and is not distilled. It is a common condiment in French cuisine and also used regularly in the United Kingdom.

- Ensure no malt vinegar as a condiment.

- Sample question: *"Can you hold the malt vinegar with my French fried potatoes order?"*

Marinades may have wheat flour as an ingredient, which adds texture to meat.

- Ensure no wheat flour in marinades.

- Sample question: *"Does the marinade for gai yang (Thai barbequed chicken) contain wheat flour?"*

Noodles or Pasta may contain gluten/wheat flour and eggs as ingredients.

- Ensure no noodles or pasta containing gluten/ wheat flour.

- Sample question: *"Are the noodles in the pad see yu made with wheat?"*

Salad Dressing that is commercially produced may contain ingredients derived from gluten/wheat, corn, dairy, eggs, fish and soy.

- Ensure no gluten/wheat in any commercially made dressings.

- Sample question: *"Does the ranch dressing identify gluten or wheat as an ingredient on the label?"*

Sauce, Dipping Sauce or Salsa may contain gluten/wheat flour as an ingredient, as well as corn, dairy, eggs, fish, peanuts, soy and tree nuts. Commercially produced sauces may contain a number of different gluten/wheat derivatives.

- Ensure no gluten/wheat or their derivatives are ingredients in sauces.

- Sample question: *"Does the peanut sauce contain wheat flour?"*

Seasonings that are commercially produced sometimes contain ingredients derived from gluten/wheat, corn, dairy and soy.

- Ensure no gluten/wheat in any commercially made seasonings.

- Sample question: *"What type of seasonings do you use to flavor the French fried potatoes?"*

Side Dishes or Accompaniments may contain gluten/wheat, as well as other ingredients such as dairy, peanuts, soy and tree nuts.

- Ensure no gluten/wheat or their derivatives are ingredients in any side dish or accompaniment.

- Sample question: *"Does the fruit compote that comes with the pork chop contain wheat flour?"*

Soy Sauce is a common ingredient in Asian and other international cuisines. In addition to being made from soy, most soy sauces also contain gluten/wheat as an ingredient. It is used in marinades or as an ingredient in sauces and soups.

- Ensure no soy sauce in marinades, sauces and soups.

- Sample question: *"Is there soy sauce in the lemon chicken?"*

Stabilizers containing gluten/wheat are commonly used in commercially produced frozen desserts.

- Ensure no stabilizers containing gluten/wheat in commercially produced frozen desserts.

- Sample question: *"Does the sorbet container identify gluten/wheat stabilizers as an ingredient on the label?"*

Thickening Agent is a term used for adding an ingredient, such as gluten/wheat flour, to soups to make the broth have a higher viscosity or thickness.

- Ensure no gluten/wheat flour is used as a thickening agent for soups.

- Sample question: *"Do you use wheat flour to thicken the broth of the egg drop soup?"*

Tortillas or Tortilla Chips may contain gluten/wheat, corn or soy and are common in Central and South American cuisines. They can be made from either corn or wheat flour and lard or vegetable oil.

- Ensure no wheat flour tortillas or tortillas chips.

- Sample question: *"Can I have corn tortillas with my carnitas (Mexican simmered pork)?"*

Wheat Flour can be used as an ingredient in the most unlikely places. Non-traditional food preparation techniques involving wheat flour are indicated throughout this book.

- Ensure no wheat flour in any dish.

- Sample question: *"Do you add wheat flour to your hollandaise sauce?"*

Yogurt, Yogurt Curd or Yogurt Sauce typically contains dairy as an ingredient and is commonly used in Mediterranean, Middle Eastern and Indian cuisines. Commercially produced yogurt may also contain gluten/wheat and soy.

- Ensure no gluten/wheat in commercially produced yogurt.

- Sample question: *"Do you use commercially produced yogurt in your raita (Indian yogurt dipping sauce) which identifies gluten or wheat as an ingredient on the label?"*

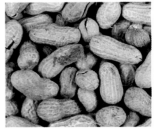

Peanuts

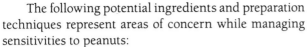

Peanuts are legumes like peas or beans and are used frequently in Asian, Central and South American cuisines. Peanut oil, also known as arachis oil in Europe, is commonly used for frying in Asian, Indian, French and French-influenced cuisines.

The following potential ingredients and preparation techniques represent areas of concern while managing sensitivities to peanuts:

- Bread or Bread Crumbs

- Cakes or Cookies

- Colors or Flavors

- Garnishes

- Peanut Oil

- Sauce or Dipping Sauce

- Side Dishes or Accompaniments

- Vegetable Bisque

- Vegetable Oil

Bread or Bread Crumbs may contain peanuts, corn, dairy, eggs, gluten/wheat flour, soy and tree nuts, as well as other ingredients and are used in many types of international cuisines.

- Ensure no bread or bread crumbs containing peanuts.

- Sample question: *"Are there peanuts in this fresh bread?"*

2

Cakes or Cookies can contain peanuts, dairy, eggs, gluten/wheat flour and tree nuts. They are included as ingredients or accompaniments to desserts in many international cuisines.

- Ensure no peanuts in cakes and cookies.

- Sample question: *"Are there any peanuts in the cookie?"*

Colors or Flavors can be made from a variety of ingredients some of which contain peanuts, corn, dairy, eggs, gluten/wheat, soy and tree nuts. These may be included in prefabricated frozen desserts.

- Ensure no colors or flavors containing peanuts are ingredients in any commercially made dessert.

- Sample question: *"Do you make your gelato fresh in the restaurant or is it from a container that identifies peanuts as an ingredient on the label?"*

Garnishes containing peanuts and tree nuts are common in Asian cuisines.

- Ensure no garnish containing peanuts is included with any dish.

- Sample question: *"Is the kang dang (Thai red curry) garnished with peanuts?"*

Peanut Oil is commonly used to fry or sauté foods in Asian, Indian, French and French-influenced restaurants.

- Ensure no peanut oil is used to fry or sauté foods.

- Sample question: *"Are the pommes frites (French fried potatoes) fried in peanut oil?"*

Sauce or Dipping Sauce may contain peanuts as an ingredient and is typically found in Asian, Central and South American cuisines. Sauces may also contain corn, dairy, eggs, fish, gluten/wheat, soy and tree nuts.

- Ensure no peanuts are used as ingredients in sauces.

- Sample question: *"Do you include peanuts in your mole sauce?"*

Side Dishes or Accompaniments may contain peanuts, as well as other ingredients such as corn, dairy, eggs, gluten/wheat, soy and tree nuts.

- Ensure no peanuts as an ingredient in any side dish or accompaniment.

- Sample question: *"Do you sauté the green beans in peanut oil?"*

Vegetable Bisque may contain peanuts and tree nuts.

- Ensure no peanuts are used as an ingredient in vegetable bisque.

- Sample question: *"Are there peanuts in the mushroom bisque?"*

Vegetable Oil can be a blend of peanuts, corn, soy and other types of oils.

- Ensure no peanut oil in vegetable oil blends.

- Sample question: *"Can I have the mushrooms sautéed in butter rather than vegetable oil?"*

Shellfish

Shellfish are divided into two categories, crustaceans and mollusks. Common crustaceans include crab, lobster and shrimp, while mollusks include abalone, escargot (snails), mussels, octopus, oysters, scallops and squid.

The following potential ingredients and preparation techniques represent areas of concern while managing sensitivities to shellfish:

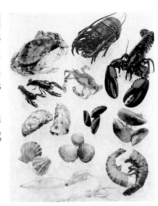

- Calamari

- Crab

- Escargot

- Lobster

- Mussels

- Oysters

- Shrimp

- Stocks and Broths

Calamari, the Italian name for squid, may be found in appetizers, entrees and soups in many international cuisines.

- Ensure no calamari is included in any dish.

- Sample question: *"Does the salmon bisque contain calamari or any other shellfish?"*

Crab may be found in appetizers, entrees and soups in many international cuisines.

- Ensure no crab is included in any dish.

- Sample question: *"Are the mushrooms stuffed with crab?"*

Escargot (snails) may be found in appetizers and entrees in some international cuisines.

- Ensure no escargot is included in any dish

- Sample question: *"Are the mushrooms stuffed with escargot (snails)?"*

Lobster may be found in appetizers, entrees and soups in many international cuisines.

- Ensure no lobster is included in any dish.

- Sample question: *"Does the risotto special contain lobster or other shellfish?"*

Mussels may be found in appetizers, entrees and soups in many international cuisines.

- Ensure no mussels are included in any dish.

- Sample question: *"Does this paella (Spansh rice dish) contain mussels or any other shellfish?"*

Oysters may be found in appetizers, entrees and soups in many international cuisines.

- Ensure no oysters are included in any dish.

- Sample question: "Does the salmon bisque contain oysters or any other shellfish?"

Shrimp may be found in appetizers, entrees and soups in many international cuisines.

- Ensure no shrimp is included in any dish.

- Sample question: *"Do your summer rolls contain shrimp?"*

Stocks and Broths may contain shellfish and fish if they are used in the preparation of seafood dishes.

- Ensure no stocks or broths made from shellfish are used in any dish.

- Sample question: *"Is your risotto special made with seafood stock?"*

Soy

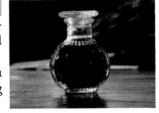

Soy is a legume like peas or beans and is used frequently in Asian cuisines. Its derivatives are contained in many commercially produced products.

The following potential ingredients and preparation techniques represent areas of concern while managing sensitivities to soy and its derivatives:

- Artificial Bacon Bits
- Artificial Mashed Potato Mix
- Bean Curd
- Bouillon
- Bread or Bread Crumbs
- Breading
- Cheese
- Chocolate

- Colors or Flavors
- Imitation Crabmeat or Seafood
- Ketchup
- Masa
- Mayonnaise
- Salad Dressing
- Sauce, Dipping Sauce or Salsa
- Seasonings
- Side Dishes or Accompaniments
- Soy Sauce
- Tofu
- Tortillas or Tortilla Chips
- Vegetable Oil
- Yogurt, Yogurt Curd or Yogurt Sauce

Artificial Bacon Bits are used as substitutes for bacon primarily in North America and may contain soy, corn and gluten/wheat, as well as other ingredients. They are typically offered with baked potatoes and in salads.

- Ensure no artificial bacon bits that contain soy are used in the preparation of baked potatoes and salads.

- Sample question: *"Is the bacon included in this salad real or artificial?"*

Artificial Mashed Potato Mix is often used as a time saving and inexpensive solution for mashed potatoes in North America and may contain soy, corn, dairy, and gluten/wheat.

- Ensure no artificial mashed potato mix that contains soy.

- Sample question: *"Are the mashed potatoes included with this entree real or artificial?"*

Bean Curd is made from soy and is similar in consistency to medium hard cheese. It is often used in Asian cuisines.

- Ensure no bean curd is included in any dish.

- Sample question: *"Is there bean curd in the kaw pad (Thai fried rice)?"*

Bouillon is often used as a time saving and inexpensive solution for soup bases and sauces. It often contains soy, corn and gluten/wheat, as well as other ingredients.

- Ensure no bouillon containing soy is used in the preparation of sauces and soups.

- Sample question: *"Is this bouillabaise (French seafood stew) made with fresh seafood stock?"*

Bread or Bread Crumbs may contain soy, corn, dairy, eggs, gluten/wheat flour, peanuts and tree nuts, as well as other ingredients and are used in many types of international cuisines.

- Ensure no bread or bread crumbs containing soy.

- Sample question. *"Do you make your bread with vegetable oil?"*

Breading may contain soy, corn, dairy, eggs and gluten/wheat flour and is used in many international cuisines.

- Ensure no soy in breading.

- Sample question: *"Is the melanzane alla griglia (Italian grilled eggplant) prepared with breading that contains vegetable oil?"*

Cheese contains dairy and possibly gluten/wheat if blue or veined cheese. Pasteurized processed cheese may also contain corn or soy depending upon the manufacturer. It is used as an ingredient in sauces, salads, entrees, side dishes and desserts.

- Ensure no pasteurized processed cheese containing soy is used in any dish.

2

- Sample question: *"Does the cheese sauce contain pasteurized processed cheese?"*

Chocolate may contain soy if made in the United States and contains dairy if it is identified as milk chocolate or listed on label. It is used as an ingredient in desserts and some sauces.

- Ensure no chocolate containing soy is used in desserts and sauces.

- Sample question: *"Can you check to see if the chocolate in the mole sauce contains soy?"*

Colors or Flavors can be made from a variety of ingredients some of which contain soy, corn, dairy, eggs, gluten/wheat, peanuts and tree nuts. These may be included in prefabricated frozen desserts, beverages and food coloring.

- Ensure no colors or flavors containing soy are ingredients in any commercially made product.

- Sample question: *"Do you make your sorbet fresh in the restaurant or is it from a container that identifies soy as an ingredient on the label?"*

Imitation Crabmeat or Seafood is also known as surimi and is commonly used in Asian cuisines. It is made of fish paste and a number of additives, then molded into a shape, usually resembling crabmeat. In addition to fish, surimi may contain soy, corn, eggs and gluten/wheat.

- Ensure no imitation crabmeat or seafood containing soy in any dish.

- Sample question: *"Do you use imitation crabmeat in your paella mariscos (Mexican seafood and rice dish)?"*

Ketchup is made from tomatoes, vinegar and many other ingredients which may include soy. It is provided as a condiment and used in some sauces.

- Ensure no ketchup with soy is used as a condiment or in sauces.

- Sample question: *"Do you prepare your cocktail sauce with ketchup that lists soy as an ingredient?"*

Masa is made from corn meal and lard or vegetable oil which may be made with soy and corn. It is used primarily in Central and South American cuisine.

- Ensure no masa made with vegetable oil containing soy is used in tamales and corn tortillas.

- Sample question: *"Is the masa in your tamales made with vegetable oil containing soy?"*

Mayonnaise contains eggs and is used as an ingredient in sauces, as well as a condiment. Commercially produced mayonnaise may also include soy.

- Ensure no mayonnaise containing soy as a condiment or in sauces.

- Sample question: *"Does the mayonnaise you use for the dipping sauce come from a container that identifies soy as an ingredient on the label?"*

Salad Dressing that is commercially produced may contain ingredients derived from soy, corn, dairy, eggs, fish and gluten/wheat. Vinaigrettes made fresh in restaurants may also include corn and soy if vegetable oil, or if less than 100% olive oil is used in the preparation.

- Ensure no soy in any commercially made dressings or fresh vinaigrettes.

- Sample question: *"Does the Russian salad dressing come from a container that identifies soy as an ingredient on the label?"*

Sauce, Dipping Sauce or Salsa may contain soy as an ingredient, as well as corn, dairy, eggs, fish, gluten/wheat flour, peanuts and tree nuts. Commercially produced sauces may contain a number of different soy derivatives.

- Ensure no soy or its derivatives as ingredients in sauces.

2

- Sample question: *"Does the chili sauce contain vegetable oil identifying soy as an ingredient?"*

Seasonings that are commercially produced sometimes contain ingredients derived from soy, corn, dairy and gluten/wheat.

- Ensure no soy in any commercially made seasonings.

- Sample question: *"What type of seasonings do you use to flavor the hash browns?"*

Side Dishes or Accompaniments may contain soy, as well as other ingredients such as corn, dairy, eggs, gluten/wheat, peanuts, soy and tree nuts.

- Ensure no soy as an ingredient in any side dish or accompaniment.

- Sample question: *"Do you sauté the broccoli rabe in vegetable oil?"*

Soy Sauce is a common ingredient in Asian and other international cuisines. In addition to being made from soy, most soy sauces also contain gluten/wheat as an ingredient. It is frequently used for marinades and in sauces.

- Ensure no soy sauce in marinades and sauces.

- Sample question: *"Does the marinade for your roasted chicken contain soy sauce?"*

Tofu is made from soy and is similar in consistency to soft cheese. It is often used in Asian cuisines.

- Ensure no tofu is included in any dish.

- Sample question: *"Does the Buddha's Feast include tofu?"*

Tortillas or Tortilla Chips may contain soy, corn or gluten/wheat and are common in Central and South American cuisines. They can be made from either corn or wheat flour and lard or vegetable oil containing corn and soy.

- Ensure no corn tortillas or tortillas chips containing soy.

- Sample question: *"Are your tortilla chips made from vegetable oil containing soy?"*

Vegetable Oil can be a blend of soy, corn, peanuts and other types of oils.

- Ensure no soy in vegetable oil blends.

- Sample question: *"Can I have the broccoli rabe sautéed in butter rather than vegetable oil?"*

Yogurt, Yogurt Curd or Yogurt Sauce typically contains dairy as an ingredient and is commonly used in Mediterranean, Middle Eastern and Indian cuisines. Commercially produced yogurt may also contain gluten/wheat and soy.

- Ensure no soy in commercially produced yogurt.

- Sample question: *"Is soy identified as an ingredient on the yogurt container?"*

Tree Nuts

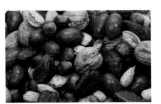

Tree nuts are considered "true nuts" and are used in many international cuisines. Some common tree nuts include almonds, Brazil nuts, cashews, chestnuts, hazelnuts, hickory nuts, macadamia nuts, pecans, pine nuts, pistachios and walnuts.

The following potential ingredients and preparation techniques represent areas of concern while managing sensitivities to tree nuts and their derivatives:

- Almonds or Almond Extract
- Breads or Bread Crumbs
- Cakes or Cookies
- Colors or Flavors
- Cashews or Cashew Powder
- Garnishes

- Pistachios

- Sauce, Dipping Sauce or Salsa

- Side Dishes or Accompaniments

- Vegetable Bisque

- Walnuts

Almonds or Almond Extract are used primarily in breads, desserts and pastries or as an ingredient in vegetable side dishes. Almond extract typically contains tree nuts and corn.

- Ensure no almonds or almond extract is used in the preparation of breads, desserts, pastries and vegetable side dishes.

- Sample question: *"Are there almonds in the haricots verts (French green beans)?"*

Bread or Bread Crumbs may contain tree nuts, corn, dairy, eggs, gluten/wheat flour, peanuts and soy, as well as other ingredients and are used in many types of international cuisines.

- Ensure no bread or bread crumbs containing tree nuts.

- Sample question: *"Are the escargots topped with bread crumbs that contains tree nuts?"*

Cakes or Cookies can contain tree nuts, dairy, eggs, gluten/wheat flour and peanuts. They are included as ingredients or accompaniments to desserts in many international cuisines.

- Ensure no tree nuts in cakes and cookies.

- Sample question: *"Are there any almonds in this cookie?"*

Cashews or Cashew Powder is often used in Middle Eastern and Indian cuisines, as well as in desserts in many other international cuisines.

- Ensure no cashews are included with any dish.

- Sample question: *"Are the kabobs made with cashew powder?"*

Colors or Flavors can be made from a variety of ingredients some of which contain tree nuts, corn, dairy, eggs, gluten/wheat, peanuts and soy. These may be included in prefabricated frozen desserts and beverages.

- Ensure no colors or flavors containing tree nuts are ingredients in any commercially made product.

- Sample question: *"Do you make your helados (Mexican ice cream, sherbet or sorbet) fresh in the restaurant or is it from a container that tree nuts are identified as an ingredient on the label?"*

Garnishes containing tree nuts and peanuts are common in Asian cuisines.

- Ensure no garnish containing tree nuts is included with any dish.

- Sample question: *"Is the kang massaman (Thai tamarind curry) garnished with cashews or any other tree nuts?"*

Pistachios are often used in Middle Eastern and Indian cuisines, as well as in desserts in many other international cuisines.

- Ensure no pistachios are included with any dish.

- Sample question: *"Does the kulfi (Indian ice cream) contain pistachios or any other tree nuts?"*

Sauce or Dipping Sauce may contain tree nuts as an ingredient. Sauces may also contain corn, dairy, eggs, fish, gluten/wheat, peanuts and soy.

- Ensure no tree nuts are used as ingredients in sauces.

- Sample question: *"Does the murg korma (Indian chicken in cream curry) contain almonds or any other tree nuts?"*

2

Side Dishes or Accompaniments may contain tree nuts, as well as other ingredients such as corn, dairy, eggs, gluten/wheat, peanuts and soy.

- Ensure no tree nuts or their derivatives are ingredients in any side dish or accompaniment.

- Sample question: *"Is there almond oil in the chutney?"*

Vegetable Bisque may contain tree nuts and peanuts.

- Ensure no tree nuts are used as an ingredient in vegetable bisque.

- Sample question: *"Are tree nuts included in the tomato bisque?"*

Walnuts are often used in breads, desserts and salads in many international cuisines.

- Ensure no walnuts are used as an ingredient in breads, desserts and salads.

- Sample question: *"Are walnuts included in the spinach salad?"*

Summary

As you can see, there is more to managing a specialized diet than simply avoiding the foundation of what you are allergic to. You will no doubt need, at some time, to return to the previous pages of this chapter to re-familiarize yourself with these potential considerations. As a reminder, if this book indicates that an ingredient may be included in a particular dish, it doesn't necessarily preclude you from ordering it. You do, however, need to confirm the possibility of its presence with the restaurant staff. If it is indicated that a dish contains an allergen you are trying to avoid, then it is best to choose another menu option or request a substitution if applicable. Armed with this knowledge, you will soon realize that there is a whole new world of food options open to you. Ask the right questions, embrace the gastronomic experience and enjoy your new freedom!

Enjoy Your Meal!

好胃口

Bon Appetit!

Buon Appetitto!

Chalo, sub khana khao!

Buen Provecho!

Gkin Kao!

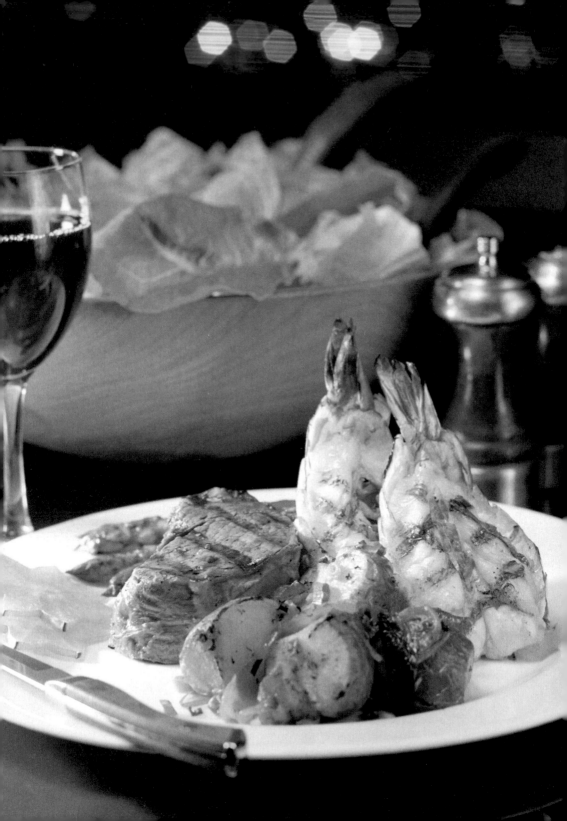

*Of all the contributions this country
has made to dining out, none is so quintessentially
American as the Steak House.*
—John Mariani

Chapter 3
Let's Eat American Steak and Seafood

Cuisine Overview

The United States of America is a nation of immigrants, whose culture is a unique mixture of international influences and home grown Americana. The US is comprised of 50 states and a number of territories. It is roughly two and a half times the size of Western Europe. It is the world's third largest nation in both population and land mass.

The Steak and Seafood restaurant is the greatest representation of the bountiful harvests of American farmers, fishermen and ranchers. At these establishments, produce, meat and seafood are prepared in a simple culinary fashion that produces a wholesome and satisfying dining experience. This is due to a belief that using good quality ingredients requires few advanced culinary preparation techniques. With this in mind, the American Steak and Seafood restaurant is one of the safer cuisines for those with food allergies or sensitivities.

The range and style of Steak and Seafood houses in America is diverse. Whether you are dining at a single independent restaurant or a large restaurant chain,

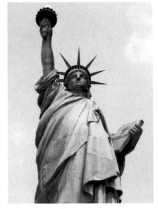
Statue of Liberty

3

each establishment has a unique atmosphere and feeling. There is the classic New York style steakhouse with its career waiters in white coats and bistro aprons or the casual wait staff at the family-oriented theme restaurants. Some restaurants choose the fusion approach of blending other international cuisines with standard steak and seafood dishes, while others give you the feeling of eating at an authentic western saloon. The quality of meat, produce and seafood is in line with the price differential between the finest steak houses and moderately priced restaurant establishments. The finest American Steak and Seafood restaurants are among the most expensive you will find in the United States. Regardless of preference, most steak and seafood restaurants can offer you a wholesome meal.

Traditional Ingredients

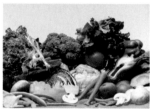

Vegetables play a big part in the American Steak and Seafood restaurant dining experience. Both in salads and in side dishes, you may see asparagus, artichokes, broccoli, carrots, green beans, hearts of palm, many types of lettuce, olives, onions, potatoes and tomatoes. Herbs include basil, garlic, rosemary, and thyme. For seasoning purposes, most restaurants simply use salt and pepper; however, some chefs incorporate exotic seasonings such as saffron into their culinary palate.

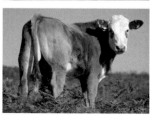

Vegetables (top). Cow (bottom).

American Steak and Seafood restaurants carry a variety of beef cuts and follow the scale of quality set forth by the U.S. government. Beef is graded for quality by U.S. Department of Agriculture (USDA) graders according to standards established by the USDA. Grades are based on the amount of marbling (flecks of fat within the cut of meat) and the age of the animal. These quality grades are an indication of palatability characteristics such as tenderness, juiciness, and flavor. While there are eight quality grades for beef, the top three grades available to most consumers are prime, choice and select. In addition to beef, you may find lamb, pork and chicken on many Steak and Seafood menus.

Many types of seafood may also be available including Maine lobster, Alaskan king crab, oysters, mussels, salmon and shrimp. Again, the preparation of these dishes is minimal and in most cases involves baking, boiling, grilling, pan frying or steaming. In some establishments, there is a special food service area generally located in the front of the restaurant where raw shellfish is prepared. This "raw bar" is a common menu section that is usually enjoyed as the appetizer portion of a meal and in some cases can serve as the entire meal all by itself.

Starch dishes available are usually potato-based, such as baked potatoes, French fried potatoes, mashed potatoes, roasted potatoes and hash browns. Rice dishes and pastas are also available. Finally, wine is a popular accoutrement in the American Steak and Seafood dining experience. Most restaurants usually feature a wine list that gives a number of varieties, both white and red, to choose from. In the finer establishments, it is likely that you will have to make a difficult decision on wines from the US and other parts of the world.

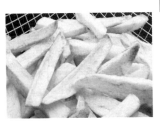

French Fried Potatoes

Gluten Awareness

Since gluten can be found in some areas of American Steak and Seafood cuisine, we have outlined 30-plus items in our sample menu. It is important to keep in mind that American food is influenced by many international culinary practices. There are seven primary points that you need to consider when dining at an American Steak and Seafood restaurant. To ensure a gluten-free experience, the areas of food preparation that you need to inquire about with your server or chef are listed below.

Sauces	Ensure the *liaison* of the sauce is butter, egg yolks or puréed vegetables—ensure no wheat flour
Flour Dusting	Wheat flour is typically used—request plain
Stocks and Broths	Ensure all stocks and broths are made fresh and not from bouillon which may contain gluten
Cooking Oil	Ensure frying oil has not been used to fry battered foods that may contain gluten
Croutons/Bread Crumbs	Wheat flour is typically used—ensure no croutons or bread crumbs
Marinades	Although uncommon, ensure marinades do not contain soy sauce or wheat flour
Cross-Contamination	Ensure all utensils and cooking surfaces have been cleaned prior to the preparation of your meal

3

Sauces

Sauces are typically served on the side at American Steak and Seafood restaurants and are often influenced by French cuisine. Of the many different sauces you may encounter, always be sure the *liaison* that binds the sauce together is not wheat flour. Other acceptable *liaisons* include egg yolks, butter and puréed vegetables. Below is a list of common and typically gluten-free sauces adapted from the French and their ingredients:

Hollandaise: A sauce that contains butter, egg yolks as its liaison and lemon juice

Béarnaise: A reduction of white wine vinegar, tarragon and shallots that is finished with egg yolks and butter

Reduction: A mixture that results from rapidly boiling a liquid (like fresh stock, wine, or a sauce without wheat flour) and causing evaporation—"reducing" the sauce—which creates a thicker sauce with a more intense flavor than the original liquid

Flour Dusting

Flour dusting is not common in American Steak and Seafood restaurants. If used, most restaurants prefer to dust meat or fish with wheat flour for texture prior to pan-frying, allowing a sauce to be evenly distributed. When meat or fish is grilled over an open flame, flour dusting is not necessary. Ensure that this practice is not used in the preparation of your meal.

Stocks and Broths

Stocks and broths are used frequently in American Steak and Seafood restaurants. They are present in sauces and soups, as well as in marinades for meats and vegetables. Ensure that stocks and broths are made fresh and not from bouillon, which may contain gluten.

Cooking Oil

Any type of oil such as canola, corn or sunflower may be used in American Steak and Seafood restaurants. Some establishments influenced by French cooking may also use peanut oil. Olive oil may be incorporated from time to time, but is rarely used for frying. Oil is used to fry or sauté foods. When ordering food that is prepared by frying, ensure that there is a dedicated fryer in the kitchen for non-battered menu items. Since battered foods may contain wheat flour, this practice minimizes the potential of gluten cross-contamination from frying.

Croutons and Bread Crumbs

Croutons and bread crumbs are used regularly as an ingredient in appetizers, soups and salads. Croutons in particular are included with most salads, while bread crumbs are used in some baked vegetable side dishes. When ordering these dishes, always be sure to request no croutons or bread crumbs. In addition, a basket of bread is usually served, so be certain to request no bread.

Marinades

Marinades are used infrequently in American Steak and Seafood restaurants. If used, ensure that the marinade does not include soy sauce, which contains wheat, or wheat flour.

Cross-Contamination

Cross-contamination occurs in two primary instances and should be considered at any restaurant you choose to dine in. One may occur when your meal is prepared in the same frying oil as foods containing other possible allergens. The second may occur when microbes or food particles are transferred from one food to another by using the same knife, cutting board, pots, pans or other utensils without washing the surfaces or tools in between uses. In the case of open flamed grills, the extreme temperature turns most food particles into carbon. Use of a wire brush designed for grill racks typically removes residual contaminants. To avoid

3

cross-contamination, restaurants need to dedicate fryers for specific foods and wash all materials that may come in contact with food in hot, soapy water prior to preparing items for those with special dietary requirements. It is important to ensure that the restaurant follows these procedures for an allergen-free dining experience.

Other Allergy Considerations

If you have other food allergies or sensitivities, it is important to remain diligent in your approach to dining out. Because American Steak and Seafood restaurants offer a wide variety of foods, there are many common food allergens used on a regular basis. Know that vegetable oil can always be substituted for any oil and may contain corn, peanuts or soy. It should be noted that unless an olive oil container specifically states 100% olive oil, it may be mixed with vegetable oil. Some restaurants may also use peanut oil for frying. If used, bouillon may contain Hydrolyzed Vegetable Protein (HVP) that can be derived from corn, soy or wheat. We have indicated the potential presence of bouillon, peanut oil and vegetable oil.

From the 30-plus items we have listed in our sample menu, we have identified each common allergen typically included in the dish as an ingredient. We have also indicated other potential allergens that may be present based upon non-traditional culinary practices. The chances of encountering common food allergens in items specific to our sample menu are outlined below.

High likelihood	Dairy, egg, fish and shellfish
Moderate likelihood	Corn, gluten, peanuts, soy and wheat
Low likelihood	Tree nuts

Dining Considerations

American Steak and Seafood restaurants generally offer a limited number of menu items. They are presented in the English language, unless you are traveling abroad. A few large restaurant chains have locations in Europe,

Central and South America and Asia. In those countries, you can expect to see menus translated into the native language.

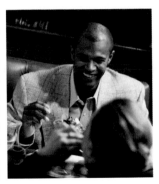

Traditionally, Americans eat two to three meals a day. Breakfast is widely considered the most important meal of the day and usually consists of breads, cereal, coffee, eggs, fruit, juice and meats. Lunch is taken between 11:30 a.m. and 1:30 p.m. and usually lasts about an hour. This meal typically consists of either a large salad, soup and sandwich or a substantial entrée. Dinner is eaten anywhere between 5 and 8 p.m. and can range from a single course to a modified course structure inspired by the French *service à la russe*, lasting from one to two hours.

Today, the standard American Steak and Seafood dining experience begins with appetizers and is followed by soup or salad, main course, and dessert. Since most American Steak and Seafood restaurants serve *à la carte*, it may be necessary to order side dishes of vegetables and starches with your entrees. The portions of these side dishes are usually quite large, so be sure to order appropriately and consider sharing them with the table. It is a rare occurrence, indeed, to leave without a full stomach. If you order too much food, you may want to leave with a doggie bag—a very American concept!

Enjoy Your Meal!

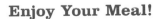

3

Sample American Steak and Seafood Menu

Appetizers
Oysters on the Half Shell
Shrimp Cocktail

Soups
Bisque (Cream Soup)

Salads
Buffalo Mozzarella and Tomato Salad
Chopped Salad
Cobb Salad
Hearts of Palm Salad
Mixed Green Salad

Meat Entrees
Hamburgers
Pork Chops
Lamb Chops
Steaks

Chicken Entrees
Grilled Chicken Breast
Roasted Chicken

Seafood Entrees
Crab
Fish Filet
Lobster

Sample American Steak and Seafood Menu

Side Dishes
Asparagus
Baked Potato
Broccoli
French Fried Potatoes
Green Beans
Hash Browns
Mashed Potatoes
Potatoes Lyonnaise
Spinach

Desserts
Chocolate Mousse
Crème Brulée (Baked Custard)
Flourless Chocolate Torte
Fresh Berries with Whipped Cream
Ice Cream
Sorbet

We would like to thank Tim Gannon, Founder and Executive Chef of Outback Steakhouse™ headquartered in Tampa, Florida and Domenica Catelli, Chef from domenica's way in Houston, Texas for their valuable contributions in reviewing the following menu items.

American Steak and Seafood Menu Item Descriptions

Appetizers
Oysters on the Half Shell
Oysters on the half shell can be served raw with lemon and a cocktail sauce made of tomato sauce, horseradish and lemon juice. They may also be baked or poached

3

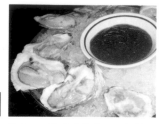

Oysters on the Half Shell served with cocktail sauce

in fresh fish stock and topped with béarnaise or hollandaise sauce.

Gluten-Free Decision Factors:
- Ensure no wheat flour in sauce
- Ensure stocks and broths are made fresh and not from bouillon which may contain gluten

Food Allergen Preparation Considerations:
- Contains shellfish from oysters
- May contain corn from bouillon and corn syrup in cocktail sauce
- May contain dairy from béarnaise or hollandaise sauce
- May contain eggs from béarnaise or hollandaise sauce
- May contain fish from fish stock
- May contain soy from bouillon

Shrimp Cocktail

Shrimp cocktail is a common appetizer in many international cuisines. Most restaurants prepare and serve this appetizer in a similar fashion. Large shrimp are steamed or boiled in water or fish stock, shelled and chilled. The shrimp are served with a cocktail sauce (tomato sauce, horseradish and lemon juice), lemon wedges and sometimes an additional mayonnaise-based sauce.

Shrimp Cocktail

Gluten-Free Decision Factors:
- Ensure stocks and broths are made fresh and not from bouillon which may contain gluten

Food Allergen Preparation Considerations:
- Contains shellfish from shrimp
- May contain corn from bouillon and corn syrup in cocktail sauce
- May contain eggs from mayonnaise-based sauce

- May contain fish from fish stock

- May contain soy from bouillon and mayonnaise-based sauce

Soups
Bisque (Cream Soup)

Bisque is a cream soup that usually features seafood, although vegetable bisques are also common. There are hundreds of recipes for this soup, but most call for standard ingredients. The base of the soup is butter, cream, some type of fresh stock or broth and wine. Onions, puréed tomatoes and potatoes are common vegetables and the soup can be seasoned with anything from sea salt to saffron. Vegetarian bisques may also include any type of ground nut. Bisques are usually garnished with parsley and sometimes may contain croutons.

Gluten-Free Decision Factors:
- Ensure no croutons

- Ensure no wheat flour as thickening agent

- Ensure stocks and broths are made fresh and not from bouillon which may contain gluten

- Ensure no imitation crabmeat or seafood which may contain gluten

Food Allergen Preparation Considerations:
- Contains dairy from butter and cream

- May contain corn from bouillon and imitation crabmeat

- May contain eggs from imitation crabmeat and croutons

- May contain fish as an ingredient, from imitation crabmeat and stock if ordered

- May contain peanuts in vegetable bisque

- May contain shellfish as an ingredient and from stock if ordered

- May contain soy from bouillon and imitation crabmeat

- May contain tree nuts in vegetable bisque

Salads

Buffalo Mozzarella and Tomato Salad

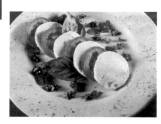

Buffalo Mozzarella and Tomato Salad

Buffalo mozzarella and tomato salad is an Italian classic that has secured a prominent place on American Steak and Seafood restaurant menus. Large slices of buffalo mozzarella are stacked with freshly cut beefsteak tomatoes. Large leafs of basil garnish this dish, which is dressed in olive oil and sometimes balsamic vinegar.

Gluten-Free Decision Factors:
- None

Food Allergen Preparation Considerations:
- Contains dairy from cheese

- May contain corn from vegetable oil

- May contains peanuts from vegetable oil

- May contain soy from vegetable oil

Chopped Salad

Think of a chopped salad as everything that is crunchy in a salad in bite sized pieces. Most chopped salads include bacon, green beans, onions and tomatoes. Some restaurants may include other crunchy vegetables, chopped nuts or add blue cheese for extra flavor. Salad dressings vary from restaurant to restaurant, but balsamic vinaigrette is typically available.

Gluten-Free Decision Factors:
- Ensure bacon bits are real—artificial bacon bits may contain gluten

- Request no croutons

- Request no blue cheese which may contain gluten

- Ensure salad dressings do not contain gluten

Food Allergen Preparation Considerations:
- May contain corn from artificial bacon bits, salad dressing and vegetable oil

- May contain dairy from cheese and salad dressing

- May contain eggs from croutons and mayonnaise-based dressing

- May contain fish from salad dressing

- May contain peanuts from vegetable oil

- May contain soy from artificial bacon bits, mayonnaise-based dressing and vegetable oil

Cobb Salad
This classic salad was invented in the late 1920's by Bob Cobb, manager of Hollywood's famous Brown Derby restaurant. Today, it is considered an American classic. Mixed greens, preferably Boston lettuce, endive and watercress, are topped with avocado, bacon, chicken breast, hard boiled eggs, tomatoes and Roquefort cheese. The traditional dressing is Dijon vinaigrette, consisting of Dijon mustard, olive oil, red wine vinegar, salt and pepper; however, other types of dressing may be available and balsamic vinaigrette can easily be substituted.

Gluten-Free Decision Factors:
- Ensure bacon bits are real - artificial bacon bits may contain gluten

- Request no blue cheese which may contain gluten

- Ensure salad dressings do not contain gluten

Food Allergen Preparation Considerations:
- Contains dairy from cheese and possibly from salad dressing

- Contains eggs from hard-boiled eggs and possibly from mayonnaise-based dressing

3

- May contain corn from artificial bacon bits, salad dressing and vegetable oil

- May contain fish from salad dressing

- May contain peanuts from vegetable oil

- May contain soy from artificial bacon bits, mayonnaise-based dressing and vegetable oil

Hearts of Palm Salad

Hearts of palm are the center of the sable palmetto, a tough-barked palm tree that grows in Central and South America. They are an important export of Brazil and Costa Rica, ending up on some menus in American Steak and Seafood restaurants. This salad usually includes hearts of palm, hard boiled eggs, olives and tomatoes. It is simply dressed in olive oil and vinegar.

Gluten-Free Decision Factors:
- None

Food Allergen Preparation Considerations:
- May contain corn from vegetable oil

- May contain eggs from hard-boiled eggs

- May contain peanuts from vegetable oil

- May contain soy from vegetable oil

Mixed Green Salad

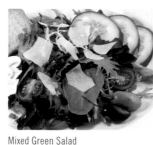

Mixed Green Salad

A mixed green salad may also be presented as the house salad. It is usually a combination of mixed greens, cucumber, onions and tomatoes. Some restaurants may add bacon bits, croutons, shredded cheese and the type of salad dressing may vary.

Gluten-Free Decision Factors:
- Ensure bacon bits are real—artificial bacon bits may contain gluten

- Request no croutons

- Ensure salad dressings do not contain gluten

Food Allergen Preparation Considerations:

- May contain corn from artificial bacon bits, salad dressing and vegetable oil

- May contain dairy from cheese and possibly from salad dressing

- May contain eggs from croutons and mayonnaise-based dressing

- May contain fish from salad dressing

- May contain peanuts from vegetable oil

- May contain soy from artificial bacon bits, mayonnaise-based dressing and vegetable oil

3

Meat Entrees
Hamburgers

Considered an American classic, the hamburger's invention has been claimed by numerous individuals in the later part of the 19th century. In actuality, the hamburger was invented by the hoards of Genghis Kahn hundreds of years before the United States was formed. Although there are many styles of hamburgers, most are made with ground meats including beef, chicken and pork. The most common is the beef hamburger, which is made of ground chuck or ground sirloin and either grilled or pan-fried. In upscale establishments you can find Kobe beef burgers, which are made from a special breed of cattle that is fed a diet of beer and corn. Some restaurants may add bread crumbs to the ground meat prior to cooking. Hamburgers are generally served on a bun with pickles, lettuce, onions and tomatoes, with French fried potatoes on the side. Ketchup, mustard and mayonnaise are usually offered as condiments.

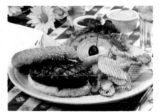

Hamburger with potato chips

Gluten-Free Decision Factors:

- Ensure no bread crumbs

- Ensure potatoes are not dusted with wheat flour or seasonings that contain gluten

3

• Ensure oil used for frying is designated for potatoes only and is not used to fry other items that may be battered or dusted with wheat flour

• Request no bun—order gluten-free bun if available

Food Allergen Preparation Considerations:
• May contain corn from bread crumbs, bun, corn syrup in ketchup, seasonings and vegetable oil

• May contain dairy from bread crumbs, bun and seasonings

• May contain eggs from bread crumbs, bun and mayonnaise

• May contain peanuts from bread crumbs, bun, peanut oil and vegetable oil

• May contain soy from bread crumbs, bun, mayonnaise, seasonings and vegetable oil

• May contain tree nuts from bread crumbs and bun

Pork Chops

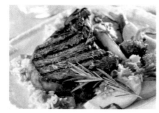

Pork chops come from the loin of the animal and there are many variations of the cut. They are generally broiled, grilled or roasted, and may be offered marinated or smoked in some restaurants. Pork chops can also be pan-fried in butter or oil. Accompaniments vary widely from restaurant to restaurant and can include fruit relish, sauerkraut and sauces.

Pork Chops are generally broiled, grilled or roasted.

Gluten-Free Decision Factors:
• Ensure pork is not dusted with wheat flour

• Ensure no soy sauce or wheat flour in marinade

• Ensure no wheat flour in sauce

• Ensure no wheat flour in accompaniments

Food Allergen Preparation Considerations:
• Food allergens may vary depending upon type of accompaniment

- May contain corn from vegetable oil

- May contain dairy from butter

- May contain peanuts from vegetable oil

- May contain soy from soy sauce in marinade and vegetable oil

Lamb Chops

The lamb chop, or whole rack of lamb where the chop is separated from, is widely considered the most flavorful cut of lamb. It is taken from the rib and has a good amount of marbling, which provides the rich flavor. The chops are usually browned on both sides in a frying pan with butter or olive oil, then roasted to perfection. They may also be marinated prior to cooking and served with a sauce. If the menu description states that the dish is herb encrusted, bread crumbs may be used. Lamb chops and rack of lamb are usually served with mint jelly on the side for dipping.

Gluten-Free Decision Factors:

- Ensure lamb is not dusted with wheat flour

- Ensure no bread crumbs

- Ensure no soy sauce or wheat flour in marinade

- Ensure no wheat flour in sauce

Food Allergen Preparation Considerations:

- May contain corn from bread crumbs and vegetable oil

- May contain dairy from bread crumbs and butter

- May contain eggs from bread crumbs

- May contain peanuts from bread crumbs and vegetable oil

- May contain soy from bread crumbs, soy sauce in marinade and vegetable oil

- May contain tree nuts from bread crumbs

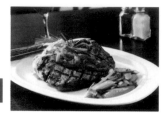

The most popular steak cuts include: filet mignon, New York strip, porterhouse and rib eye.

Steaks

Steaks come in a variety of cuts, the most popular being filet mignon, New York strip, porterhouse and rib eye. Steaks are generally broiled or grilled and seasoned with salt and pepper. They may also be pan-fried in butter or oil. Some restaurants may marinate their steaks or serve them with a sauce, usually a béarnaise, hollandaise or a reduction.

Gluten-Free Decision Factors:

- Ensure beef is not dusted with wheat flour
- Ensure no soy sauce or wheat flour in marinade
- Ensure no wheat flour in sauce

Food Allergen Preparation Considerations:

- May contain corn from vegetable oil
- May contain dairy from butter, béarnaise or hollandaise sauce
- May contain eggs from béarnaise or hollandaise sauce
- May contain peanuts from vegetable oil
- May contain soy from soy sauce in marinade and vegetable oil

Chicken Entrees
Grilled Chicken Breast

Grilled chicken breast is a relatively common menu item in American Steak and Seafood restaurants. In addition to grilled, chicken breasts may also be pan-fried in butter or oil. Occasionally, they may be marinated and come with a sauce. Fortunately, you can usually order a plain grilled chicken breast without any sauce. This entrée is typically accompanied by one or two side vegetables, even though many restaurants serve à la carte.

Gluten-Free Decision Factors:

- Ensure chicken is not dusted with wheat flour

- Ensure no soy sauce or wheat flour in marinade

- Ensure no wheat flour in sauce

Food Allergen Preparation Considerations:
- Food allergens may vary depending upon type of accompaniment

- May contain corn from vegetable oil

- May contain dairy from butter

- May contain peanuts from vegetable oil

- May contain soy from soy sauce in marinade and vegetable oil

Roasted Chicken

Chicken is typically roasted on a spit or in a pan with butter or oil. The chicken may be buttered, rubbed with herbs and oil or marinated prior to cooking. A reduction sauce may also be served in some restaurants. The common portion served is half a chicken, complete with breast, wing and thigh on the bone. This entrée is typically accompanied by one or two side vegetables, even though many restaurants serve à la carte.

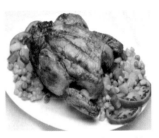
Roasted Chicken with a side vegetable.

Gluten-Free Decision Factors:
- Ensure chicken is not dusted with wheat flour

- Ensure no soy sauce or wheat flour in marinade

- Ensure no wheat flour in sauce

Food Allergen Preparation Considerations:
- Food allergens may vary depending upon type of accompaniment

- May contain corn from vegetable oil

- May contain dairy from butter

- May contain peanuts from vegetable oil

- May contain soy from soy sauce in marinade and vegetable oil

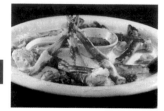

Crab Legs

3

Seafood Entrees
Crab

Alaskan king crab, Maryland blue crab, snow crab and stone crab are the most common varieties of this crustacean offered. Crabs are usually baked or boiled in water or fish stock. The smaller crabs, like Maryland blue crab and stone crab, may be stuffed prior to baking and may contain bread crumbs. Crabs are usually served with drawn butter (melted butter and vegetable oil) and lemon wedges. Unless you are dining at the source of the catch, you may find that your crab has been frozen prior to preparation.

Gluten-Free Decision Factors:
- Ensure no bread crumbs if baked

- Ensure stocks and broths are made fresh and not from bouillon which may contain gluten

Food Allergen Preparation Considerations:
- Contains shellfish from crab

- May contain corn from bouillon, bread crumbs and vegetable oil in drawn butter

- May contain dairy from bread crumbs and drawn butter

- May contain eggs from bread crumbs

- May contain fish from fish stock

- May contain peanuts from bread crumbs and vegetable oil

- May contain soy from bouillon, bread crumbs, and vegetable oil in drawn butter

- May contain tree nuts from bread crumbs

Fish Filet

Most restaurants offer a fish of the day, which usually revolves around what is in season. Halibut, salmon and sea bass are very common, with many restaurants also offering fresh water fish such as rainbow trout. Fish filets are usually grilled, poached or steamed. They may also be pan-fried with butter or oil and topped with a number of different sauces.

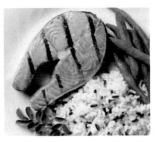

Grilled Salmon

3

Gluten-Free Decision Factors:
- Ensure no wheat flour in sauce

- Ensure stocks and broths are made fresh and not from bouillon which may contain gluten if poached

Food Allergen Preparation Considerations:
- Contains fish

- May contain corn from bouillon and vegetable oil

- May contain dairy from butter

- May contain peanuts from vegetable oil

- May contain soy from bouillon and vegetable oil

Lobster
There are two types of lobster typically served at American Steak and Seafood restaurants: Australian and Maine. Australian lobster is known for its large flavorful tail and is usually frozen prior to preparation. Maine lobsters are widely considered to have the sweetest flavor and are typically fresh or live prior to cooking. Lobster tails are usually baked or grilled; whereas, whole Maine lobster is traditionally boiled in water or fish stock. Most lobster is generally served with drawn butter and lemon wedges. Baked Maine Lobster is often halved and topped with bread crumbs and fresh herbs.

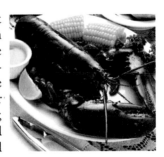

Lobster with butter and lemon

Gluten-Free Decision Factors:
- Ensure no bread crumbs if baked

- Ensure stocks and broths are made fresh and not from bouillon which may contain gluten

Food Allergen Preparation Considerations:
- Contains shellfish from lobster

3

- May contain corn from bouillon, bread crumbs and vegetable oil in drawn butter

- May contain dairy from bread crumbs and drawn butter

- May contain eggs from bread crumbs

- May contain fish from fish stock

- May contain peanuts from bread crumbs and vegetable oil

- May contain soy from bouillon, bread crumbs, and vegetable oil in drawn butter

- May contain tree nuts from bread crumbs

Side Dishes
Asparagus

Asparagus is usually prepared in the French style, steamed until they are cooked and still crisp. They are often sautéed in butter or oil, with garlic or onions sometimes added. Some restaurants offer béarnaise or hollandaise sauce on top or on the side for dipping.

Gluten-Free Decision Factors:

- Ensure no wheat flour in sauce

Food Allergen Preparation Considerations:

- May contain corn from vegetable oil

- May contain dairy from butter, béarnaise and hollandaise sauce

- May contain eggs from béarnaise and hollandaise sauce

- May contain peanuts from vegetable oil

- May contain soy from vegetable oil

Baked Potato

A baked potato is typically a safe choice in any restaurant. The accompaniments vary from restaurant to restaurant, but can include bacon bits, butter, cheese, chives and sour cream. Cheese sauce may also be offered. Mix and match what you like or have it plain. Almost all baked potatoes are made to order.

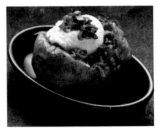

Gluten-Free Decision Factors:

- Ensure bacon bits are real—artificial bacon bits may contain gluten

Baked Potato with sour cream, chives and bacon bits

- Ensure no wheat flour in cheese sauce

Food Allergen Preparation Considerations:

- May contain corn from artificial bacon bits and cheese sauce

- May contain dairy from butter, cheese and sour cream

- May contain soy from artificial bacon bits and cheese sauce

Broccoli

In most cases, broccoli is steamed at American Steak and Seafood restaurants. You may also request it sautéed with butter or olive oil and garlic. In some establishments, the option of cheese sauce may also be available.

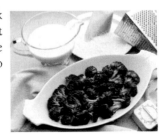

Gluten-Free Decision Factors:

- Ensure no wheat flour in cheese sauce

Broccoli with cheese sauce

Food Allergen Preparation Considerations:

- May contain corn from cheese sauce and vegetable oil

- May contain dairy from butter and cheese sauce

- May contain peanuts in vegetable oil

- May contain soy from cheese sauce and vegetable oil

3

French Fried Potatoes

French fried potatoes come in many different shapes and sizes. Once cut, the potatoes are fried in oil. Some restaurants may season their fries, while others prefer salting. Ketchup is usually served on the side.

Gluten-Free Decision Factors:

- Ensure potatoes are not dusted with wheat flour or seasonings that contain gluten

- Ensure oil used for frying is designated for potatoes only and is not used to fry other items that may be battered or dusted with wheat flour

Food Allergen Preparation Considerations:

- May contain corn from corn syrup in ketchup, seasonings and vegetable oil

- May contain dairy from seasonings

- May contain peanuts from peanut oil and vegetable oil

- May contain soy from ketchup, seasonings and vegetable oil

Green Beans

Green Beans

Green beans are usually served in the French style, steamed until they are cooked and still crisp. They are typically served plain or sautéed in butter or oil. Other ingredients such as almonds, garlic and onions may also be included. Green beans may be served with béarnaise or hollandaise sauce on the side.

Gluten-Free Decision Factors:

- Ensure no wheat flour in sauce

Food Allergen Preparation Considerations:

- May contain corn from vegetable oil

- May contain dairy from butter, béarnaise and hollandaise sauce

- May contain eggs from béarnaise and hollandaise sauce

- May contain peanuts from vegetable oil

- May contain soy from vegetable oil

- May contain tree nuts from almonds

Hash Browns

Hash browns are a classic side dish. Julienned potatoes are simply pan fried with butter or vegetable oil, very much like a pancake. They are fried on one side and then carefully flipped over to brown on the other side. Occasionally, they may have sliced onions added to them. Hash browns are usually only seasoned with salt and pepper.

Gluten-Free Decision Factors:
- Ensure no wheat flour or seasonings that contain gluten

Food Allergen Preparation Considerations:
- May contain corn from seasonings and vegetable oil

- May contain dairy from butter and seasonings

- May contain peanuts from vegetable oil

- May contain soy from seasonings and vegetable oil

Mashed Potatoes

Mashed Potatoes are made a variety of ways, most of which include butter and milk to add a creamy texture. The potatoes can be mashed, smashed or whipped with or without the skins left on the spud. Chives and onions are often added to the mix, with garlic mashed potatoes and parmesan cheese mashed potatoes growing in popularity. Salt and pepper are the standard seasonings used; however, some chefs may add fresh herbs to enhance the flavor.

3

Gluten-Free Decision Factors:
- Ensure no wheat flour as ingredient
- Ensure no artificial mashed potato mix which may contain gluten

Food Allergen Preparation Considerations:
- May contain corn from artificial mashed potato mix
- May contain dairy from artificial mashed potato mix, butter, cheese and milk
- May contain soy from artificial mashed potato mix

Potatoes Lyonnaise

Potatoes Lyonnaise are a French potato side dish, very similar to American hash browns. Potatoes are sliced or cubed and then pan fried with sliced onions, butter, salt and pepper. Some restaurants may choose to bake this dish or substitute vegetable oil for butter.

Gluten-Free Decision Factors:
- Ensure no wheat flour as ingredient

Food Allergen Preparation Considerations:
- May contain corn from vegetable oil
- May contain dairy from butter
- May contain peanuts from vegetable oil
- May contain soy from vegetable oil

Spinach

Spinach is full of vitamins and makes a great side dish. It is typically steamed or sautéed in olive oil with garlic or onions. Creamed spinach is also usually available; however, most recipes indicate wheat flour as an ingredient.

Gluten-Free Decision Factors:
- Ensure no wheat flour in creamed spinach

Food Allergen Preparation Considerations:

- May contain corn from vegetable oil

- May contain dairy from butter and cream

- May contain peanuts from vegetable oil

- May contain soy from vegetable oil

3

Desserts
Chocolate Mousse

Chocolate mousse has become a popular dessert and can be found on the menus of many international cuisines. There are a number of variations, but the preparation is typically consistent with the following recipe. Chocolate is melted in a double-boiler with milk and sugar. Whipped eggs are then carefully folded into the chocolate sauce after it has cooled. Next, whipped heavy cream is added to the mixture, which is allowed to sit for a few minutes before the mousse is poured into a container and chilled. Some styles incorporate liqueurs such as coffee, orange and peppermint for a distinctive flavor. Chocolate mousse may be served with whipped cream and a cookie.

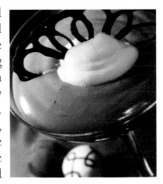
Chocolate Mousse

Gluten-Free Decision Factors:

- Ensure no flavors containing gluten

- Ensure no wheat flour as ingredient

- Request no cookie

Food Allergen Preparation Considerations:

- Contains dairy from cream, milk and possibly from chocolate and cookie

- Contains eggs as an ingredient and possibly from cookie

- May contain corn from colors or flavors in liqueurs

- May contain peanuts from cookie and various flavors

- May contain soy from colors or flavors in liqueurs and chocolate

3

• May contain tree nuts from cookie and various flavors

Crème Brulée (Baked Custard)

Crème Brulée is one of the most popular French desserts and is equally popular in American Steak and Seafood restaurants. The custard is made with heavy cream, egg yolks, sugar and vanilla. The whisked ingredients are then baked. After it has cooled, it is topped with brown sugar that is caramelized by placing the custard in a broiler or torched by hand. There are many different types of *Crème Brulée,* some of which may contain different flavors such as almond, chocolate or fresh berries.

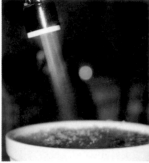
Caramelizing Crème Brulée by hand torch

Gluten-Free Decision Factors:
• Ensure no wheat flour as ingredient

Food Allergen Preparation Considerations:
• Contains dairy from cream

• Contains eggs from egg yolks

• May contain corn from almond or vanilla extract

• May contain soy from chocolate

• May contain tree nuts from almond extract

Flourless Chocolate Torte

Yes, there is such a thing as flourless chocolate torte...even if some pastry chefs forget the title. Butter, chocolate, eggs and sugar are the standard ingredients and ground nuts may also be added to make up for the lack of flour which would normally hold everything together. Some pastry chefs may use bread crumbs or flour, even though the title suggests they are omitted.

Flourless Chocolate Torte

Gluten-Free Decision Factors:
• Ensure no wheat flour as ingredient

• Ensure no bread crumbs

3

Food Allergen Preparation Considerations:

- Contains dairy from butter, chocolate and possibly from bread crumbs

- Contains eggs as an ingredient and possibly from bread crumbs

- May contain corn from bread crumbs

- May contain peanuts from bread crumbs

- May contain soy from chocolate and bread crumbs

- May contain tree nuts from bread crumbs

Fresh Berries with Whipped Cream

Fresh berries in season usually include blueberries, raspberries and strawberries. Depending on your location, other types such as blackberries, boysenberries and loganberries may be available. They are served chilled and are usually topped with whipped cream.

Gluten-Free Decision Factors:

- None

Food Allergen Preparation Considerations:

- Contains dairy from whipped cream

Ice Cream

Ice cream is typically available at American Steak and Seafood restaurants. Some restaurants serve pre-fabricated ice cream, while others choose to make their own. Many ice cream brands are gluten-free and they come in big containers with clear labels. Ask your server to read the ingredients listed on the container and keep your flavor choices simple.

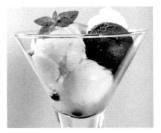

Ice Cream may be pre-fabricated, or made by the restaurant.

Gluten-Free Decision Factors:

- Ensure no flavors containing gluten

- Ensure no malt and wheat as ingredients

- Ensure no stabilizers which may contain gluten

- Request no cookie

3

Food Allergen Preparation Considerations:

- Contains dairy as an ingredient and possibly from chocolate and colors or flavors

- May contain corn from colors or flavors and malt

- May contain eggs from cookie

- May contain peanuts from cookie and various flavors

- May contain soy from colors or flavors, chocolate and cookie

- May contain tree nuts from cookie and various flavors

Sorbet

Sorbet is puréed fruit and sugar that is frozen and served like ice cream. Raspberry, lemon and lime sorbets are the most common, though you may encounter many other fruit flavors or chocolate. Occasionally, sorbet is served with a Pirouline, other type of cookie or wafer.

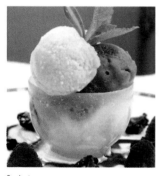

Sorbet

Gluten-Free Decision Factors:

- Ensure no stabilizers which may contain gluten

- Ensure no wheat as ingredient

- Request no cookie

Food Allergen Preparation Considerations:

- May contain corn from colors or flavors

- May contain dairy from chocolate, colors or flavors and cookie

- May contain eggs from cookie

- May contain peanuts from cookie and various flavors

- May contain soy from colors or flavors, chocolate and cookie

- May contain tree nuts from cookie and various flavors

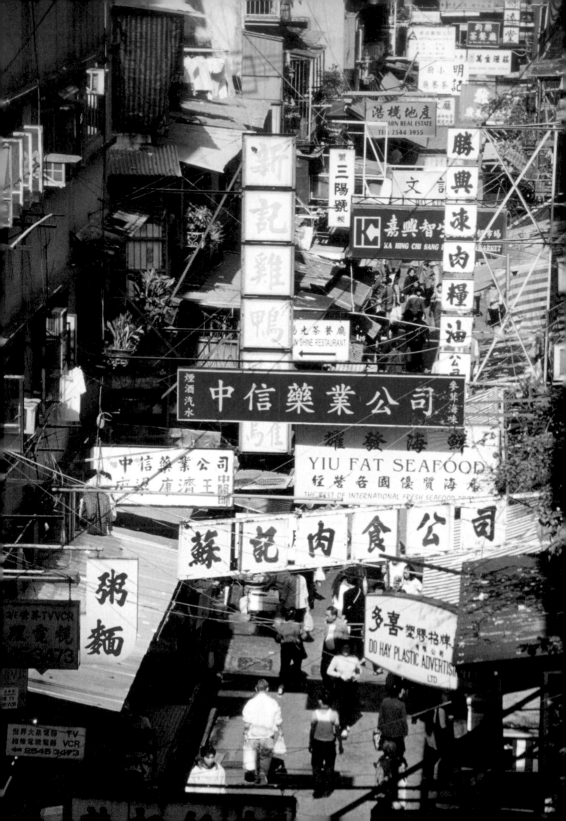

Eating is the utmost important part of life.
—Confucius

Chapter 4
Let's Eat Chinese Cuisine

Cuisine Overview

China has the world's largest population with 1.3 billion people and is the third largest country in land mass. As can be expected given these facts, ingredients in Chinese cuisine vary greatly from region to region. All across China, though, food is divided into two categories: *Fan* (starches) and *T'sai* (meat and vegetables).

The Chinese believe that a well-balanced meal can create harmony in one's life and improve mental and physical well being. A traditional Chinese meal consists of many dishes that contain vegetables, meat and starch, which are prepared the way they have been for thousands of years. These dishes feature bite-sized pieces of food, so cutlery is not necessary. In fact, when the Mongols conquered China, they were considered quite barbaric for using knives to cut their meat.

The Chinese technique of preparing food in this fashion grew out of an economic need rather than an aesthetic aspiration, as there were periods of famine and fuel shortage in the nation's history. Stir frying eliminated food waste and reduced the amount of fuel necessary to produce a meal, which ultimately solved two problems at the same time. Cooking foods for a short time at a high temperature also allows vegetables

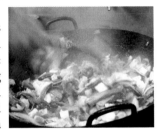
Cooking in a Wok

to remain crisp, thereby retaining a greater amount of their raw nutritional value. This cooking technique, combined with a balanced approach of including the flavors of bitter, sour, hot, salty and sweet, create a cuisine that is enjoyed by billions of people around the world.

Traditional Ingredients

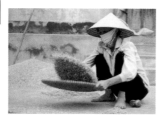

Woman Harvesting Rice

The vegetables consumed are based upon what is available from region to region and include amaranth, cabbage, carrots, different types of green beans, numerous mushrooms, mustard greens, onions, radishes, and turnips. Many spices are incorporated into Chinese cooking, such as cinnamon, ginger, garlic, malva, mint and red pepper. Curry powder also plays an important role in southern Chinese cooking. Soy sauce is the main ingredient used to season dishes, most of which contain wheat.

As far as protein is concerned, the Chinese eat almost everything, including: beef, chicken, duck, goose, mutton, pheasant, pork, seafood and venison. Another popular source of protein is tofu, which is derived from soybeans. It is worth mentioning that there are a number of other animal proteins consumed in Asia, such as dog, which you can find in markets and restaurants in China. Luckily, these items are conspicuously missing from restaurant menus in the Western world.

Common forms of starch eaten include buckwheat, maize, millet, *kao-liang* (sorghum), potato, rice, sweet potato and wheat (in breads, dumpling skins and pancakes). The Northern region is cold and not conducive to the cultivation of rice, so breads and pancakes serve as the starch portion of meals there. In the South, rice is abundant and is eaten as either a whole grain or in rice flour that can be used for dumpling dough and noodles. Tea is the national drink of China and in almost every Chinese dialect is called *cha*. Tea has also played a vital role in Chinese history as it is considered a national treasure, and has even been used as a state currency. There are more than a thousand varieties of tea, with the three main types being oolong, green and black, known as red tea in China. Tea is to the Chinese what wine is to the French. Most people drink it as part of their daily routine, preserving a nationalistic sense of decorum as part of the Chinese culture.

Gluten Awareness

Since gluten is present in most areas of Chinese cuisine, we have outlined eight items in our sample menu. There are seven primary points that you need to consider when dining at a Chinese restaurant. To ensure a gluten-free experience, the areas of food preparation that you need to inquire about with your server or chef are listed below.

Soy Sauce	Ensure no soy sauce is used. Request gluten-free soy sauce, gluten-free tamari or Bragg's liquid aminos if available
Flour Dusting	Corn or potato starch is typically used—ensure no wheat flour
Stocks and Broths	Ensure all stocks and broths are made fresh and not from bouillon which may contain gluten
Cooking Oil	Ensure frying oil has not been used to fry battered foods that may contain gluten
Noodles and Dumplings	Wheat flour is typically used—ensure no wheat flour
Battering	Request plain-cooked food—ensure no batter
Cross-Contamination	Ensure all utensils and cooking surfaces have been cleaned prior to the preparation of your meal

Soy Sauce

From a gluten perspective, your choices will be extremely limited in traditional Chinese restaurants for a number of reasons, due mostly to the abundant use of soy sauce. Soy sauce is used in most Chinese dishes and is present in almost every Chinese sauce such as hoi sin, duck sauce and Chinese style barbecue sauce. Soy sauce is made from soybeans, which are considered one of the "seven necessities" of life in China, along with oil, rice, salt, tea, vinegar and firewood. Today, more than 90% of all soy sauces produced contain wheat. Gluten-free soy sauce, gluten-free tamari or Bragg's liquid aminos are featured at some restaurants such as P.F. Chang's China Bistro®.

4

However, the demand for these products has not necessitated their production and distribution on a global basis as of yet.

Flour Dusting

Flour dusting is common in Chinese cuisine. Most restaurants prefer to dust using corn or potato starch —rather than wheat flour—to texture meats or fish before frying, thereby allowing a sauce to be evenly distributed.

Stocks and Broths

Stocks and broths are used frequently in Chinese cuisines and are present in sauces and soups. Ensure that stocks and broths are made fresh and not from bouillon, which may contain gluten.

Cooking Oil

Canola oil is typically used in Chinese restaurants; however other oils such as corn, peanut, sesame or vegetable may be used from time to time. Oil is used to fry or sauté foods. When ordering food that is prepared by frying, ensure that there is a dedicated fryer in the kitchen for non-battered menu items. Since battered foods may contain wheat flour, this practice minimizes the potential of gluten cross-contamination from frying.

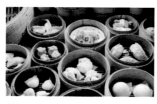

Wheat flour is used for most dumpling skins, pancakes and noodles, and precludes these dishes for those with gluten allergies or sensitivities.

Noodles and Dumplings

Wheat flour is used for most dumpling skins, pancakes and noodles, and precludes the majority of *Fan* dishes for those with gluten allergies or sensitivities. Although rice flour based noodles and dumpling skins are used in Southern Chinese cuisine and Asian fusion restaurants, soy sauce is present in most of these dishes.

Battering

Battering of meats is common in Chinese cuisine and in some geographic regions, such as the United States, it is especially prevalent. Wheat flour is typically used for batter in Chinese restaurants. Request that your order is plain-cooked or steamed.

Cross-Contamination

Cross-contamination occurs in two primary instances and should be considered at any restaurant you choose to dine in. One may occur when your meal is prepared in the same frying oil as foods containing other possible allergens. The second may occur when microbes or food particles are transferred from one food to another by using the same knife, cutting board, pots, pans or other utensils without washing the surfaces or tools in between uses. In the case of open flamed grills, the extreme temperature turns most food particles into carbon. Use of a wire brush designed for grill racks typically removes residual contaminants. To avoid cross-contamination, restaurants need to dedicate fryers for specific foods and wash all materials that may come in contact with food in hot, soapy water prior to preparing items for those with special dietary requirements. It is important to ensure that the restaurant follows these procedures for an allergen-free dining experience.

Other Allergy Considerations

If you have other food allergies or sensitivities, it is important to remain diligent in your approach to dining out. Because Chinese cuisine utilizes a multitude of food products, there are many common food allergens used on a regular basis. As previously noted, canola oil is typically used in Chinese restaurants; however, corn, peanut and vegetable oil (which may contain corn, peanuts or soy) can also be used. If used, bouillon may contain Hydrolyzed Vegetable Protein (HVP) that can be derived from corn, soy or wheat. We have indicated the potential presence of bouillon and oils.

From the eight menu items we have listed in our sample menu, we have identified each common allergen typically included in the dish as an ingredient. We have also indicated other potential allergens that may be present based upon varied culinary practices. The chances of encountering common food allergens in items specific to our sample menu are outlined on the next page.

High Likelihood	Corn, gluten, soy and wheat
Moderate Likelihood	Eggs, fish, peanuts, shellfish and tree nuts
Low Likelihood	Dairy

4

Dining Considerations

Menus in Chinese restaurants tend to be presented in the language of the country you are dining in. This is due to the fact that most diners can neither read the Chinese alphabet, nor understand the spoken language. The names of many dishes serve as a description of the menu item itself, such as lemon chicken. Although, the recipes of these dishes may vary from restaurant to restaurant, the preparation styles remain relatively consistent. There are many dishes that are ubiquitous and can be found in virtually every Chinese restaurant; however, most of these dishes contain soy sauce.

Chopsticks and Chinese-style soup spoons are the only necessary tools needed to enjoy a Chinese meal. Additionally, most Chinese restaurants have adapted Western style cutlery for their guests who prefer to use knives and forks. Whatever utensils you decide to use, they are inconsequential to your enjoyment of Chinese cuisine.

As is the case with most Asian cuisines, Chinese food is designed to be enjoyed family style. Finding a balance between many dishes and sharing them with your table is a very important part of Chinese culture. This grew out of the Chinese idea of incorporating the *ying* and *yang* in every facet of daily life. *Fan* (starch) and *Tsai* (meat and vegetable) dishes must be balanced in every meal and the five flavors of bitter, sour, hot, salty and sweet should also be evenly distributed. This creates harmony at the dinner table and is believed to fortify the body and the soul.

好胃口

(This is Chinese for Bon Appetit!)

Sample Chinese Menu

Soup
Egg Drop Soup
Sizzling Rice Soup

Chicken Entrees
Lemon Chicken
Steamed Chicken and Broccoli

Seafood Entrees
Steamed Fish

Vegetarian Entrees
Buddha's Feast

Noodle and Rice Dishes
Steamed Rice

Desserts
Fresh Tropical Fruits

4

*We would like to thank P.F. Chang's China Bistro®
headquartered in Scottsdale, Arizona and Sueson
Vess, Founder and President of Special Eats™ in
Chicago, Illinois for their valuable contributions in
reviewing the following menu items.*

Chinese Menu Item Descriptions

Soups
Egg Drop Soup
If it is prepared in the traditional fashion, the base of the
soup is fresh chicken stock and is typically thickened
with corn or potato starch. Sliced button mushrooms,
green onion and spinach are the standard vegetables

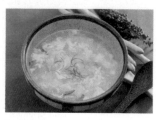

Egg Drop Soup

and the soup is seasoned with salt and pepper. Tofu may also be added. The ingredients may be sautéed in oil, prior to being added to the chicken stock. As its name would suggest, the soup has whisked eggs dropped into the broth, which look like white ribbons. Chinese soups are often garnished with fried noodles or wonton strips.

Gluten-Free Decision Factors:

- Ensure no soy sauce—order gluten-free sauce if available

- Ensure stocks and broths are made fresh and not from bouillon which may contain gluten

- Ensure no wheat flour as thickening agent

- Request no fried noodles or wonton strips

Food Allergen Preparation Considerations:

- Contains eggs as an ingredient

- May contain corn from bouillon, corn starch and vegetable oil

- May contain peanuts from peanut oil and vegetable oil

- May contain soy from bouillon, soy sauce, tofu and vegetable oil

Sizzling Rice Soup

Sizzling rice soup is a menu item with the final preparation of the dish done tableside. The base of the soup is fresh chicken stock or broth that has been thickened with corn starch or potato starch and seasoned with salt and pepper. Strips of chicken and sometimes shrimp are combined with bamboo shoots, eggs, mushrooms and water chestnuts in the broth. Tofu may also be added. At your table, your server adds rice to the soup that has been fried in oil, thus creating the famous "sizzle." Chinese soups are often garnished with fried noodles or wonton strips.

Gluten-Free Decision Factors:
- Ensure no soy sauce—order gluten-free sauce if available
- Ensure stocks and broths are made fresh and not from bouillon which may contain gluten
- Ensure no wheat flour as thickening agent
- Request no fried noodles or wonton strips

Food Allergen Preparation Considerations:
- May contain corn from bouillon, corn starch and vegetable oil
- May contain eggs as an ingredient
- May contain peanuts from peanut oil and vegetable oil
- May contain shellfish from shrimp
- May contain soy from bouillon, soy sauce, tofu and vegetable oil

Chicken Entrees
Lemon Chicken

Lemon chicken is a sweet and tangy dish found on most Chinese restaurant menus. Slices of chicken breast are dusted in corn or potato starch and wok fried in oil. Once the chicken is cooked, it is added to a sauce made up of fresh chicken stock, lemons, lemon juice, rice wine vinegar and sugar. Lemon chicken is usually only seasoned with salt and pepper, but some recipes call for ginger. The traditional recipe calls for no vegetables, but many restaurants will add green peppers, mushrooms and onions.

Gluten-Free Decision Factors:
- Ensure no soy sauce—order gluten-free sauce if available
- Ensure chicken is not battered or dusted with wheat flour

- Ensure stocks and broths are made fresh and not from bouillon which may contain gluten

- Ensure oil used for frying has not been used to fry other items which may be battered or dusted with wheat flour

Food Allergen Preparation Considerations:

- May contain corn from bouillon, corn starch and vegetable oil

- May contain eggs from batter

- May contain peanuts from peanut oil and vegetable oil

- May contain soy from bouillon, soy sauce and vegetable oil

Steamed Chicken and Broccoli

Chicken and broccoli are common ingredients found in almost every Westernized Chinese restaurant. You must specifically request the dish steamed, as it is typically served in a soy-based sauce. Sliced chicken breast and broccoli are simply steamed and served plain.

Gluten-Free Decision Factors:

- Ensure no soy sauce—order gluten-free sauce if available

Food Allergen Preparation Considerations:

- May contain soy from soy sauce

Seafood Entrees
Steamed Fish

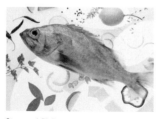

Steamed Fish

Chinese restaurants generally offer a steamed fish, which can be any fish available. Some restaurants may serve whole steamed fish; however, it is much more common to have a fish filet. The fish is usually accompanied by one of a number of different sauces, most of which contain soy sauce. It may also be served with steamed vegetables, but in many cases you need to order a vegetable dish separately.

Gluten-Free Decision Factors:
- Ensure no soy sauce—order gluten-free sauce if available

Food Allergen Preparation Considerations:
- Contains fish

- May contain soy from soy sauce

Vegetarian Entrees
Buddha's Feast
This mixed Asian vegetable dish is either steamed or stir-fried. If it is stir-fried, the dish is tossed in a wok with fresh vegetable or chicken stock and oil. Many restaurants will also add soy sauce to season the dish, so it is typically easier to order the Buddha's Feast steamed. The vegetables of the dish vary, but you can usually expect to see some combination of baby corn, bamboo shoots, bok choy, broccoli, cabbage, Chinese broccoli, carrots, shitake mushrooms and water chestnuts. Garlic and ginger are usually included for flavor and bean curd or tofu may also be included to add extra protein to the dish.

Gluten Free Decision Factors:
- Ensure no soy sauce—order gluten-free sauce if available

- Ensure stocks and broths are made fresh and not from bouillon which may contain gluten

Food Allergen Preparation Considerations:
- May contain corn from baby corn, bouillon and vegetable oil

- May contain peanuts from peanut oil and vegetable oil

- May contain soy from bean curd, bouillon, soy sauce, tofu and vegetable oil

Noodle and Rice Dishes
Steamed Rice

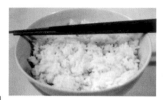

Plain steamed rice is usually safe to eat. Chinese restaurants typically offer steamed white rice and many now offer steamed brown rice. Since the rice is steamed in a designated rice cooker, the chances of it coming into contact with any foods during cooking are minimal.

4 | Steamed Rice

Gluten-Free Decision Factors:
  • None

Food Allergen Preparation Considerations:
  • None

Desserts
Fresh Tropical Fruits

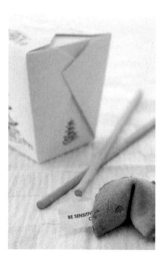

Fresh tropical fruit makes a light choice for dessert. Bite-sized chunks of pineapple, guava, papaya and banana are the most common fruits served.

Gluten-Free Decision Factors:
  • None

Food Allergen Preparation Considerations:
  • None

One final note: Be sure to read your fortune—just don't eat the cookie!

4

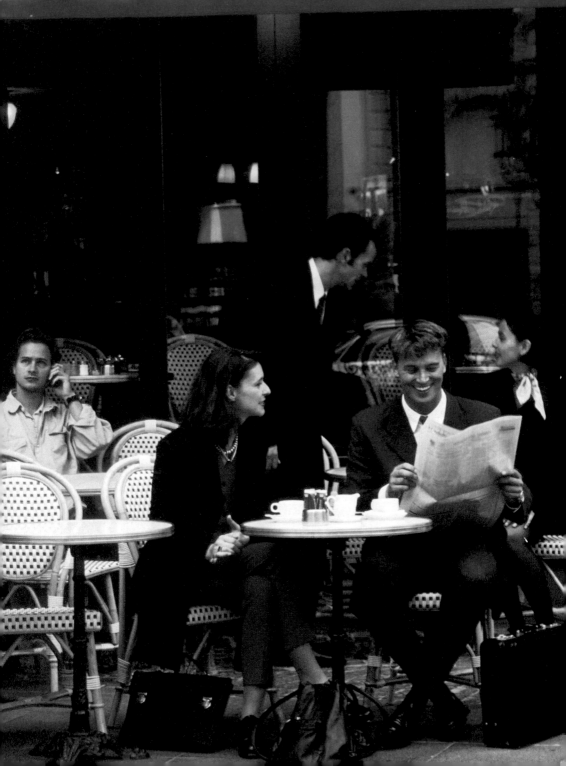

Eating is a serious venture,
if not a patriotic duty, in France.
—Patricia Roberts

Chapter 5
Let's Eat French Cuisine

Cuisine Overview

With a population of just over 60 million and a land mass roughly twice the size of Colorado, France is the largest nation in Western Europe. Although its history can be traced back some 30,000 years, most historians agree that the formal history of France began when Clovis, King of the Franks, brought Christianity to the country with his baptism in the 5th century. France is divided into 22 regions, including the island of Corsica and is further represented in territories around the world.

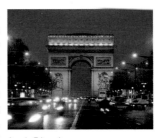

Arc de Triomphe

French cuisine is dynamic to say the least. The food preparation techniques used in France are arguably some of the most sophisticated from a culinary perspective. Chefs must master these techniques, as French food is a passion for millions of people around the world. French cooking is not unified by one school of thought, but rather by regional influences including geography, climate and other international cultures. In the regions of Brittany and Normandy, local culinary specialties revolve around seafood, beef and cheese, as they are coastal regions and cattle is the dominant livestock raised in that area. In the south, Provençal cuisine is influenced by Italy, with

5

its use of olive oil and herbs. The foods of Alsace on the German border feature sweet wines and sausages of a distinctly Germanic flavor. Each region is known for its specific culinary delights, which are assembled on menus around the world under one classification: French!

"*Les Champs de Blé*" (the fields of wheat) is an important symbol of the French culture. Wheat is a big part of the French gastronomic experience and is present in everything from baguettes to beignets. Be that as it may, there are many French menu items that are traditionally gluten-free.

Traditional Ingredients

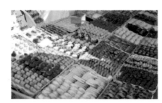

The French are adventurous eaters and vegetables play a huge role in French dining.

The French are certainly adventurous eaters. Their creative and innovative culinary palate includes everything from saffron to snails. Vegetables play a huge role in French dining along with meat and poultry, but exotic ingredients like frog legs, calf brains and foies gras are just as important. In fact, the most unusual menu items you will encounter in a restaurant are usually quite common to the French.

Asparagus, artichokes, green beans, many types of lettuce, leeks, olives, onions, potatoes and tomatoes are common vegetables. Herbs include basil, fennel, laurel, lavender, marjoram, rosemary, savory, tarragon and thyme.

Beef, chicken, duck, lamb, pork and seafood provide the majority of protein in French food and their desserts are widely considered some of the best in the world. Cheese is a big part of the French diet and plays an important role in their cuisine. There are more varieties of cheese in France than there are days in the year! Brie and Camembert are well known soft cheeses. Chèvre is cheese made from goats' milk that is sweet and creamy when fresh, yet grows to be salty and hard as it ages. Roquefort is one of the more common blue cheeses. When traveling in France, every area you visit will have a local specialty cheese that is prized by its inhabitants.

Like the Italians, the French have been drinking wine for hundreds of years. Wine is to the French what tea is to the English. Most people drink it as part of their daily routine, preserving a nationalistic sense of decorum as part of the French culture. Not only do the French drink wine with most meals, but it is used regularly in food preparation. Wines in France are classified by appellation, a term that refers to a viticulture region distinguished by geographical features which produce wines with shared characteristics. The Bordeaux region is held in high regard for its production of some of the world's finest red wine. The wines of Alsace are sweeter and generally revolve around white grape varietals. Champagne is known, of course, for its production of sparkling wines, while wines of Burgundy display a lighter viscosity and subtle flavors.

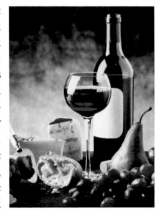

Cheese and Wine

5

Gluten Awareness

Although gluten is present in many areas of French cuisine, we have outlined 30 items in our sample menu. There are seven primary points that you need to consider when dining at a French restaurant. To ensure a gluten-free experience, the areas of food preparation that you need to inquire about with your server or chef are listed below.

Sauces	Ensure the *liaison* of the sauce is butter, egg yolks or puréed vegetables ensure no wheat flour
Flour Dusting	Wheat flour is typically used—request plain
Stocks and Broths	Ensure all stocks and broths are made fresh and not from bouillon which may contain gluten
Cooking Oil	Ensure frying oil has not been used to fry battered foods that may contain gluten
Croutons, Bread Crumbs and Bread	Wheat flour is typically used—ensure no croutons, bread crumbs or bread
Malt Vinegar	Ensure no malt vinegar as a condiment
Cross-Contamination	Ensure all utensils and cooking surfaces have been cleaned prior to the preparation of your meal

Sauces

Of the many different sauces you may encounter in French cuisine, always be sure the *liaison* that binds the sauce together is not wheat flour. Other acceptable *liaisons* include egg yolks, butter and puréed vegetables. Below is a list of common and typically gluten-free French sauces and their ingredients:

Hollandaise	A sauce that contains butter, egg yolks as its liaison and lemon juice
Béarnaise	A reduction of white wine vinegar, tarragon and shallots that is finished with egg yolks and butter
Reduction	A mixture that results from rapidly boiling a liquid (like fresh stock, wine, or a sauce without wheat flour) and causing evaporation—"reducing" the sauce—which creates a thicker sauce with a more intense flavor than the original liquid
Rémoulade	A sauce that contains mayonnaise, mustard, capers, chopped gherkins (French pickles), herbs, and anchovies

Other common French sauces include wheat flour as a *liaison* or thickening agent. Below are three common French sauces that you need to avoid:

Roux	A sauce made of flour, fat and butter —a roux can be white, blond, or brown, depending on ingredients and cooking time *Note: Roux is typically not included as part of a menu description*
Béchamel	A white roux with milk
Velouté	A white roux with a light chicken or veal stock added

Flour Dusting

Flour dusting is common in French cuisine. Most restaurants prefer to dust meat or fish with wheat flour for texture prior to pan frying, allowing a sauce to be evenly distributed. Ensure that this practice is not used in the preparation of your meal.

Stocks and Broths

Stocks and broths are used frequently in French cuisine. They are present in sauces and soups, as well as in marinades for meats and vegetables. Ensure that stocks and broths are made fresh and not from bouillon, which may contain gluten.

Cooking Oil

5

The French use mostly peanut, corn and sunflower oil for the purpose of frying. Olive oil can also be used for cooking, but rarely for frying. Outside of France, other oils such as corn or vegetable may be substituted from time to time. Oil is used to fry or sauté foods. When ordering food that is prepared by frying, ensure that there is a dedicated fryer in the kitchen for non-battered menu items. Since battered foods may contain wheat flour, this practice minimizes the potential of gluten cross-contamination from frying.

Croutons, Bread Crumbs and Bread

Croutons and bread crumbs are used regularly as an ingredient in appetizers, soups and salads. The French generally do not waste any food product, especially old bread. When ordering these dishes, always be sure to request no croutons or bread crumbs. In addition, a basket of bread is usually served, so be certain to request no bread.

Vinegars

Malt vinegar is a common table condiment in French restaurants and is a popular accoutrement for *pommes frites* (French fried potatoes). It is fermented from barley and not distilled; therefore, it contains gluten and must be avoided.

Cross-Contamination

Cross-contamination occurs in two primary instances and should be considered at any restaurant you choose to dine in. One may occur when your meal is prepared in the same frying oil as foods containing other possible allergens. The second may occur when microbes or food particles are transferred from one food to another by using the same knife, cutting board, pots, pans or other utensils without washing the surfaces or tools in between uses. In the case of open flamed grills, the extreme temperature turns most food particles into carbon. Use of a wire brush designed for grill racks typically removes residual contaminants. To avoid cross-contamination, restaurants need to dedicate fryers for specific foods and wash all materials that may come in contact with food in hot, soapy water prior to preparing items for those with special dietary requirements. It is important to ensure that the restaurant follows these procedures for an allergen-free dining experience.

Other Allergy Considerations

If you have other food allergies or sensitivities, it is important to remain diligent in your approach to dining out. Because French cuisine is complex, there are many common food allergens used on a regular basis. While in France, be aware that peanut oil is often used to fry foods. Know that vegetable oil can always be substituted for any oil and may contain corn, peanuts or soy. It should be noted that unless an olive oil container specifically states 100% olive oil, it may be mixed with vegetable oil. If used, bouillon may contain Hydrolyzed Vegetable Protein (HVP) that can be derived from corn, soy or wheat. We have indicated the potential presence of bouillon and non-traditional cooking oils.

From the 30 menu items we have listed in our sample menu, we have identified each common allergen typically included in the dish as an ingredient. We have also indicated other potential allergens that may be present based upon non-traditional culinary practices. The chances of encountering common food allergens in items specific to our sample menu are outlined below.

High Likelihood	Dairy, eggs, fish and shellfish
Moderate Likelihood	Corn, gluten, peanuts, soy and wheat
Low Likelihood	Tree nuts

Dining Considerations

French menu items are usually presented in the French language. You often find menu descriptions in the language of the country you are in following the name of the French menu item. While traveling, be sure to familiarize yourself with the common French culinary terms included in this chapter to assist you in your dining experience.

French restaurants serve their cuisine in a style known as *service à la russe,* which is the practice of serving a meal in many courses. Previously, the French dined in a fashion much closer to our modern buffets. Today, the standard French lunch or dinner begins with *hors d'oeuvres* and is followed by soup, main course, salad, cheese and dessert. This multi-course plan was adapted from the Russian culture during the Napoleonic wars in the 19th century and remains the standard for our modern French gastro-nomic experience.

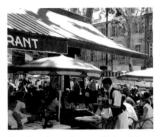

French restaurants serve their cuisine in a style known as *service à la russe,* which is the practice of serving a meal in many courses.

The French generally eat three meals a day. *Le petit déjeuner* is a light breakfast and usually consists of bread, cereals, fruit and coffee. *Le déjeuner* takes place between noon and 2 p.m. and is a larger meal, often consisting of three courses including soup, salad and a main dish. *Le goûter* is a snack sometimes taken in the late afternoon. The French dinner or *le dîner* is preceded by *l'apéritif,* a national custom that involves setting aside half an hour or so before a meal to share a drink, small appetizers and conversation with family, friends, neighbors or colleagues. *Le dîner* is a long affair, complete with many courses and lasts two to four hours; thereby allowing ample time to enjoy and savor the meal. It is also a time for the whole family to gather together and talk about their day. Wine is enjoyed throughout the evening, with after dinner drinks such as *calvados*, *cognac* and *eaux de vie* reserved for the end of the meal.

Bon Appetit!

Sample French Menu

Appetizers
Crevette Cocktail (Shrimp Cocktail)
Escargot (Snails)
Foies Gras (Fat Liver)
Les Huîtres (Oysters on the Half Shell)
Steak Tartare (Beef Tartar)
Tartare de Saumon (Salmon Tartar)

Soups
Bisque (Cream Soup)
Vichyssoise (Potato Leek Soup)

Salads
Artichauts à la Vinaigrette (Artichoke Salad)
Asperge à la Vinaigrette (Asparagus Salad)
Mesclun de Salade (Mixed Green Salad)
Salade Niçoise (Nice Style Salad)

Egg Entrees
Les Oeufs (Fried Eggs)
Les Omelettes (Omelets)

Beef Entrees
Filet de Boeuf (Beef Filet)
Fondue Bourguignon (Beef Fondue)
Steak au Poivre (Peppered Steak)
Steak Frites (Steak and French Fried Potatoes)

Chicken Entrees
Poulet Provençal (Roasted Chicken with Herbs)

Seafood Entrees
Bouillabaise (Seafood Stew)
Moules Frites (Mussels and French Fried Potatoes)
Saumon en Papillote (Baked Salmon)

Sample French Menu

Side Dishes
Gratin Dauphinois (Creamed Potatoes)
Haricots Verts (French Green Beans)
Pommes Frites (French Fried Potatoes)
Ratatouille (Vegetable Stew)

Desserts
Assiette de Fromage (Cheese Plate)
Crème Brulée (Baked Custard)
Fruits à la Crème (Fresh Fruit with Cream)
Mousse au Chocolat (Chocolate Mousse)
Les Sorbets (Sorbet)

5

We would like to thank Nicolas Bergerault, Founder and President of L'atelier des Chefs in Paris, France and Stephane Tremolani, former Executive Chef de Cuisine at the French Embassy in Rome, Italy for their valuable contributions in reviewing the following menu items.

French Menu Item Descriptions

Appetizers
Crevette Cocktail (Shrimp Cocktail)
Shrimp cocktail is a common appetizer across many international cuisines. *Crevette Cocktail* usually refers to medium sized shrimp. *Les Gambas*, large shrimp or prawns, may also be seen on some menus in France. Most restaurants prepare and serve this appetizer in a similar fashion. The shrimp are boiled in water or fish stock, shelled and chilled. They are traditionally served with a cocktail sauce (tomato sauce, horseradish and lemon juice), lemon wedges and sometimes an additional mayonnaise-based sauce.

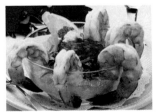

Crevette Cocktail (Shrimp Cocktail) with Cocktail Sauce

Gluten-Free Decision Factors:
- Ensure stocks and broths are made fresh and not from bouillon which may contain gluten
- Ensure no wheat flour in sauce

Food Allergen Preparation Considerations:
- Contains shellfish from shrimp
- May contain corn from bouillon and corn syrup in cocktail sauce
- May contain eggs from mayonnaise-based sauce
- May contain fish from fish stock
- May contain soy from bouillon and mayonnaise-based sauce

Escargot (Snails)

Escargot (Snails)

Escargot is a delicacy that has been enjoyed in Europe since the time of the ancient Romans. The French have carried on this tradition for hundreds of years and have developed many different recipes for the common garden snail. The texture of prepared escargot is very similar to that of a portabella mushroom and the traditional French preparation is very simple. The snails are removed from the shell and salted for a period of usually three days. Next, a purée of butter, garlic, parsley and shallots is placed in the shell. The snails are returned to the shell and topped with the remainder of the purée. They are then baked and garnished with chopped parsley, pepper and salt before serving. Rather than using shells, some recipes call for mushroom caps or a special ceramic dish to hold the ingredients.

Gluten-Free Decision Factors:
- Ensure no bread crumbs

Food Allergen Preparation Considerations:
- Contains dairy from butter and possibly from bread crumbs
- Contains shellfish from escargot (snails)

- May contain corn from bread crumbs

- May contain eggs from bread crumbs

- May contain peanuts from bread crumbs

- May contain soy from bread crumbs

- May contain tree nuts from bread crumbs

Foies Gras (Fat Liver)

Directly translated *foies gras* or *foie gras* means fat liver. Duck (*le canard*) or goose (*l'oie*) liver is predominantly used in French cuisine and is served three different ways: whole, in a pâté or in a mousse. French law requires that any product labeled foies gras must be 80% liver, the other 20% can be other meat from chicken, duck, goose or pork. For whole foies gras, the liver is usually marinated overnight in milk or salt water. After being marinated, the liver is thinly sliced, so that all the nerves can be removed. It is then cooked in a terrine with salt, pepper and cognac. Finally, it is set aside for three to four days before being served. Outside of France, you may encounter foies gras that is roasted or pan seared and then served plain or with various vegetables. Pâté de foies gras differs from mousse de foies gras in the consistency of its texture. Both pâté and mousse may contain dairy, eggs and truffles.

Gluten-Free Decision Factors:
- Request no bread

Food Allergen Preparation Considerations:
- May contain corn from bread

- May contain dairy from bread and milk

- May contain eggs as an ingredient and from bread

- May contain peanuts from bread

- May contain soy from bread

- May contain tree nuts from bread

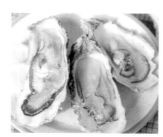

Les Huîtres (Oysters on the Half Shell)

Les Huîtres (Oysters on the Half Shell)

Oysters on the half shell can be served raw with lemon and cocktail sauce. They may also be baked or poached in fresh fish stock and topped with béarnaise or hollandaise sauce.

Gluten-Free Decision Factors:

- Ensure stocks and broths are made fresh and not from bouillon which may contain gluten

- Ensure no wheat flour in sauces

Food Allergen Preparation Considerations:

- Contains shellfish from oysters

- May contain corn from bouillon and corn syrup in cocktail sauce

- May contain dairy from béarnaise and hollandaise sauce

- May contain eggs from béarnaise and hollandaise sauce

- May contain fish from fish stock

- May contain soy from bouillon

Steak Tartare (Beef Tartar)

Steak tartare is a traditional appetizer prepared in French restaurants with many variations. In France, raw ground filet mignon, ground round or ground top sirloin are the common cuts of choice used in this dish. Chopped shallots and capers are served on the side along with lemon, olive oil and white wine vinegar. This allows the guest to pick and choose what ingredients to mix. Outside of France, the dish is usually pre-mixed with the above ingredients and may also include anchovies, garlic and mayonnaise; however, this in uncommon in France. Many recipes also call for a raw egg and white wine. There are a variety of seasonings used including *Herbs de Provence* (marjoram, thyme, summer savory, basil, rosemary, fennel seeds and lavender), mustard powder, pepper and salt. In France, some restaurants may serve Dijon

5

mustard, ketchup (yes, ketchup) and hot pepper sauce on the side.

Gluten-Free Decision Factors:
- None

Food Allergen Preparation Considerations:
- May contain corn from corn syrup in ketchup and vegetable oil
- May contain eggs from mayonnaise and raw egg
- May contain fish from anchovies
- May contain peanuts from vegetable oil
- May contain soy from mayonnaise and vegetable oil

Tartare de Saumon (Salmon Tartar)
There are hundreds of recipes for Salmon Tartar and most are very similar. Raw salmon is either minced or finely cubed. Capers, lemon juice, olive oil, diced scallions and diced shallots are mixed with the salmon and the dish is usually garnished with fresh dill or parsley. In some regions of France, Dijon mustard or mayonnaise may be included.

Gluten-Free Decision Factors:
- None

Food Allergen Preparation Considerations:
- Contains fish from salmon
- May contain corn from vegetable oil
- May contain eggs from mayonnaise
- May contain peanuts from vegetable oil
- May contain soy from mayonnaise and vegetable oil

Soups
Bisque (Cream Soup)
Bisque is a cream soup that usually features seafood, although vegetable bisques are also common. There

Bisque (Cream Soup) Featuring an Oyster

are hundreds of recipes for this soup, but most call for standard ingredients. The base of the soup is butter, cream, some type of fresh stock or broth and wine. Onions, puréed tomatoes and potatoes are common vegetables and the soup can be seasoned with anything from sea salt to saffron. Vegetarian bisques may also include any type of ground nut. Bisques are usually garnished with parsley and sometimes may contain croutons.

Gluten-Free Decision Factors:

- Ensure no croutons

- Ensure no wheat flour as thickening agent

- Ensure stocks and broths are made fresh and not from bouillon which may contain gluten

- Ensure no imitation crabmeat or seafood which may contain gluten

Food Allergen Preparation Considerations:

- Contains dairy from butter and cream

- May contain corn from bouillon and imitation crabmeat

- May contain eggs from croutons and imitation crabmeat

- May contain fish as ingredient and from seafood stock and imitation crabmeat if ordered

- May contain peanuts in vegetable bisque

- May contain shellfish as ingredient and from seafood stock if ordered

- May contain soy from bouillon and imitation crabmeat

- May contain tree nuts in vegetable bisque

Vichyssoise (Potato Leek Soup)

Vichyssoise is a chilled vegetable soup. It was created by Chef Louis Diat at New York's Ritz-Carlton Hotel in

1917, but it is a very common menu item in French restaurants. The base of the soup is butter, fresh chicken broth, cream and white wine. Chives, leeks, onions and potatoes are typically included and the soup is seasoned with basil, bay leaf, chervil, pepper, salt and thyme. The soup is usually garnished with chopped chives or parsley.

Gluten-Free Decision Factors:
- Ensure stocks and broths are made fresh and not from bouillon which may contain gluten
- Ensure no wheat flour as thickening agent

Food Allergen Preparation Considerations:
- Contains dairy from butter and cream
- May contain corn from bouillon
- May contain soy from bouillon

Salads
Artichauts à la Vinaigrette (Artichoke Salad)

Artichokes with vinaigrette are a popular French salad. There are a number of different recipes that either call for whole artichokes or artichoke hearts, which are steamed first to make the meat of the vegetable tender. Of all the different types of vinaigrettes used to dress the artichokes, most usually contain chives, garlic, olive oil, shallots, wine or sherry vinegar and wine. From time to time, you may encounter vinaigrette made with Dijon mustard.

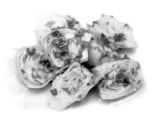

Artichauts à la Vinaigrette (Artichoke Salad)

Gluten-Free Decision Factors:
- None

Food Allergen Preparation Considerations:
- May contain corn from vegetable oil
- May contain peanuts from vegetable oil
- May contain soy from vegetable oil

5

5

Asperge à la Vinaigrette (Asparagus Salad)

Asparagus with vinaigrette can be prepared many different ways. After the asparagus has been steamed and chilled, chopped onions, tomatoes, shallots and chives can be added. The vinaigrette will usually contain garlic, olive oil, shallots, tarragon, wine or sherry vinegar and wine. From time to time, you may encounter vinaigrette made with Dijon mustard or a vinaigrette that contains hard-boiled eggs.

Gluten-Free Decision Factors:
- None

Food Allergen Preparation Considerations:
- May contain corn from vegetable oil
- May contain eggs from hard-boiled eggs in vinaigrette
- May contain peanuts from vegetable oil
- May contain soy from vegetable oil

Mesclun de Salade (Mixed Green Salad)

Mesclun is a green salad made from several types of young leaves, typically including arugula, dandelion, radicchio, and endive. Some recipes call for fresh berries, carrots, cucumbers, onions, tomatoes, and walnuts. When presented as *Mesclun de Salade*, the dish is usually just the greens tossed in varying types of vinaigrette. From time to time, you may encounter vinaigrette made with Dijon mustard.

Gluten-Free Decision Factors:
- None

Food Allergen Preparation Considerations:
- May contain corn from vegetable oil
- May contain peanuts from vegetable oil
- May contain soy from vegetable oil
- May contain tree nuts from walnuts

Salade Niçoise (Nice Style Salad)

Salade Niçoise comes from the south of France and is a favorite at French restaurants. There are many different recipes, but most usually contain anchovies, hard boiled eggs, green beans, mixed greens, potatoes, olives, onions and tomatoes. Seared tuna is a popular ingredient and you may also encounter salmon. The salad is always accompanied by some type of vinaigrette and may contain Dijon mustard.

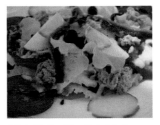

Salade Niçoise (Nice Style Salad)

5

Gluten-Free Decision Factors
- None

Food Allergen Preparation Considerations:
- Contains eggs from hard-boiled eggs

- Contains fish from anchovies, salmon or tuna

- May contain corn from vegetable oil

- May contain peanuts from vegetable oil

- May contain soy from vegetable oil

Eggs Entrees
Les Oeufs (Fried Eggs)

Eggs are usually eaten at *le déjeuner* (lunch) and are typically fried in butter in the north of France or olive oil in the south. *Oeuf dur* means "hard boiled eggs," but their consistency in France can sometimes be between soft and hard boiled. Eggs are often accompanied with *jambon* (ham) or *lardon* (fatty bacon).

Gluten-Free Decision Factors:
- Ensure oil used for frying has not been used to fry other items which may be battered or dusted with wheat flour

Food Allergen Preparation Considerations:
- Contains eggs

- May contain corn from vegetable oil

- May contain dairy from butter

- May contain peanuts from peanut oil and vegetable oil

- May contain soy from vegetable oil

5

Les Omelettes (Omelets)

Omelets are also eaten at *le déjeuner* (lunch) and are usually fried in butter in the north of France or olive oil in the south. Omelets are offered with a variety of ingredients including *nature* (plain), *jambon* (ham), *fromage* (cheese), *aux fines herbes* (mixed herbs) and *provençal* (mixed vegetables).

Gluten-Free Decision Factors:

- Ensure oil used for frying has not been used to fry other items which may be battered or dusted with wheat flour

- Ensure no wheat flour as fluffing agent

Food Allergen Preparation Considerations:

- Contains eggs

- May contain corn from vegetable oil

- May contain dairy from butter and cheese

- May contain peanuts from peanut oil and vegetable oil

- May contain soy from vegetable oil

Beef Entrees
Filet de Boeuf (Beef Filet)

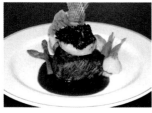

Filet de Boeuf (Beef Filet)

Filet de Boeuf is known to most as filet mignon. It is usually seasoned with salt and pepper and may sometimes be seasoned with other herbs. The beef may be pan seared in butter or olive oil or grilled over an open flame. It is often accompanied with béarnaise or hollandaise sauce. It should be noted that *Filet de Boeuf en Croute,* also known as *Filet de Boeuf Wellington*, is wrapped in puff pastry which contains wheat flour.

Gluten-Free Decision Factors:

- Ensure no wheat flour in sauce

- Ensure beef is not dusted with wheat flour

- Ensure beef is not breaded

Food Allergen Preparation Considerations:

- May contain corn from breading and vegetable oil

- May contain dairy from breading, butter, béarnaise and hollandaise sauce

- May contain eggs from breading, béarnaise and hollandaise sauce

- May contain peanuts from vegetable oil

- May contain soy from breading and vegetable oil

5

Fondue Bourguignon (Beef Fondue)

Fondue Bourguignon is classic beef fondue. Raw cubes of beef, usually filet mignon or rump steak, are served with a pot of hot vegetable oil. With fondue forks, a diner simply dips the beef into the hot oil until the desired temperature is reached. The dish is accompanied with a variety of dipping sauces and may include béarnaise, hollandaise, mayonnaise and ketchup.

Gluten-Free Decision Factors:

- Ensure no wheat flour in sauce

- Ensure beef is not dusted with wheat flour

Food Allergen Preparation Considerations:

- May contain corn from corn syrup in ketchup and vegetable oil

- May contain dairy from butter, béarnaise and hollandaise sauce

- May contain eggs from mayonnaise, béarnaise and hollandaise sauce

- May contain peanuts from peanut oil and vegetable oil

- May contain soy from mayonnaise and vegetable oil

5

Steak au Poivre (Peppered Steak)

Steak au Poivre is a standard French beef dish. Strip or sirloin steak is salted and pan fried with a little olive oil or butter. The French prefer the cooking temperature to be rare (bleu) or medium rare (à point). The steak is removed and a reduction of butter, red wine and cracked peppercorn is made in the pan using the fat or jus that remains. Garlic and shallots are sometimes used in the sauce. The dish is usually served with a side of *haricots verts* (French green beans) and carrots.

Gluten-Free Decision Factors:

- Ensure no wheat flour in sauce

- Ensure beef is not dusted with wheat flour

Food Allergen Preparation Considerations:

- Contains dairy from butter

- May contain corn from vegetable oil

- May contain peanuts from vegetable oil

- May contain soy from vegetable oil

Steak Frites (Steak and French Fried Potatoes)

Steak Frites can be many cuts of meat including porterhouse, sirloin, rib eye, shell steak or filet mignon. The steak is usually pan fried in butter or oil and seasoned with salt and pepper. Once the steak is done, a reduction can be made with butter, shallots and red wine. The steak is always accompanied by *pommes frites* (French fried potatoes) and may come with herb butter, ketchup, mayonnaise, béarnaise or hollandaise sauce. Malt vinegar is a common table condiment used for *pommes frites* in French restaurants and contains gluten.

Steak Frites (Steak and French Fried Potatoes)

Gluten-Free Decision Factors:

- Ensure no wheat flour in sauce

- Ensure beef is not dusted with wheat flour

- Ensure potatoes are not dusted with wheat flour

- Ensure oil used for frying is designated for potatoes only and is not used to fry other items that may be battered or dusted with wheat flour

- Request no malt vinegar

Food Allergen Preparation Considerations:
- May contain corn from corn syrup in ketchup and vegetable oil

- May contain dairy from butter, béarnaise and hollandaise sauce

- May contain eggs from mayonnaise, béarnaise and hollandaise sauce

- May contain peanuts from peanut oil and vegetable oil

- May contain soy from mayonnaise and vegetable oil

Chicken Entrees
Poulet Provençal (Roasted Chicken with Herbs)
Poulet Provençal is a marinated chicken dish that is either roasted in a special rotisserie oven or baked. This dish is a variation of the ubiquitous *Poulet Roti* (roasted chicken) found all over France. The whole chicken is marinated with garlic, *Herbs de Provence* (marjoram, thyme, summer savory, basil, rosemary, fennel seeds and lavender), lemon juice, olive oil, pepper and salt. After it is roasted, the chicken is served with vegetables which may include roasted potatoes with rosemary and salt or *haricots verts* (French green beans).

Gluten-Free Decision Factors:
- Ensure no soy sauce or wheat flour in marinade

Food Allergen Preparation Considerations:
- May contain dairy from butter in side vegetables

- May contain soy from soy sauce in marinade

- May contain tree nuts in side vegetables

Seafood Entrees
Bouillabaise (Seafood Stew)

More than just a soup or stew, *Bouillabaise* is a French gastronomic tradition. In a clear fresh fish stock or broth, many types of seafood are combined including clams, crab, any fish, lobster, mussels, oysters, scallops and shrimp. The vegetables usually included are carrots, celery, leeks, onions and potatoes. *Bouillabaise* is typically seasoned with garlic, pepper, salt and saffron, but may also be seasoned with a *bouquet garni* (cheese cloth bag full of herbs) containing *Herbes de Provence*. Some recipes call for croutons or toasted bread on the side.

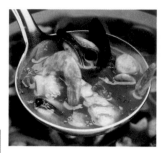

Bouillabaise (Seafood Stew)

5

Gluten-Free Decision Factors:

- Ensure no croutons or bread

- Ensure no wheat flour as thickening agent

- Ensure stocks or broths are made fresh and not from bouillon which may contain gluten

Food Allergen Preparation Considerations:

- Contains fish as an ingredient

- Contains shellfish as an ingredient

- May contain corn from bouillon and bread

- May contain dairy from bread

- May contain eggs from bread and croutons

- May contain peanuts from bread

- May contain soy from bouillon and bread

- May contain tree nuts from bread

Moules Frites (Mussels and French Fried Potatoes)

Steamed mussels are very popular in Belgium and France. They are served both as an appetizer and as an entrée and are typically accompanied with *pommes frites*. The mussels are steamed or boiled in fresh fish stock, then topped with a sauce that contains butter, onions or shallots, white wine and sometimes garlic. Occasionally, the mussels may be topped with bread crumbs. *Pommes frites* may come with herb butter, ketchup, mayonnaise, béarnaise or hollandaise sauce. Malt vinegar is a common table condiment used for *pommes frites* in French restaurants and contains gluten.

Gluten-Free Decision Factors:
- Ensure no wheat flour in sauce
- Ensure no bread crumbs
- Ensure stocks and broths are made fresh and not from bouillon which may contain gluten
- Ensure potatoes are not dusted with wheat flour
- Ensure oil used for frying is designated for potatoes only and is not used to fry other items that may be battered or dusted with wheat flour
- Request no malt vinegar

Food Allergen Preparation Considerations:
- Contains dairy from butter and possibly from bread crumbs, béarnaise and hollandaise sauce
- Contains shellfish from mussels
- May contain corn from bouillon, bread crumbs, corn syrup in ketchup and vegetable oil
- May contain eggs from bread crumbs, mayonnaise, béarnaise and hollandaise sauce
- May contain peanuts from bread crumbs, peanut oil and vegetable oil
- May contain soy from bouillon, bread crumbs and vegetable oil
- May contain tree nuts from bread crumbs

Saumon en Papillote (Baked Salmon)
The term *"en Papillote"* refers to the French style of cooking in a parchment paper bag. This is an excellent way to cook, as it allows all the flavors inside to permeate the fish. You may find any fish made *"en Papillote."* A filet of salmon is placed in the center of a large piece of parchment paper that has been brushed with butter or olive oil. Blanched vegetables including julienned car-

rots, leeks and green beans are added to garlic, onions and shallots that are sautéed in butter or olive oil. The dish can be seasoned with various herbs including coriander, fennel, pepper and salt. The parchment paper is then folded in the shape of a bag and baked until brown. Egg whites are sometimes used to seal the parchment paper bag.

Gluten-Free Decision Factors:
- Ensure fish is not dusted with wheat flour

Food Allergen Preparation Considerations:
- Contains fish from salmon

- May contain corn from vegetable oil

- May contain dairy from butter

- May contain eggs from the sealing of parchment paper bag

- May contain peanuts from peanut oil and vegetable oil

- May contain soy from vegetable oil

Side Dishes
Gratin Dauphinois (Creamed Potatoes)
A creamed potato casserole, *Gratin Dauphinois* is a common French side dish. Thinly sliced potatoes are baked in a cream sauce with butter, crème fraîche and milk. It is seasoned with garlic, salt, pepper and may also contain nutmeg. Some recipes call for grated gruyère cheese and bread crumbs; however the traditional style omits these ingredients.

Gluten-Free Decision Factors:
- Ensure no wheat flour as ingredient

- Ensure no bread crumbs

Food Allergen Preparation Considerations:
- Contains dairy from butter, crème fraîche, milk and possibly from bread crumbs and cheese

- May contain corn from bread crumbs

- May contain eggs from bread crumbs

- May contain peanuts from bread crumbs

- May contain soy from bread crumbs

- May contain tree nuts from bread crumbs

Haricots Verts (French Green Beans)

The French prepare green beans by steaming them until they are cooked, yet still crisp. *Haricots verts* can be served plain, in butter or olive oil and may contain almonds, garlic and onions. They may also be topped with béarnaise or hollandaise sauce.

Gluten-Free Decision Factors:
- Ensure no wheat flour in sauce

Food Allergen Preparation Considerations:
- May contain corn from vegetable oil

- May contain dairy from butter, béarnaise or hollandaise sauce

- May contain eggs from béarnaise or hollandaise sauce

- May contain peanuts from peanut oil and vegetable oil

- May contain soy from vegetable oil

- May contain tree nuts from almonds

Pommes Frites (French Fried Potatoes)

Pommes Frites are classic French fried potatoes, although many give credit to the Belgians for creating this dish. The potatoes are typically sliced very thin and fried in peanut or vegetable oil. They are seasoned with salt, but some recipes call for a butter, garlic and parsley sauce on the side for dipping. The French also like to dip them in herb butter, ketchup, mayonnaise, béarnaise or hollandaise sauce. Malt vinegar is a common table condiment used for *pommes frites* in French restaurants and contains gluten.

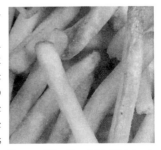
Pommes Frites (French Fried Potatoes)

5

Gluten-Free Decision Factors:

- Ensure potatoes are not dusted with wheat flour prior to frying

- Ensure oil used for frying is designated for potatoes only and is not used to fry other items that may be battered or dusted with wheat flour

- Request no malt vinegar

Food Allergen Preparation Considerations:

- May contain corn from corn syrup in ketchup and vegetable oil

- May contain dairy from butter, béarnaise and hollandaise sauce

- May contain eggs from mayonnaise, béarnaise and hollandaise sauce

- May contain peanuts from peanut oil and vegetable oil

- May contain soy from mayonnaise and vegetable oil

Ratatouille (Vegetable Stew)

Ratatouille is a traditional vegetable dish from the south of France that can be served as a side dish as well as an entrée. It resembles a vegetable stew and includes bell peppers, eggplant, onions, tomatoes and zucchini. The vegetables are cooked in olive oil and white wine, then seasoned with garlic, *Herbs de Provence*, pepper and salt. Although uncommon, some recipes call for grated cheese. *Ratatouille* can be served hot or chilled.

Gluten-Free Decision Factors:

- Ensure no wheat flour as ingredient

- Ensure stocks and broths are made fresh and not from bouillon which may contain gluten

Food Allergen Preparation Considerations:

- May contain corn from bouillon and vegetable oil

- May contain dairy from cheese

- May contain peanuts from vegetable oil
- May contain soy from bouillon and vegetable oil

Desserts
Assiette de Fromage (Cheese Plate)

Generally speaking, cheese is eaten with salad prior to the dessert course in France and is typically listed in the dessert section of the menu. In most cases, you are offered a variety of different cheeses including brie, camembert and chèvre; however, the types may vary based upon location and availability. Cheese is usually served with bread or crackers and sometimes sliced fruit.

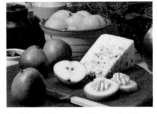

Assiette de Fromage (Cheese Plate) with Fruit

5

Gluten-Free Decision Factors:

- Request no bread or crackers

- Request no blue or veined cheese which may contain gluten

Food Allergen Preparation Considerations:

- Contains dairy from cheese and possibly from bread

- May contain corn from bread

- May contain eggs as ingredient and from bread

- May contain peanuts from bread

- May contain soy from bread

- May contain tree nuts from bread

Crème Brulée (Baked Custard)

Crème Brulée is one of the most popular French desserts. The custard is made with heavy cream, egg yolks, sugar and vanilla. The whisked ingredients are then baked. After it has cooled, it is topped with brown sugar that is caramelized by placing the custard in a broiler or torching it by hand. There are many different types of crème brulée, some of which may contain different flavors such as almond, chocolate and fresh berries.

Gluten-Free Decision Factors:
- Ensure no wheat flour as ingredient

Food Allergen Preparation Considerations:
- Contains dairy from cream
- Contains eggs from egg yolks
- May contain corn from almond and vanilla extract
- May contain soy from chocolate
- May contain tree nuts from almond extract

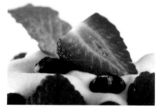

Fruits à la Crème (Fresh Fruit with Cream)

Fruits à la Crème (Fresh Fruit with Cream)

Crème fraîche is a slightly tangy and nutty thick cream that is naturally fermented. The French adore this cream as a dessert with fresh fruit. Mixed berries are usually the fruit of choice, but you can find it with other fruits such as apples and melons.

Gluten-Free Decision Factors:
- None

Food Allergen Preparation Considerations:
- Contains dairy from cream

Mousse au Chocolat (Chocolate Mousse)

Chocolate mousse has become a popular dessert and can be found on the menus of many international cuisines. There are a number of variations, but the preparation is typically consistent with the following recipe. Chocolate is melted in a double-boiler with milk and sugar. Whipped eggs are then carefully folded into the chocolate sauce after it has cooled. Next, whipped heavy cream is added to the mixture, which is allowed to sit for a few minutes before the mousse is poured into a container and chilled. Some styles incorporate liqueurs such as coffee, orange and peppermint for a distinctive flavor. Chocolate mousse may be served with whipped cream and a cookie.

Gluten-Free Decision Factors:
- Ensure no wheat flour as ingredient

- Request no cookie

Food Allergen Preparation Considerations:
- Contains dairy from cream, milk and possibly from chocolate and cookie

- Contains eggs as an ingredient and possibly from cookie

- May contain peanuts from cookie and various flavors

- May contain tree nuts from cookie and various flavors

Mousse au Chocolat (Chocolate Mousse)

5

Les Sorbets (Sorbet)

Sorbet is puréed fruit and sugar that is frozen and served like ice cream. If the restaurant uses *service à la russe,* sorbet may be offered in between courses to cleanse your palate. Raspberry, lemon and lime sorbets are the most common. You may also encounter many other fruit flavors or chocolate. Occasionally, sorbet is served with some kind of cookie or pirouline.

Gluten-Free Decision Factors:
- Ensure no wheat flour as ingredient

- Ensure no stabilizers which may contain gluten

- Request no cookie

Food Allergen Preparation Considerations:
- May contain corn from colors or flavors

- May contain dairy from cookie

- May contain eggs from cookie

- May contain peanuts from cookie and various flavors

- May contain soy from chocolate, colors or flavors and cookie

- May contain tree nuts from cookie and various flavors

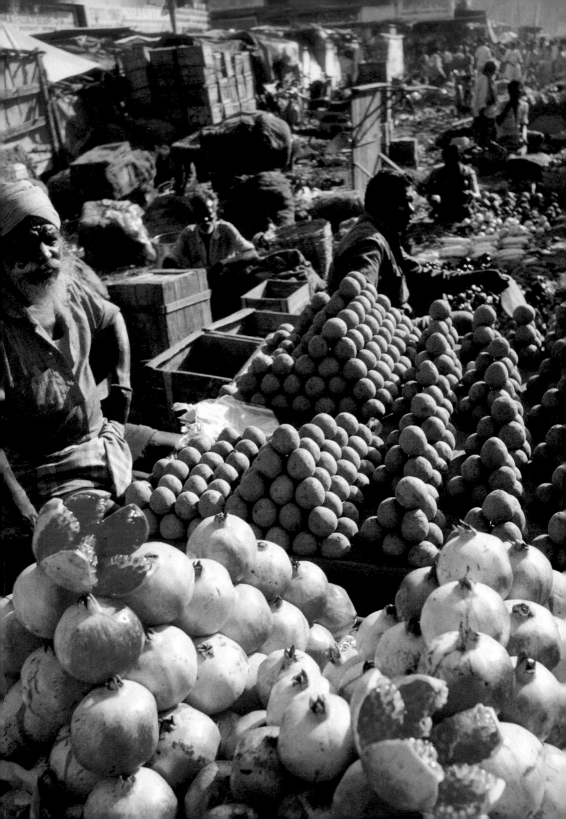

Far more indispensable than food for the
physical body is spiritual nourishment for the soul.
One can do without food for a considerable time,
but a man of the spirit cannot exist for a single
second without spiritual nourishment.
—Gandhi

CHAPTER 6
Let's Eat Indian Cuisine

Cuisine Overview

With over a billion inhabitants, India is second only to China in population. The 35 states and territories of India occupy a landmass roughly the size of Europe. The cultural identity of India is extraordinarily complex due to the conquest of its lands: From the Aryans, Mongolians and Persians to the Greeks, Portuguese and the British. This is further complicated by the fact that there are 40-plus languages and dialects spoken, most of which have their own alphabet and script. How then can one classify the culinary identity of a country with over a billion people, speaking over 40 languages and dialects who have been conquered or occupied by at least 10 different civilizations? One word: *Masala!*

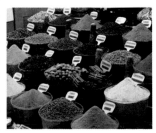

Masala is the Hindi word for spice and is the single unifying factor of the 16 major schools of Indian cooking. Regional cuisines in the North include *Avahd, Kashmiri, Lucknow, Punjabi, Rajasthan* and *Uttar Pradesh.* Southern cooking is represented by the *Andhra* or *Hyderabad, Kerala* and *Tamil Nadu* cooking styles, while *Bengali* is the predominant Eastern Indian cuisine. In the West, *Goan, Gujarati, Konkani, Maharashtrian* and *Parsi* cuisines hold the greatest prominence.

In addition to its conquerors, the original indig-

6

enous civilization, the Dravidians, have had a large impact on traditional cuisine. The Dravidians were responsible for the creation and development of the *Ayurveda*, one of the first examples of life sciences in early civilization. The *Ayurveda* was the first documentation of thought that recognized the importance of nutrition and its impact on physical, mental and spiritual health. These early discoveries still remain in practice and are relevant today, serving as the basis for many Indian culinary principles.

Vegetarianism has long been a part of India's culinary history. It is widely believed that the early civilizations of the Indian sub-continent were vegetarian, but this has yet to be confirmed by archeologists. The first documented evidence of vegetarianism in India was in the 6th century BC, through the teachings of both Buddha and Mahavir Jain, the two greatest spiritual influences in Indian culture. The Emperor Ashoka, further popularized the virtue of vegetarianism during his rule in the 2nd century BC. Today, vegetarian dishes hold a prominent place in the Indian gastronomic experience.

Familiarity with Indian cuisine varies greatly depending upon your geographic location. In the United Kindom, for example, there are over 9,000 Indian restaurants and the cuisine itself has become as common as Mexican food in California. Indian neighborhoods can be found in cities all over the world; this is where you will find the most authentic cuisine outside the Indian sub-continent.

Traditional Ingredients

Like many cuisines in Asia, Indian culinary ingredients are directly related to the availability of products in each region. Since the country is so large, there is a cornucopia of food products used in the many schools of Indian cooking. Dairy products, legumes, spices and vegetables are regularly consumed at most Indian meals. Breads, crepes and pancakes made from chickpea, lentil, potato, rice and wheat flours are also a daily staple of their diet.

Since the number of vegetarians in Indian is substantial, there is obviously an extensive variety

Legumes, such as lentils, are often used as ingredients (left). Chili peppers are a common Indian spice (right).

of vegetables used regularly. Cabbage, carrots, cauliflower, corn, onions, potatoes, pumpkin, shallots, spinach, tomatoes and turnips are common vegetables found across Indian cuisine. Legumes such as black gram, chick peas and lentils are often used as ingredients, as well as ground into flours for bread. Nuts play a big part, with almonds, cashews, peanuts, pistachios and walnuts frequently incorporated into dishes. In addition, Indian cuisine utilizes many different types of fruit such as coconut, mango and raisins as ingredients in their dishes and in chutney, the famous spiced fruit spread.

Masala (spice) is used in the majority of dishes. Although the exact spices for a specific dish vary from chef to chef, their choices for what spices to include are standard across Indian cuisine. These common Indian herbs and spices include bay leaves, black pepper, cardamom, chili pepper, cinnamon, cloves, coriander, cumin, fennel, fenugreek, garlic, ginger, mustard seed and turmeric.

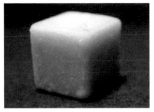

6

Paneer, a soft Indian cheese, is used in vegetarian dishes and desserts.

Because the cow is sacred to Hindus, dairy products are prevalent far more often than beef in Indian cooking; although, you may find beef in non-Hindu Indian restaurants. *Ghee* (clarified butter) is traditionally used to cook food, in addition to peanut, seed and other vegetable oils. Yogurt is often included in curry dishes, with buttermilk, cream and milk incorporated from time to time. *Paneer,* a soft Indian cheese, is used in vegetarian dishes and desserts.

Sources of protein in Indian restaurants are directly reflective of each restaurant owner's religious beliefs. Generally speaking, most Indian restaurants offer chicken, fish and lamb dishes, with *paneer* (Indian cheese), lentils and yogurt serving as the major sources of protein for vegetarians. A Hindu restaurant would never serve beef; whereas, one would expect to find it in a Muslim restaurant, where you would not find pork or shellfish. In fact, it is rare to see pork on a typical Indian menu.

The Indian culture is known for its consumption of non-alcoholic specialty beverages. Tea is considered a national treasure, with the orange pekoe blend being the most common. Because of India's geographic location, thousands of tea varieties are available including red, green and black. *Masala Chai* is a popular Indian beverage enjoyed around the world that is made with black tea, cardamom, hot milk and sugar. Another non-alcoholic specialty beverage is *Lassi*. It is made with yogurt and salt or sugar, which can be requested plain or with a variety of natural flavors such as mint, mango or strawberry.

Gluten Awareness

Although gluten is present in some areas of Indian cuisine, we have outlined 25-plus items in our sample menu. There are six primary points that you need to consider when dining at an Indian restaurant. To ensure a gluten-free experience, the areas of food preparation that you need to inquire about with your server or chef are listed below.

Sauces	Ensure sauces do not contain wheat flour
Stocks and Broths	Ensure all stocks and broths are made fresh and not from bouillon which may contain gluten
Cooking Oil	Ensure frying oil has not been used to fry battered foods that may contain gluten
Bread and Pancakes	Wheat flour is typically used—ensure no wheat flour
Marinades	Although uncommon, ensure marinades do not contain wheat flour or soy sauce
Cross-Contamination	Ensure all utensils and cooking surfaces have been cleaned prior to the preparation of your meal

Sauces

Culinary practices vary in Indian restaurants. Although it is uncommon, some sauces may have wheat flour added to them as a thickening agent. Many standard Indian condiments such chutney, Indian pickles or *raita* resemble sauces. Chutneys are spicy fruit or vegetable spreads and are very common in Indian restaurants. Indian pickles are made with fruit or vegetables in oil with aromatic spices and differ from western pickles in that they resemble relish. They almost never contain vinegar and are not made from cucumbers. *Raita* is a yogurt dipping sauce.

Although ingredients will vary widely from restaurant to restaurant, below is a list of common and typically gluten-free condiments and their ingredients.

Coconut Chutney	Coconut, chili pepper, vegetable oil, yogurt, Indian herbs and spices
Mango Chutney	Mango, ginger, onions, raisins, Indian herbs and spices
Mint Chutney	Mint, chili pepper, lemon juice, onions, salt, sugar, oil, Indian herbs and spices
Tamarind Chutney	Tamarind pulp, sugar, oil, water, Indian herbs and spices
Tomato Chutney	Tomato, chili pepper, cilantro, garlic, salt, sugar, tamarind juice, Indian herbs and spices
Indian Pickles	Any type of fruit or vegetable with Indian herbs and spices in oil
Raita	A yogurt sauce with Indian herbs and spices, which may also contain sliced onions and tomatoes

Stocks and Broths

Stocks and broths are used frequently in Indian cuisine and are present in sauces and soups. Ensure that stocks and broths are made fresh and not from bouillon, which may contain gluten.

Cooking Oil

Indians sometimes use *ghee* (clarified butter) to fry foods because of its perceived health benefits and high smoking point. The flavor is rather strong, so many chefs prefer to use other types of oils including: canola, coconut, corn, mustard seed, olive, peanut, sesame and sunflower. Outside of India, vegetable oil may be substituted from time to time. Oil is used to fry or sauté foods. When ordering food that is prepared by frying, ensure that there is a dedicated fryer in the kitchen for non-battered menu items. Since battered foods may contain wheat flour, this practice minimizes the potential of gluten cross-contamination from frying.

Bread and Pancakes

Dosas, a South Indian version of the crepe or pancake, are usually stuffed with a filling and served with chutneys. In some cases, they resemble a pizza, with the ingredients placed on the top of the crepe or pancake. *Dosas* are often made with black gram, lentil, potato or rice flour. If ordered, ensure that *dosas* do not contain wheat flour.

With the exception of many *dosas,* most breads and pancakes are made with wheat flour in Indian restaurants. At left is a list of common breads and pancakes made with wheat flour that should be avoided.

Marinades

Marinades are used frequently in Indian restaurants and differ from most cuisines in that they are typically citrus or yogurt based. Although uncommon, other types of marinades may be used in restaurants that incorporate non-traditional culinary practices. If this is the case, ensure that the marinade does not include soy sauce, which contains wheat, or wheat flour.

Cross-Contamination

Cross-contamination occurs in two primary instances and should be considered at any restaurant you choose to dine in. One may occur when your meal is prepared in the same frying oil as foods containing other possible allergens. The second may occur when microbes or food particles are transferred from one food to another by using the same knife, cutting board, pots, pans or other utensils without washing the surfaces or tools in between uses. In the case of open flamed grills, the extreme temperature turns most food particles into carbon. Use of a wire brush designed for grill racks typically removes residual contaminants. To avoid cross-contamination, restaurants need to dedicate fryers for specific foods and wash all materials that may come in contact with food in hot, soapy water prior to preparing items for those with special dietary requirements. It is important to ensure that the restaurant follows these procedures for an allergen-free dining experience.

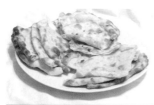

Common bread and pancakes with wheat flour that should be avoided:

Bhatura	Poori
Chappati	Puri
Kulcha	Rava Dosa
Naan	Roti
Paratha	

6

Other Allergy Considerations

If you have other food allergies or sensitivities, it is important to remain diligent in your approach to dining out. Because Indian cuisine is complex, there are many common food allergens used on a regular basis. While in India, be aware that *ghee* (clarified butter) is often used to fry foods. Know that vegetable oil can always be substituted for any oil and may contain corn, peanuts or soy. Peanuts and tree nuts are frequently used both as an ingredient and in cooking oils. If used, bouillon may contain Hydrolyzed Vegetable Protein (HVP) that can be derived form corn, soy or wheat. We have indicated the potential presence of bouillon and cooking oils.

From the 25-plus items we have listed in our sample menu, we have identified each common allergen typically included in the dish as an ingredient. We have also indicated other potential allergens that may be present based upon non-traditional culinary practices. The chances of encountering common food allergens in items specific to our sample menu are outlined below.

High likelihood	Corn, dairy, fish, peanuts and soy
Moderate likelihood	Gluten, shellfish, tree nuts and wheat
Low likelihood	Eggs

In addition, your sensitivity to spice levels can be an important concern. Indian food is often extremely spicy due to the use of chili peppers and powders. *Tandoor* dishes tend to be far less spicy than curries. In most cases, you can order dishes mild. Keep in mind that mild to an Indian chef may still be quite spicy. If you are especially sensitive, it is important to discuss these concerns with your server or chef.

Dining Considerations

Menus in Indian restaurants tend to be presented in the language of the country you are dining in. This is due to the fact that most people neither read the Indian language alphabets, nor understand the 40-

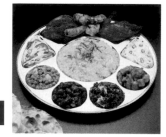

Indian Meal Tray

6

plus languages and dialects spoken in India. Since Indian languages have different alphabets than the English language, menus may have the name of a dish spelled phonetically in English. With this in mind, you will soon realize that there are many different ways to phonetically spell an Indian dish. Kabobs, whether it is spelled kababs, kebobs or kebabs, is the same skewered meat dish.

Depending on where you are dining, it may be acceptable to eat with your hands; however, most restaurants offer Western cutlery for your convenience. As is the case with most Asian cuisines, Indian food is designed to be enjoyed "family style." Finding a balance between many dishes and sharing them with your table is a very important part of the Indian culture.

Dining schedules in India vary according to religious practices. The customary eating schedule for many Hindus includes a light meal in the morning, a heavier meal in the afternoon and another light meal in the evening. For Muslims, the dining schedule is similar; however, during the month of Ramadan, fasting is observed during daylight hours.

Chalo, sub khana khao!
(Bon Appetit in Hindi.
It literally means
"Come, let's start eating!")

Sample Indian Menu

Appetizers
Aloo Tikki (Potato Patty)
Kabobs (Skewered Meat)
Pakoras (Vegetable Fritters)
Papadam (Spicy Crackers)

Sample Indian Menu

Soups
Curried Coconut Soup
Mulligatawny (Chicken and Vegetable Soup)
Sambar (Lentil and Vegetable Stew)

Salad
Kachumber (Chopped Salad)

Curry Entrees
Channa Masala (Chickpeas in Tomato Curry)
Gosht Vindaloo (Spicy Lamb Curry)
Jhinga Masala (Shrimp in Coconut Curry)
Malai Kofta (Vegetarian Croquettes in Mild Curry)
Murg Korma (Chicken in Cream Curry)
Murg Tikki Masala (Chicken in Tomato Curry)
Rogan Josh (Mild Lamb Curry)
Saag Paneer (Indian Cheese and Spinach Curry)

Tandoor Specialties
Boti Kabob (Skewered Lamb)
Murg Tandoori (Tandoori Barbeque Chicken)
Murg Tikka (Yogurt Marinated Chicken)
Seekh Kabob (Skewered Minced Lamb)

Dosas (South Indian Specialties)
Masala Dosa (Spicy Vegetable Filled Crepe)
Sada Dosa (Lentil and Rice Crepe)
Uthappam (Lentil and Rice Pancake)

Desserts
Kheer (Rice Pudding)
Kulfi (Indian Ice Cream)
Rasmalai (Cheese Balls in Sweet Cream)

6

*We would like to thank Samir Majmudar, owner
of Rani Indian Bistro in Brookline, Massachusettes
and Tariq Zaman, owner of The Spice Company
in Moseley, United Kingdom for their valuable
contributions in reviewing the following menu items.*

Indian Menu Item Descriptions

Appetizers
Aloo Tikki (Potato Patty)

Aloo Tikki is a popular North Indian appetizer. The preparation involves combining slightly mashed potatoes with vegetable flour, usually chickpea *(besan)*, corn *(makai)* or water chestnut *(singara)*. Some chefs may also add yogurt curd. The potato mixture is seasoned with spices, which vary from kitchen to kitchen and usually include chili powder, cumin, salt and pepper. The resulting mixture is then formed into balls or patties and pan fried in *ghee* (clarified butter) or oil. *Aloo Tikki* is typically garnished with coriander leaves (cilantro), chopped green chili peppers, onions, tomatoes and some type of chutney on the side for dipping.

Gluten-Free Decision Factors:

- Ensure no wheat flour—chickpea, corn or water chestnut flour is typically used

- Ensure no wheat flour in chutney

Food Allergen Preparation Considerations:

- May contain corn from corn flour and vegetable oil

- May contain dairy from butter and yogurt curd

- May contain peanuts from peanut oil and vegetable oil

- May contain soy from vegetable oil

6

Kabobs (Skewered Meat)

Indian *Kabobs* are usually offered with chicken or lamb; however, fish, shrimp and vegetarian *Kabobs* are available in some restaurants. In most cases, the ingredients are marinated in a yogurt sauce with Indian spices, which usually include chili powder, cumin, coriander, garlic, ginger and turmeric. The marinade may also include lime juice or vegetable oil. The meat is then skewered and grilled over an open flame or baked in a tandoori oven. *Kabobs* may be served with some type of chutney or *raita* (a yogurt sauce) on the side for dipping.

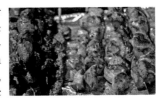
Kabobs (Skewered Meat)

6

Gluten-Free Decision Factors:

• Ensure no wheat flour in chutney

• Ensure no soy sauce or wheat flour in marinade

Food Allergen Preparation Considerations:

• Contains dairy from yogurt sauce

• May contain corn from vegetable oil

• May contain fish if ordered

• May contain peanuts from peanut oil and vegetable oil

• May contain shellfish if ordered

• May contain soy from soy sauce in marinade and vegetable oil

Pakoras (Vegetable Fritters)

Pakoras are popular hot appetizers eaten in India, enjoyed especially during the rainy season. A thick batter is made with chickpea flour (*besan*), chili powder, cumin, salt and pepper. Chopped cabbage, cauliflower, chili pepper, coriander leaves, mint leaves, onions, potatoes and spinach are added. The resulting mixture is then formed into balls or patties and pan fried in *ghee* or oil. *Pakoras* are usually garnished with coriander or mint leaves and served with some type of chutney on the side for dipping.

Gluten-Free Decision Factors:
- Ensure no wheat flour—chickpea, corn or water chestnut flour is typically used
- Ensure no wheat flour in chutney

Food Allergen Preparation Considerations:
- May contain corn from corn flour and vegetable oil
- May contain dairy from butter
- May contain peanuts from peanut oil and vegetable oil
- May contain soy from vegetable oil

6

Papadam (Spicy Crackers)

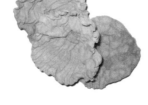

Papadam (Spicy Crackers)

Papadam are crackers made out of lentil (*urad daal*) or chickpea (*besan*) flour and are eaten very much like tortilla chips in Mexico. The dough is lentil or chickpea flour with salt, water and may include other Indian spices. They come in many flavors, including black or red pepper, garlic or plain and can be pan fried in *ghee* or oil or baked. *Papadam* are then served with dipping sauces which usually include *raita* and some type of chutney.

Gluten-Free Decision Factors:
- Ensure no wheat flour—chickpea, corn or water chestnut flour is typically used
- Ensure no wheat flour in chutney

Food Allergen Preparation Considerations:
- May contain corn from corn flour and vegetable oil
- May contain dairy from butter and yogurt sauce
- May contain peanuts from peanut oil and vegetable oil
- May contain soy from vegetable oil

Soups
Curried Coconut Soup

Curried coconut soup is very common in Indian restaurants and can be served chilled or hot. The base of the soup consists of coconut milk, milk, water and sometimes egg yolks or *ghee*. In most cases, the soup is seasoned with a curry powder consisting of cardamom, chili powder, cloves, and cumin. It may also contain various spices such as nutmeg or fennel. Although ingredients vary, almonds, coconut flakes, onions and pistachios are typically included. The soup is usually garnished with toasted coconut flakes.

Gluten-Free Decision Factors:
- Ensure no wheat flour as thickening agent

Food Allergen Preparation Considerations:
- Contains dairy from milk and possibly from butter

- May contain eggs from egg yolks

- May contain tree nuts from almonds and pistachios

Mulligatawny (Chicken and Vegetable Soup)

Mulligatawny is the most common version of spicy chicken soup found in Indian restaurants. There are hundreds of variations, but most follow a basic recipe. Fresh chicken stock is the base of the soup, with standard ingredients including carrots, celery, chicken, chili peppers, lentils, lemon juice, onions, potatoes, tomatoes and rice. Some chefs include coconut milk and milk. The ingredients of the soup are sautéed in *ghee* or oil with various types of Indian spices and then added to the fresh chicken stock. *Mulligatawny* can be garnished with cream or coconut cream, chopped coriander leaves or parsley and toasted almonds or pistachios.

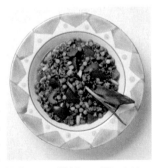

Mulligatawny (Chicken and Vegetable Soup)

Gluten-Free Decision Factors:
- Ensure stocks and broths are made fresh and not from bouillon which may contain gluten

- Ensure no wheat flour as thickening agent

Food Allergen Preparation Considerations:
- May contain corn from bouillon and vegetable oil

- May contain dairy from butter, cream or milk

- May contain peanuts from peanut oil and vegetable oil

- May contain soy from bouillon and vegetable oil

- May contain tree nuts from almonds and pistachios

6

Sambar (Lentil and Vegetable Stew)

Sambar is a South Indian vegetable stew. The base of the stew is a fresh vegetarian stock made with water, tamarind juice or paste and *sambar* powder (ground black pepper, chili powder, coconut, coriander, cumin, fenugreek seed, lentils, mustard seed and tumeric). Many types of chopped vegetables, which usually include onions, potatoes, shallots, tomatoes and turnips, are sautéed in *ghee* or oil. The vegetables are then added to the fresh stock with lentils or rice. It is served as a stew or a side dish with *dosas* (South Indian crepes or pancakes).

Gluten-Free Decision Factors:
- Ensure stocks and broths are made fresh and not from bouillon which may contain gluten

- Ensure no wheat flour as thickening agent

- Ensure no wheat flour in *dosas*

Food Allergen Preparation Considerations:
- May contain corn from bouillon, corn flour in *dosas* and vegetable oil

- May contain dairy from butter

- May contain peanuts from peanut oil and vegetable oil

- May contain soy from bouillon and vegetable oil

Salads
Kachumber (Chopped Salad)

Kachumber is an Indian chopped salad which is common with every meal. A salad in an Indian restaurant serves only as an accompaniment rather than a course in itself. This salad usually consists of chopped carrots, chili peppers, cucumbers, onions, radishes and tomatoes. It is seasoned with chopped coriander leaves, cumin, red chili powder and salt. These ingredients are then tossed in a bowl with lemon juice and sometimes oil.

Gluten-Free Decision Factors:

- None

Food Allergen Preparation Considerations:

- May contain corn from vegetable oil

- May contain peanuts from peanut oil and vegetable oil

- May contain soy from vegetable oil

Curry Entrees
Channa Masala (Chickpeas in Tomato Curry)

Channa Masala is usually a vegetarian dish, however fresh chicken stock is used from time to time. Chopped chili, garlic, ginger and onions are sautéed in *ghee* or oil. Chopped or crushed tomatoes are then added with water or occasionally chicken stock. Boiled and drained chickpeas are then added with *garam masala* powder (a spice mixture which varies, but typically includes black pepper, cloves, coriander, cumin and red chili powder). The dish is usually garnished with chopped coriander leaves.

Gluten-Free Decision Factors:

- Ensure stocks and broths are made fresh and not from bouillon which may contain gluten

- Ensure no wheat flour in sauce

Food Allergen Preparation Considerations:
- May contain corn from bouillon and vegetable oil
- May contain dairy from butter
- May contain peanuts from peanut oil and vegetable oil
- May contain soy from bouillon and vegetable oil

6

Gosht Vindaloo (Spicy Lamb Curry)

Gosht Vindaloo is a spicy lamb curry dish. Cubed lamb is marinated in a paste made of black pepper, cinnamon, cloves, coriander, cumin, garlic, ginger, red chili powder, turmeric and cider or wine vinegar for a period of up to 24 hours. Chopped onions and potatoes are sautéed in *ghee* or oil. The lamb and the marinade are then added with diced chili peppers and crushed tomatoes and all the ingredients are simmered for about a half an hour. The dish is usually served with basmati rice and garnished with chopped coriander leaves or bay leaves.

Gluten-Free Decision Factors:
- Ensure no wheat flour in sauce
- Ensure no soy sauce or wheat flour in marinade

Food Allergen Preparation Considerations:
- May contain corn from vegetable oil
- May contain dairy from butter
- May contain peanuts from peanut oil and vegetable oil
- May contain soy from soy sauce in marinade and vegetable oil

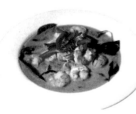

Jhinga Masala
(Shrimp in Coconut Curry)

Jhinga Masala (Shrimp in Coconut Curry)

Jhinga Masala is one of the most common shrimp dishes found in Indian restaurants. The base of the curry is typically coconut milk; however, this ingredient may be omitted in some restaurants. *Garam masala* powder, garlic, ginger and tamarind are sautéed in *ghee* or oil. Chopped onions, crushed tomatoes and shrimp are then added and the entire mixture is brought to a boil. Once the shrimp is cooked, coconut milk and salt are added. Sometimes lemon or tamarind juice may also be used. The dish is usually served with basmati rice and garnished with chopped coriander leaves or bay leaves.

Gluten-Free Decision Factors:
- Ensure no wheat flour in sauce

Food Allergen Preparation Considerations:
- Contains shellfish from shrimp

- May contain corn from vegetable oil

- May contain dairy from butter

- May contain peanuts from peanut oil and vegetable oil

- May contain soy from vegetable oil

Malai Kofta (Vegetarian Croquettes in Mild Curry)
Malai Kofta is a traditional vegetarian dish that may be traced back to the Muslim Moghul Empire which once controlled most of the Indian subcontinent. The croquettes are made with mashed potatoes or rice, cashews, chopped green chili, coriander, *paneer* and raisins. They are dusted with corn, lentil (*urad daal*) or chickpea (*besan*) flour and pan fried in *ghee* or oil. The croquettes are then added to a mild curry sauce made with *garam masala* powder, cream or yogurt, garlic, ginger, onions, *paneer,* puréed tomatoes and *ghee* or oil. The dish is usually served with basmati rice and garnished with chopped coconut.

Gluten-Free Decision Factors:
- Ensure no wheat flour—chickpea, corn or lentil flour is typically used

- Ensure croquettes are not dusted with wheat flour

- Ensure no wheat flour in sauce

Food Allergen Preparation Considerations:
- Contains dairy from cheese, cream, yogurt and possibly from butter

- Contains tree nuts from cashews

- May contain corn from vegetable oil

- May contain peanuts from peanut oil and vegetable oil

- May contain soy from vegetable oil

Murg Korma (Chicken in Cream Curry)

Murg Korma (Chicken in Cream Curry)

Murg Korma is a popular curry dish made in Indian restaurants all over the world. Garlic and onions are sautéed in *ghee* or oil with cardamom, cloves, coriander, ginger and salt. Yogurt is then stirred in, along with other spices such as *garam masala* powder and often almonds. Cubed boneless chicken is added and the dish is simmered for about twenty minutes. Milk or cream is then added a few minutes prior to serving. The dish is usually served with basmati rice and garnished with chopped coriander leaves (cilantro).

Gluten-Free Decision Factors:
- Ensure no wheat flour in sauce

Food Allergen Preparation Considerations:
- Contains dairy from cream, yogurt and possibly butter

- May contain corn from vegetable oil

- May contain peanuts from peanut oil and vegetable oil

- May contain soy from vegetable oil

- May contain tree nuts from almonds

Murg Tikka Masala (Chicken in Tomato Curry)

Murg Tikka Masala may be the most popular dish found in Indian restaurants across the globe. In fact, it is estimated that over 23 million portions are sold annually in restaurants in the United Kingdom alone. Although recipes for this dish vary widely, the basic preparation of the dish remains consistent. Cubed boneless chicken is marinated in yogurt, lemon juice, cumin, cinnamon, red chili powder, black pepper, ginger and salt for a period of up to 24 hours. It is then grilled over an open flame or baked in a tandoori oven. To prepare the tomato curry sauce, onions are sautéed in *ghee* or oil. Tomato purée and crushed tomatoes are added along with garlic paste, ginger paste and *garam masala* powder. Occasionally, almonds or cashews may be included. To give the dish a red color, red food coloring may also be added. The chicken is then added to the tomato curry and finished with cream. The dish is usually served with basmati rice and garnished with sliced almonds, chopped coriander leaves (cilantro) or shaved coconut.

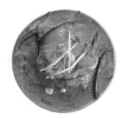

Murg Tikka Masala (Chicken in Tomato Curry)

6

Gluten-Free Decision Factors:

- Ensure no wheat flour in sauce

- Ensure no soy sauce or wheat flour in marinade

Food Allergen Preparation Considerations:

- Contains dairy from cream, yogurt and possibly from butter

- May contain corn from food coloring and vegetable oil

- May contain peanuts from peanut oil and vegetable oil

- May contain soy from food coloring, soy sauce in marinade and vegetable oil

- May contain tree nuts from almonds and cashews

Rogan Josh (Mild Lamb Curry)

Rogan Josh is a popular lamb dish that is typically less spicy than *Gosht Vindaloo*. Cubed lamb is marinated in a paste made of cardamom, cinnamon, coriander, cumin, red chili powder, turmeric and yogurt for a period of up to 24 hours. Puréed garlic, ginger, onions and tomatoes are then mixed with *garam masala* powder. This mixture is brought to a boil with a touch of *ghee* or oil. The lamb and the marinade are then added and all the ingredients are simmered for about a half an hour or until the curry is reduced to a thick sauce. The dish is usually served with basmati rice and garnished with chopped coriander leaves (cilantro).

Gluten-Free Decision Factors:
- Ensure no wheat flour in sauce
- Ensure no soy sauce or wheat flour in marinade

Food Allergen Preparation Considerations:
- Contains dairy from yogurt and possibly from butter
- May contain corn from vegetable oil
- May contain peanuts from peanut oil and vegetable oil
- May contain soy from soy sauce in marinade and vegetable oil

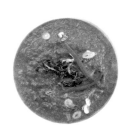

Saag Paneer (Indian Cheese and Spinach Curry)

Saag Paneer (Indian Cheese and Spinach Curry)

Saag Paneer is a common Indian vegetarian dish. A paste is made of garlic, onions and ginger, then sautéed in a pan with *ghee* or oil. Buttermilk or cream, chili powder, *garam masala* powder, spinach and yogurt are added and simmered for 20 to 30 minutes. *Paneer* is added and all the ingredients are cooked for approximately five minutes. The dish is usually served with basmati rice.

Gluten-Free Decision Factors:
- Ensure no wheat flour in sauce

Food Allergen Preparation Considerations:
- Contains dairy from buttermilk or cream, cheese, yogurt and possibly from butter
- May contain corn from vegetable oil

- May contain peanuts from peanut oil and vegetable oil

- May contain soy from vegetable oil

Tandoor Specialties
Boti Kabob (Skewered Lamb)

Boti Kabobs are a direct influence of the Muslim culture on traditional Indian culinary practices. Cubed lamb is marinated in yogurt with cardamoms, cinnamon, coriander seeds, garlic, lemon juice and red chili powder for a period of up to 24 hours. The lamb is then skewered and grilled over an open flame or baked in a tandoori oven. While cooking, the *Kabobs* are continually basted with the marinade which has had vegetable oil added to it. The dish is usually served with basmati rice, a variety of grilled vegetables and garnished with cucumber, lemon wedges, lettuce and sliced onions.

Gluten-Free Decision Factors:
- Ensure no soy sauce or wheat flour in marinade

Food Allergen Preparation Considerations:
- Contains dairy from yogurt

- May contain corn from vegetable oil

- May contain peanuts from peanut oil and vegetable oil

- May contain soy from soy sauce in marinade and vegetable oil

Murg Tandoori (Tandoori Barbeque Chicken)

Murg Tandoori is the typical Indian version of barbequed chicken. Quartered chicken or boneless cubed chicken are marinated in yogurt, chili powder, garlic, ginger, *garam masala* powder, lemon juice and mustard oil for a period of up to 24 hours. The chicken is then skewered and grilled over an open flame or baked in a tandoori oven. While cooking, the chicken is continually basted with the marinade which has had *ghee* or oil added to it. The dish is usually served with basmati rice and garnished with lemon wedges and sliced onions.

Gluten-Free Decision Factors:
- Ensure no soy sauce or wheat flour in marinade

Food Allergen Preparation Considerations:
- Contains dairy from yogurt and possibly from butter

- May contain corn from vegetable oil

- May contain peanuts from peanut oil and vegetable oil

- May contain soy from soy sauce in marinade and vegetable oil

Murg Tikka (Yogurt Marinated Chicken)

Murg Tikka is prepared exactly the same way as *Murg Tikka Masala,* except it is served without the tomato curry sauce. Cubed boneless chicken is marinated in yogurt, lemon juice, cumin, cinnamon, black pepper, ginger, red chili powder and salt for a period of up to 24 hours and grilled over an open flame or baked in a tandoori oven. To give the chicken a red color, red food coloring or tomato sauce may also be added. While cooking, the chicken is continually basted with *ghee* or oil. The dish is usually served with basmati rice and garnished with lemon wedges and sliced onions.

Gluten-Free Decision Factors:
- Ensure no soy sauce or wheat flour in marinade

Food Allergen Preparation Considerations:
- Contains dairy from yogurt and possibly from butter

- May contain corn from food coloring and vegetable oil

- May contain peanuts from peanut oil and vegetable oil

- May contain soy from food coloring, soy sauce in marinade and vegetable oil

Seekh Kabob (Skewered Minced Lamb)

Like *Boti Kabobs, Seekh Kabobs* are a direct influence of the Muslim culture on traditional Indian culinary practices. They are similar to sausage, without the sausage casings or skins. Lamb is ground or minced with cashew powder, chickpea flour *(besan)*, caraway seeds, coriander, eggs, fenugreek, garlic paste, ginger paste, *garam masala* powder, green chili pepper, nutmeg powder, onions, papaya pulp and tomato paste or red food coloring. The mixture is then formed around skewers and grilled over an open flame or baked in a tandoori oven. The dish is usually served with basmati rice and dipping sauces, usually *raita* and some type of chutney. It is typically garnished with lemon wedges and sliced onions.

6

Gluten-Free Decision Factors:
- Ensure no wheat flour in chutney

Food Allergen Preparation Considerations:
- Contains eggs as an ingredient
- Contains tree nuts from cashew powder
- May contain corn from food coloring
- May contain dairy from yogurt sauce
- May contain soy from food coloring

Dosas (South Indian Specialties)
Masala Dosa (Spicy Vegetable Filled Crepe)

Masala Dosas are a spicy version of this South Indian specialty. A fermented dough is made with a combination of chickpea *(besan)*, lentil *(dal)* or rice flour and salt. A vegetable filling is prepared by sautéing sliced chili peppers, onions, peas and sometimes garlic in *ghee* or oil. Cooked cubed potatoes are then added with Indian spices, usually *garam masala* powder. Once fermented, the batter is placed on a griddle which has been lightly brushed with *ghee* or oil to make a thin crepe or pancake. The vegetable filling is then placed in the center and the crepe is wrapped around it like a small burrito. *Dosas* are usually served with common Indian condiments such as chutney, Indian pickles, *raita* and *sambar.*

Gluten-Free Decision Factors:

- Ensure no wheat flour—chickpea, lentil or rice flour are typically used

- Ensure no wheat flour in chutney and *sambar*

- Ensure stocks and broths are made fresh and not from bouillon which may contain gluten—if *sambar* is served

Food Allergen Preparation Considerations:

- May contain corn from bouillon and vegetable oil

- May contain dairy from butter and yogurt sauce

- May contain peanuts from peanut oil and vegetable oil

- May contain soy from bouillon and vegetable oil

Sada Dosa (Lentil and Rice Crepe)

Sada Dosas are the perfect substitute for bread when available in Indian restaurants. A fermented dough is made using a combination of lentil (*dal*) and rice flour with salt. Once fermented, the batter is placed on a griddle which has been lightly brushed with *ghee* or oil to make a thin crepe or pancake. *Dosas* are usually served with common Indian condiments such as chutney, Indian pickles, *raita* and *sambar.*

Gluten-Free Decision Factors:

- Ensure no wheat flour—lentil and rice flour are typically used

- Ensure no wheat flour in chutney and *sambar*

- Ensure stocks and broths are made fresh and not from bouillon which may contain gluten—if *sambar* is served

Food Allergen Preparation Considerations:

- May contain corn from bouillon and vegetable oil

- May contain dairy from butter and yogurt sauce

- May contain peanuts from peanut oil and vegetable oil

- May contain soy from bouillon and vegetable oil

Uthappam (Lentil and Rice Pancake)

Uthappam is an Indian version of the Italian favorite: pizza. A fermented dough is made using a combination of lentil (*dal*) and rice flour with salt. Once fermented, chopped onions, tomatoes, green chili, cashews and coriander (cilantro) are added to the batter. The resulting mixture is then placed on a griddle which has been lightly brushed with *ghee* or oil to make a pancake. *Uthappam* is usually served with common Indian condiments such as chutney, pickles, *raita* and *sambar.*

Gluten-Free Decision Factors:

- Ensure no wheat flour   lentil and rice flour are typically used

- Ensure no wheat flour in chutney and *sambar*

- Ensure stocks and broths are made fresh and not from bouillon which may contain gluten—if *sambar* is served

Food Allergen Preparation Considerations:

- Contains tree nuts from cashews

- May contain corn from bouillon and vegetable oil

- May contain dairy from butter and yogurt sauce

- May contain peanuts from peanut oil and vegetable oil

- May contain soy from bouillon and vegetable oil

Desserts
Kheer (Rice Pudding)

Kheer is one of the more popular Indian desserts. Milk is brought to a boil with basmati rice, cardamom and sugar. Once the liquid is reduced in half, sliced nuts are added such as almonds, cashews or pistachios and the mixture is allowed to cool. Saffron and raisins may also be added from time to time. *Kheer* is usually topped with sliced tree nuts.

Gluten-Free Decision Factors:
- Ensure no wheat flour as ingredient

Food Allergen Preparation Considerations:
- Contains dairy from milk

- Contains tree nuts from almonds, cashews or pistachios

Kulfi (Indian Ice Cream)

Kulfi is an Indian ice cream made with a mixture of sweet condensed milk, cream and ground cardamom. For different flavors, fresh fruit purée, ground nuts and occasionally, a touch of saffron may be added. The mixture is then poured into molds and frozen for 12 hours. *Kulfi* can be garnished with rose water or ground nuts.

Gluten-Free Decision Factors:
- Ensure no wheat flour as ingredient

Food Allergen Preparation Considerations:
- Contains dairy from cream and milk

- May contain tree nuts from ground nuts

Rasmalai (Cheese Balls in Sweet Cream)

Rasmalai is a common Indian dessert. *Paneer* and powdered sugar are mixed together and shaped into flat balls similar to a biscuit. They are then cooked in a light syrup made of sugar and water until they have a spongy consistency. In another pan, cardamom, cream, saffron, sugar and vanilla are brought a boil. The cheese balls are then added to the sweet cream and allowed to cool. *Rasmalai* is garnished with sliced tree nuts such as almonds, cashews or pistachios.

Gluten-Free Decision Factors:
- None

Food Allergen Preparation Considerations:
- Contains dairy from cheese and cream
- Contains tree nuts from almonds, cashews or pistachios
- May contain corn from vanilla extract

6

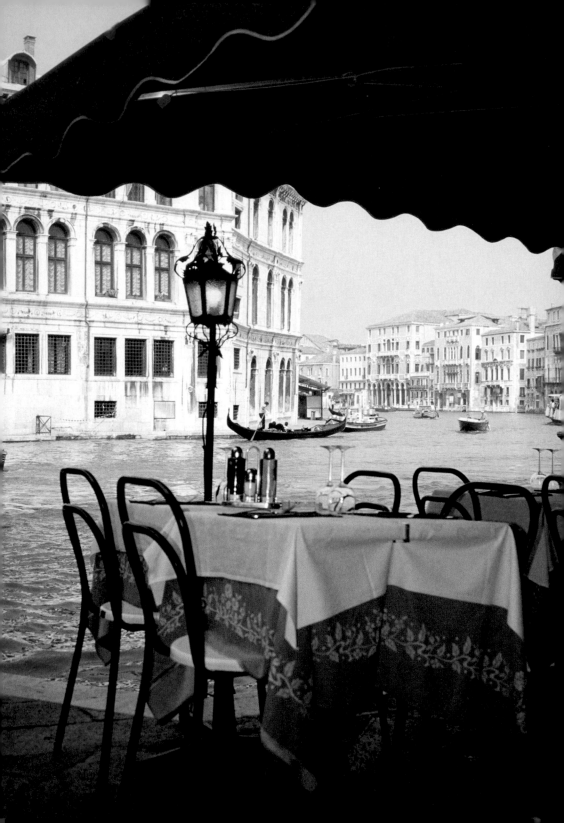

*One of the very nicest things about life
is the way we must regularly stop whatever it is we
are doing and devote our attention to eating.*
—Luciano Pavarotti

Chapter 7
Let's Eat Italian Cuisine

7

Cuisine Overview

Italy has a population of over 58 million and is slightly larger than the United Kingdom or the state of California. There are 20 different regions or states, each of which has developed its own culinary practices. For classification purposes, these regions can be divided into three categories of cuisine: Northern, Central and Southern. Climate and environment have been the greatest influences to culinary practices in these regions and their respective diets have remained virtually unchanged for centuries.

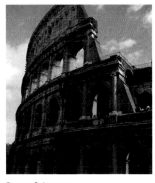
Roman Colosseum

What one eats really depends on where one is located in Italy. Northern Italian cuisine is famous for polenta and risotto, as well as popular cheeses and pesto sauce. Pasta, red wine and carbonara sauce are indicative of Central Italian cuisine. Southern Italian cuisine is known for seafood dishes, pizza and dark rich olive oil.

The foods of Italy are perhaps the most common ethnic cuisine found around the world. Restaurants, regardless of location, generally offer dishes that represent a number of the regional specialties found in Italy. Although some staples of the Italian diet contain gluten, there are numerous gluten-free dishes available at restaurants.

Traditional Ingredients

The Italian diet is rich in carbohydrates and vegetables; yet surprisingly limited in its use of meats. Vegetables, bread, pasta, cheese and olive oil are the hallmarks of Italian cuisine. The use of these traditional ingredients, in a variety of styles represented by the three major regions of Italy, is the essence of their national cuisine.

Italy is known for its bounty of bright vegetables. Artichokes, asparagus, cauliflower, eggplant, legumes, olives, peppers, porcini mushrooms, spinach, tomatoes and zucchini are abundant. Fresh herbs such as bay leaves, basil, garlic, mint, oregano, parsley, pepper, rosemary, sage, salt and thyme are regularly used, with olive oil prominently positioned in most kitchens.

Cheeses are a big part of the Italian diet and there are wide variety of choices. *Asiago, bel paese, fontina, crescienza, gorgonzola, mascarpone, pecorino sardo, provolone, ricotta, robiola* and *taleggio* are Italian table cheeses. *Mozzarella* and *provatura* are cooking cheeses, whereas, *parmigiano reggiano* and *pecorino romano* are cheeses that are usually grated and used to top dishes.

Although meats are used in limited quantities, most meals include protein of some kind. Prosciutto (cured ham) and salami are usually eaten during the appetizer portion of the meal. Chicken, fish, beef and lamb are typically featured in entrées and shellfish may be available with every course.

Like the French, Italians have been drinking wine for hundreds of years. Most Italians drink wine as part of their daily routine. Not only do they drink wine with most meals, but it is used regularly in food preparation. Each individual state or region produces its own style of wine. Italians produce twice as much red wine annually as they do white, most prominently in the Northern and Central regions of Tuscano, Piemonte and Veneto. These red wines include *Barolo, Barbaresco, Brunello di Montalcino, Chianti* and *Vallpolicella*. White wines, which are produced all over Italy, include *Asti Spumanti, Marsala, Pinot Grigio* and *Soave*.

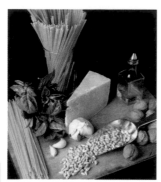

Although some staples of the Italian diet contain gluten, there are numerous gluten-free dishes available at restaurants.

7

Gluten Awareness

Although gluten is present in many areas of Italian cuisine, we have outlined 25-plus items in our sample menu. There are seven primary points that you need to consider when dining at an Italian restaurant. To ensure a gluten-free experience, the areas of food preparation that you need to inquire about with your server or chef are listed below

Sauces	Ensure sauces do not contain wheat flour
Flour Dusting	Wheat flour is typically used—request plain
Stocks and Broths	Ensure all stocks and broths are made fresh and not from bouillon which may contain gluten
Cooking Oil	Ensure frying oil has not been used to fry battered foods that may contain gluten
Pasta	Wheat flour is typically used—ensure no pasta; request gluten-free pasta or substitute polenta, if available
Battering, Bread & Breading	Wheat flour is typically used—request plain-cooked food. Ensure no batter, bread or breading
Cross-Contamination	Ensure all utensils and cooking surfaces have been cleaned prior to the preparation of your meal

Sauces

Of the many different sauces you may encounter in Italian cuisine, always be sure the sauce is not thickened with wheat flour. Below is a list of common and typically gluten-free Italian sauces and their ingredients:

Alfredo	A white sauce made of butter, cream and parmesan cheese
Bolognese	A meat sauce made with pancetta, ground meat, tomatoes, onions and garlic
Carbonara	A white sauce made with butter, eggs, pancetta, pecorino and parmesan cheese
Marinara	A red sauce made with basil, garlic, olive oil, onions, oregano and tomatoes

7

Pesto	A garlic and olive oil sauce made with basil and pine nuts
Piccata	A lemon and caper sauce made with white wine and butter
Pomodoro	Translated from Italian, pomodoro means tomato and can be any type of tomato sauce

Some Italian sauces include bread crumbs or wheat flour. Below are two common Italian sauces that you need to avoid:

Agliata	A garlic sauce made with bread crumbs, olive oil and vinegar
Pesto Ericino	A Sicilian pesto sauce made with almonds, basil, bread crumbs, garlic, olive oil and tomatoes

Flour Dusting

Flour dusting is common in Italian cuisine. Most restaurants prefer to dust using wheat flour to texture meats or fish prior to pan frying, thereby allowing a sauce to be evenly distributed. Ensure that this practice is not used in the preparation of your meal.

Stocks and Broths

Stocks and broths are used frequently in Italian cuisine. They are used in sauces and soups, as well as in marinades for meats and vegetables. Ensure that stocks and broths are made fresh and not from bouillon, which may contain gluten.

Cooking Oil

Olive oil is typically used in Italian restaurants, but rarely used for frying. Outside of Italy, other oils such as corn or vegetable may be substituted from time to time. Oil is used to fry or sauté foods. When ordering food that is prepared by frying, ensure that there is a dedicated fryer in the kitchen for non-battered menu items. Since battered foods may contain wheat flour,

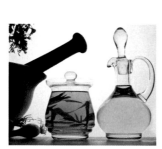

Olive oil is typically used in Italian restaurants. Outside of Italy, other oils such as corn or vegetable may be substituted from time to time.

this practice minimizes the potential of gluten cross-contamination from frying.

Pasta

There are over 400 different types of pasta produced in Italy, the vast majority of which are made from wheat flour. Depending upon your geographic location, gluten-free pasta may be available at restaurants. In Italy, for example, there are over 450 restaurants that offer gluten-free alternatives to wheat flour pasta. Polenta may also be available as a gluten-free alternative to wheat flour pasta.

Battering, Bread & Breading

Battering is used for frying foods like calamari and breading is used for meat cutlets. Wheat flour is typically used for battering and breading in Italian restaurants. Bread crumbs are used regularly as an ingredient in appetizers, soups and entrées. When ordering these dishes, request that your order is plain-cooked to ensure no battering, breading or bread crumbs. In addition, a basket of bread is usually served with most meals, so be certain to request no bread.

Cross-Contamination

Cross-contamination occurs in two primary instances and should be considered at any restaurant you choose to dine in. One may occur when your meal is prepared in the same frying oil as foods containing other possible allergens. The second may occur when microbes or food particles are transferred from one food to another by using the same knife, cutting board, pots, pans or other utensils without washing the surfaces or tools in between uses. In the case of open flamed grills, the extreme temperature turns most food particles into carbon. Use of a wire brush designed for grill racks typically removes residual contaminants. To avoid cross-contamination, restaurants need to dedicate fryers for specific foods and wash all materials that may come in contact with food in hot, soapy water prior to preparing items for those with special dietary requirements. It is important to

7

ensure that the restaurant follows these procedures for an allergen-free dining experience.

Other Allergy Considerations

If you have other food allergies or sensitivities, it is important to remain diligent in your approach to dining out. Because Italian cuisine is complex, there are many common food allergens used on a regular basis. Know that vegetable oil can always be substituted for any oil and may contain corn, peanut or soy. It should be noted that unless an olive oil container specifically states 100% olive oil, it may be mixed with vegetable oil. If used, bouillon may contain Hydrolyzed Vegetable Protein (HVP) that can be derived form corn, soy or wheat. We have indicated the potential presence of bouillon and non-traditional cooking oils.

From the 25-plus items we have listed in our sample menu, we have identified each common allergen typically included in the dish as an ingredient. We have also indicated other potential allergens that may be present based upon non-traditional culinary practices. The chances of encountering common food allergens in our sample menu are outlined below.

High likelihood   Dairy, egg, fish, gluten, shellfish and wheat

Moderate likelihood Corn and soy

Low likelihood   Peanuts and tree nuts

Dining Considerations

Italian menu items are usually presented in the Italian language. You may often find menu descriptions in the language of the country you are in following the name of the Italian menu item. While traveling, be sure to familiarize yourself with the common Italian culinary terms included in this chapter to assist you in your dining experience.

Italians generally eat two meals a day. In the morning, they usually drink coffee with warm milk and may have a *biscotti* or sweet biscuit. The first big meal of the day happens between 1 p.m. and 3 p.m. and is called *pranzo*. This is usually the largest meal of the day and consists of four to five courses. The evening meal or *cena* is usually a quick affair when eaten at home with the family, beginning at 8 p.m. and ending before nine. As a special meal, *cena* can be enjoyed later than many people are used to, sometimes beginning at 9 or 10 p.m. It is a lighter meal than the afternoon *pranzo*. When dining out or entertaining guests in the home, Italians like to eat slowly and savor their food. Most meals typically last between two to three hours. Wine and conversation are a must at an Italian table, so it is best to relax and enjoy the experience.

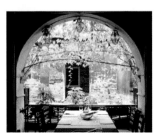

There are generally four courses to a meal: *antipasto* (soups, salads or appetizers), *primo* (pasta), *secondo* (entrées) and *dolce* (desserts). Occasionally, an additional vegetable course may be added after the *secondo* and is called the *contorno*. Wine is served continually throughout the meal, with sweet dessert wines enjoyed at the end of the meal.

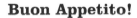

Buon Appetito!

Sample Italian Menu

Appetizers
Calamari alla Griglia (Grilled Calamari)
Carpaccio di Manzo (Beef Carpaccio)
Carpaccio di Salmone (Salmon Carpaccio)
Cocktail di Gamberi (Shrimp Cocktail)
Cozze al Vapore (Steamed Mussels)
Prosciutto e Melone (Cured Ham and Melon)

Soups
Gazpaccio

Salads
Insalata Caprese (Mozzarella Tomato Salad)
Insalata Mista (Mixed Green Salad)

Italian Specialties
Risotto ai Frutti di Mare (Arborio Rice and Seafood Dish)
Risotto ai Funghi (Arborio Rice and Mushroom Dish)
Risotto ai Quattro Formaggi (Arborio Rice and Cheese Dish)
Risotto al Pollo (Arborio Rice and Chicken Dish)

Meat Entrees
Costatella D'Agnello (Rack of Lamb)
Fileto di Manzo (Filet Mignon)
Medalione di Manzo (Beef Tenderloin Medallions)
Vitello (Veal)

Chicken Entrees
Petti di Pollo (Chicken Breast)
Pollo Arrosto Rosmarino (Rosemary Roasted Chicken)

Seafood Entrees
Salmone alla Griglia (Grilled Salmon)
Scampi (Prawns)

Sample Italian Menu

Side Dishes

Broccoli Rabe (Broccoli Florets)

Funghi all' Aglio e Olio (Mushrooms in Garlic and Olive Oil)

Melanzane alla Griglia (Grilled Eggplant)

Polenta (Boiled Corn Meal)

Desserts

Frutti di Stagione (Fresh Fruit in Season)

Gelato (Italian Ice Cream or Sherbet)

Granita (Italian Ice)

Zabaglione (Italian Custard)

7

We would like to thank Arber Murici of Lumi in New York, New York and Stephane Tremolani, former Executive Chef de Cuisine of the French Embassy in Rome, Italy for their valuable contributions in reviewing the following menu items.

Italian Menu Item Descriptions

Appetizers
Calamari alla Griglia (Grilled Calamari)

Many Italian restaurants offer grilled calamari; however, it is more commonly fried. Slices of calamari are marinated in lemon juice or olive oil then cooked on a grill over an open flame. Lemon wedges and marinara sauce for dipping are usually served on the side.

Gluten-Free Decision Factors:

- Ensure no wheat flour in sauce

- Ensure calamari is not battered

- Ensure calamari is not dusted with wheat flour

- Ensure no bread crumbs

Food Allergen Preparation Considerations:
- Contains shellfish from calamari

- May contain corn from batter, bread crumbs, dipping sauce and vegetable oil

- May contain dairy from bread crumbs and dipping sauce

- May contain eggs from batter, bread crumbs and dipping sauce

- May contain peanuts from bread crumbs, dipping sauce and vegetable oil

- May contain soy from bread crumbs and vegetable oil

- May contain tree nuts from bread crumbs and dipping sauce

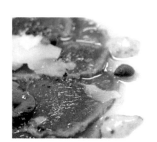

Carpaccio di Manzo (Beef Carpaccio)

Carpaccio di Manzo (Beef Carpaccio)
Beef Carpaccio is thinly sliced rare beef lightly dressed with olive oil and sometimes balsamic vinegar. Shaved *parmigiano reggiano,* capers and dried herbs top the beef. This dish is generally garnished with fresh basil.

Gluten-Free Decision Factors:
- None

Food Allergen Preparation Considerations:
- Contains dairy from cheese

- May contain corn from vegetable oil

- May contain peanuts from vegetable oil

- May contain soy from vegetable oil

Carpaccio di Salmone (Salmon Carpaccio)

Like Beef Carpaccio, Salmon Carpaccio is thinly sliced raw salmon marinated in olive oil and lemon. There are many different recipes for this dish, however they are all similar. In some variations, balsamic vinegar, shallots, fresh dill and capers can be present. You may encounter a version of *Carpaccio di Salmone* at a restaurant that includes fava beans. The preparation of the fava beans most likely contains wheat flour.

Gluten-Free Decision Factors:
- Ensure no wheat flour in fava beans

Food Allergen Preparation Considerations:
- Contains fish from salmon

- May contain corn from vegetable oil

- May contain corn from vegetable oil

- May contain soy from vegetable oil

7

Cocktail di Gamberi (Shrimp Cocktail)

Shrimp cocktail is a common appetizer in many international cuisines. Most restaurants prepare and serve this appetizer in a similar fashion. Large shrimp are boiled in water or fish stock, shelled and chilled. The shrimp are served with a cocktail sauce (tomato sauce, horseradish and lemon juice) and lemon wedges. Italians prefer a mayonnaise-based cocktail sauce made with ketchup, a dash of pepper sauce and a touch of liquor such as whiskey or cognac.

Gluten-Free Decision Factors:
- Ensure stocks and broths are made fresh and not from bouillon which may contain gluten

Food Allergen Preparation Considerations:
- Contains shellfish from shrimp

- May contain corn from bouillon and corn syrup in cocktail sauce

- May contain eggs from mayonnaise-based sauce

- May contain fish from fish stock

- May contain soy from bouillon and mayonnaise-based sauce

Cozze al Vapore (Steamed Mussels)

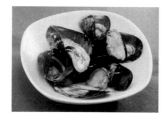

Cozze al Vapore (Steamed Mussels)

7

Steamed mussels are a very popular appetizer in Italian restaurants. They are served both as an appetizer or as an entrée, which is usually accompanied with pasta. The mussels are steamed or boiled in fish stock, then topped with a sauce that contains butter, onions or shallots, white wine and sometimes garlic. Occasionally, the mussels may be topped with bread crumbs.

Gluten-Free Decision Factors:

- Ensure no bread crumbs

- Ensure no wheat flour pasta—order gluten-free pasta or polenta if available

- Ensure stocks and broths are made fresh and not from bouillon which may contain gluten

Food Allergen Preparation Considerations:

- Contains dairy from butter and possibly from bread crumbs

- Contains shellfish from mussels

- May contain corn from bouillon and bread crumbs

- May contain eggs from bread crumbs and pasta

- May contain peanuts from bread crumbs

- May contain soy from bread crumbs and bouillon

- May contain tree nuts from bread crumbs

Prosciutto e Melone (Cured Ham and Melon)

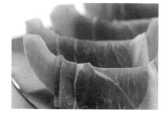

Prosciutto e Melone (Cured Ham and Melon)

Prosciutto e Melone is a common dish found in many Italian restaurants. It is fresh cantaloupe or honey dew wrapped with *prosciutto di parma*, an Italian cured ham. Sometimes the dish contains aged hard cheese such as *parmigiano reggiano*.

Gluten-Free Decision Factors:
- None

Food Allergen Preparation Considerations:
- May contain dairy from cheese

Soups
Gazpaccio
This chilled soup usually consists of puréed tomatoes, onions, peppers and garlic, but may contain any fresh vegetable. It is seasoned with salt and pepper and may also contain other fresh Italian herbs. The popularity of gazpaccio has allowed this soup to be adapted into many regional cuisines in Europe. Although it is uncommon in Italy, restaurants outside the country may add wheat flour and croutons.

Gluten-Free Decision Factors:
- Ensure no croutons
- Ensure no wheat flour as thickening agent

Food Allergen Preparation Considerations:
- May contain corn as ingredient
- May contain eggs from croutons

Salads
Insalata Caprese (Mozzarella Tomato Salad)
Buffalo mozzarella and tomato salad is an Italian classic. Large slices of buffalo mozzarella are stacked with freshly sliced tomatoes. It is usually seasoned with salt and pepper and potentially other dried herbs on occasion. Large leafs of basil garnish this dish, which is lightly dressed in olive oil and sometimes balsamic vinegar.

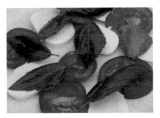

Insalata Caprese (Mozzarella Tomato Salad)

Gluten-Free Decision Factors:
- None

Food Allergen Preparation Considerations:
- Contains dairy from cheese

- May contain corn from vegetable oil

- May contain peanuts from vegetable oil

- May contain soy from vegetable oil

Insalata Mista (Mixed Green Salad)

A mixed green salad in Italy is usually a combination of mixed greens, cucumbers, onions and tomatoes. Some Italian restaurants may add anchovies or croutons and the type of salad dressings may vary.

Gluten-Free Decision Factors:

- Request no croutons

Food Allergen Preparation Considerations:

- May contain corn from vegetable oil

- May contain eggs from croutons

- May contain fish from anchovies

- May contain peanuts from vegetable oil

- May contain soy from vegetable oil

Italian Specialties
Risotto ai Frutti di Mare (Arborio Rice and Seafood Dish)

Risotto is a Northern Italian dish with seafood being one of the common varieties. The preparation techniques of *risotto* dishes are usually similar, but the ingredients vary depending on the type of *risotto* that you order. In *Risotto ai Frutti di Mare,* arborio rice is boiled in fresh stock, usually chicken, fish or shrimp. In a separate pan, white wine is simmered with garlic, olive oil, onions or shallots, salt and pepper. Mushrooms such as porcini or portabella are often added. Mixed seafood (usually calamari, clams, fish, oysters, mussels, scallops and shrimp) is then cooked in the wine until its temperature is somewhere between rare and medium rare. The seafood is then added to the rice, which has had fresh stock continually added to it as the moisture evaporates. As the moisture continues to evaporate, butter, *parmigiano reggiano* and *romano* cheese are added. The dish is usually garnished with parsley.

Gluten-Free Decision Factors:
- Ensure stocks and broths are made fresh and not from bouillon which may contain gluten

Food Allergen Preparation Considerations:
- Contains dairy from butter and cheese

- Contains fish as ingredient

- Contains shellfish as ingredient

- May contain corn from bouillon and vegetable oil

- May contain peanuts from vegetable oil

- May contain soy from bouillon and vegetable oil

7

Risotto ai Funghi (Arborio Rice and Mushroom Dish)

In *Risotto ai Funghi,* arborio rice is boiled in fresh stock, usually chicken or mushroom. In a separate pan, white wine is simmered with garlic, olive oil, onions or shallots, salt and pepper. Mushrooms such as cremini, porcini and portabella are added. Some recipes may even call for *tartufi,* which are black or white truffles. The mushrooms are then added to the rice, which has had fresh stock continually added to it as the moisture evaporates. As the moisture continues to evaporate, butter, *parmigiano reggiano* and *romano* cheese are added. The dish is usually garnished with parsley.

Gluten-Free Decision Factors:
- Ensure stocks and broths are made fresh and not from bouillon which may contain gluten

Food Allergen Preparation Considerations:
- Contains dairy from butter and cheese

- May contain corn from bouillon and vegetable oil

- May contain peanuts from vegetable oil

- May contain soy from bouillon and vegetable oil

Risotto ai Quattro Formaggi (Arborio
Rice and Cheese Dish)

Risotto ai Quattro Formaggi (Arborio Rice and Cheese Dish)

In *Risotto ai Quattro Formaggi,* arborio rice is boiled in fresh stock, usually chicken or vegetable. In a separate pan, white wine is simmered with garlic, olive oil, onions or shallots, salt and pepper. This is then added to the rice, which has had fresh stock continually added to it as the moisture evaporates. As the moisture continues to evaporate, butter, *fontina, parmigiano reggiano, pecorino* and *romano* cheese are added. The dish is usually garnished with parsley.

Gluten-Free Decision Factors:
- Ensure stocks and broths are made fresh and not from bouillon which may contain gluten

Food Allergen Preparation Considerations:
- Contains dairy from butter and cheese
- May contain corn from bouillon and vegetable oil
- May contain peanuts from vegetable oil
- May contain soy from bouillon and vegetable oil

Risotto al Pollo (Arborio Rice and Chicken Dish)

In *Risotto al Pollo,* arborio rice is boiled in fresh chicken stock. In a separate pan, white wine is simmered with garlic, olive oil, onions or shallots, salt and pepper. Slices of chicken are then added, sometimes with aromatic herbs such as anise, fennel or rosemary. The chicken is then added to the rice, which has had fresh stock continually added to it as the moisture evaporates. As the moisture continues to evaporate, butter, *parmigiano reggiano* and *romano* cheese are added. The dish is usually garnished with parsley.

Gluten-Free Decision Factors:
- Ensure stocks and broths are made fresh and not from bouillon which may contain gluten

Food Allergen Preparation Considerations:
- Contains dairy from butter and cheese

- May contain corn from bouillon and vegetable oil

- May contain peanuts from vegetable oil

- May contain soy from bouillon and vegetable oil

Meat Entrees
Costatella D'Agnello (Rack of Lamb)

Costatella (rack) or *costoletta* (chop) are widely considered the most flavorful cut of lamb. They are taken from the rib and have a good amount of marbling, which provides the rich flavor. Italians traditionally roast lamb with olive oil, rosemary, salt, pepper and plenty of garlic. If the menu description states that the dish is herb encrusted, bread crumbs are usually used. The dish is typically served with a side vegetable or pasta.

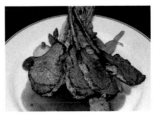

Costoletta D'Agnello (Lamb Chops)

7

Gluten-Free Decision Factors:

- Ensure lamb is not dusted with wheat flour

- Ensure no wheat flour pasta—order gluten-free pasta or polenta if available

- Ensure no bread crumbs

Food Allergen Preparation Considerations:

- Food allergens may vary in side vegetables

- May contain corn from bread crumbs and vegetable oil

- May contain dairy from bread crumbs

- May contain eggs from bread crumbs and pasta

- May contain peanuts from bread crumbs and vegetable oil

- May contain soy from bread crumbs and vegetable oil

- May contain tree nuts from bread crumbs

Fileto di Manzo (Filet Mignon)

Fileto di Manzo is the classic dish known to most as filet mignon. It is usually seasoned with salt and pepper and may sometimes be seasoned with other Italian herbs. The beef may be pan seared in butter or olive oil; it can also be grilled over an open flame. The dish is typically served with a side vegetable or pasta.

Gluten-Free Decision Factors:
- Ensure beef is not dusted with wheat flour
- Ensure no wheat flour pasta—order gluten-free pasta or polenta if available

Food Allergen Preparation Considerations:
- Food allergens may vary in side vegetables
- May contain corn from vegetable oil
- May contain dairy from butter
- May contain eggs from pasta
- May contain peanuts from vegetable oil
- May contain soy from vegetable oil

Medalione di Manzo (Beef Tenderloin Medallions)

Slices of beef tenderloin are pan seared in butter or olive oil, or they can be grilled over an open flame. The medallions are usually seasoned with salt and pepper and may also be seasoned with other Italian herbs. It is common for the medallions to be served in *marinara* or *pomodoro* sauce. The dish is typically served with a side vegetable or pasta.

Gluten-Free Decision Factors:
- Ensure no wheat flour in sauce
- Ensure beef is not dusted with wheat flour
- Ensure no wheat flour pasta—order gluten-free pasta or polenta if available

Other Potential Allergens
- Food allergens may vary in side vegetables
- May contain corn from vegetable oil
- May contain dairy from butter and sauce
- May contain eggs from pasta
- May contain peanuts from vegetable oil
- May contain soy from vegetable oil
- May contain tree nuts from sauce

Vitello (Veal)

Veal is a very popular type of meat served in Italian restaurants. It is meat from a young calf, usually eight months in age, and considered more tender and flavorful than regular beef. The most common cuts of veal you may encounter are *scallopine* (cutlet), *costatella* (rack of rib) and *costoletta* (chop). Veal can be prepared a number of different ways and is usually grilled, pan seared or roasted. When offered as *scallopine,* it is typically served in a sauce like *parmigiana* (a tomato sauce with *parmigiano reggiano* cheese) or *piccata* (a lemon and caper sauce made with white wine and butter). In the case of *parmigiana* or *piccata*, the veal may be breaded or flour dusted. If the menu description states that the veal is herb encrusted, bread crumbs are typically used. Veal is usually served with a side vegetable or pasta in restaurants outside of Italy. However, pasta with veal in Italy is uncommon.

Gluten-Free Decision Factors:
- Ensure no wheat flour in sauce
- Ensure no breading
- Ensure veal is not dusted with wheat flour
- Ensure no bread crumbs
- Ensure no wheat flour pasta—order gluten-free pasta or polenta if available

Food Allergen Preparation Considerations:
- Food allergens may vary in side vegetables

- May contain corn from bread crumbs, breading and vegetable oil

- May contain dairy from bread crumbs, breading, butter, cheese and sauce

- May contain eggs from bread crumbs, breading and pasta

- May contain peanuts from bread crumbs and vegetable oil

- May contain soy from bread crumbs, breading and vegetable oil

- May contain tree nuts from bread crumbs and sauce

Chicken Entrees
Petti di Pollo (Chicken Breast)
Grilled chicken breast is a relatively common menu item in Italian restaurants. Chicken breasts can be prepared many different ways and usually come topped with a sauce. Some chicken breast entrées with sauces include; *all' anice* (a cream sauce with anise and fennel), *al limone* (*piccata* style in a lemon and caper sauce made with white wine and butter) and *parmigiana*. In the case of *al limone* or *parmigiana*, the chicken may be breaded or flour dusted. If the menu description states that the chicken is herb encrusted, bread crumbs are typically used. Chicken breast entrées are usually accompanied by a side vegetable or pasta.

Gluten-Free Decision Factors:
- Ensure no wheat flour in sauce

- Ensure no breading

- Ensure chicken is not dusted with wheat flour

- Ensure no bread crumbs

- Ensure no wheat flour pasta—order gluten-free pasta or polenta if available

Food Allergen Preparation Considerations:
- Food allergens may vary in side vegetables

- May contain corn from bread crumbs, breading and vegetable oil

- May contain dairy from bread crumbs, breading, butter, cheese, cream and sauce

- May contain eggs from bread crumbs, breading and pasta

- May contain peanuts from bread crumbs and vegetable oil

- May contain soy from bread crumbs, breading and vegetable oil

- May contain tree nuts from bread crumbs and sauce

7

Pollo Arrosto Rosmarino (Rosemary Roasted Chicken)

Italian restaurants serve many different styles of roasted chicken, with rosemary being the most commonly used herb. A whole chicken is rubbed with olive oil, fresh rosemary, salt, pepper and possibly anise, fennel, garlic, oregano and thyme. It is then roasted in an oven or over an open flame. Half a roasted chicken is the common portion. If the menu description states that the chicken is herb encrusted, bread crumbs are typically used. The dish is usually served with a side vegetable or pasta.

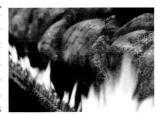

Pollo Arrosto Rosmarino (Rosemary Roasted Chicken)

Gluten-Free Decision Factors:
- Ensure no bread crumbs

- Ensure no wheat flour pasta—order gluten-free pasta or polenta if available

Food Allergen Preparation Considerations:
- Food allergens may vary in side vegetables

- May contain corn from bread crumbs and vegetable oil

- May contain dairy from bread crumbs

- May contain eggs from bread crumbs and pasta

- May contain peanuts from bread crumbs and vegetable oil

- May contain soy from bread crumbs and vegetable oil

- May contain tree nuts from bread crumbs

Seafood Entrees
Salmone alla Griglia (Grilled Salmon)

Grilled salmon is popular in Italian restaurants in the coastal areas of Italy, as well outside of the country. Salmon filets are grilled and seasoned with fresh lemon juice and herbs, usually dill or rosemary. Once cooked, the filet may be served *al limone* or with lemon wedges. The dish is typically served with a side vegetable or pasta.

Gluten-Free Decision Factors:

- Ensure no wheat flour in sauce

- Ensure no wheat flour pasta—order gluten-free pasta or polenta if available

Food Allergen Preparation Considerations:

- Food allergens may vary in side vegetables

- Contains fish from salmon

- May contain corn from vegetable oil

- May contain dairy from butter and sauce

- May contain eggs from pasta

- May contain peanuts from vegetable oil

- May contain soy from vegetable oil

- May contain tree nuts from sauce

Scampi (Prawns)

Scampi simply means prawns; extremely large ones called *mazzancolle* are very popular in Rome. In most cases, they are sautéed in butter or olive oil with white wine, garlic, salt, pepper and topped with minced basil or parsley. Cream and lemon juice are other ingredients used occasionally when prepared in this style. *Fra diavolo* (sautéed in a spicy tomato sauce) and *al forno* (baked in tomato sauce and topped with cheese) are other common variations. If baked, although uncommon, bread crumbs may be present. Scampi is often served with pasta as a side dish.

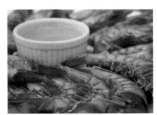

Scampi simply means prawns; extremely large ones called mazzancolle are very popular in Rome.

Gluten-Free Decision Factors:
- Ensure no wheat flour in sauce
- Ensure no bread crumbs
- Ensure no wheat flour pasta—order gluten-free pasta or polenta if available

Food Allergen Preparation Considerations:
- Contains shellfish from shrimp
- May contain corn from bread crumbs and vegetable oil
- May contain dairy from bread crumbs, butter, cheese, cream and sauce
- May contain eggs from bread crumbs and pasta
- May contain peanuts from bread crumbs and vegetable oil
- May contain soy from bread crumbs and vegetable oil
- May contain tree nuts from bread crumbs and sauce

Side Dishes
Broccoli Rabe (Broccoli Florets)
Broccoli Rabe is a slightly bitter tasting relative of broccoli. It is also called *brocoletti di rape, rape* and *rapini*. It resembles the leafy flower of regular broccoli and is very popular in Southern Italy. Outside of Italy, many restaurants may substitute *broccoli rabe* with regular broccoli. The Italian preference is to boil *broccoli rabe* for a few minutes to take out the bitterness, then sauté it in olive oil with garlic, salt and chili peppers.

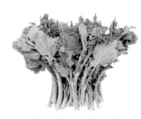

Broccoli Rabe (Broccoli Florets)

In Northern Italian restaurants, butter may be added along with various Italian herbs. The dish is usually garnished with chopped parsley and sometimes lemon wedges.

Gluten-Free Decision Factors:
- None

Food Allergen Preparation Considerations:
- May contain corn from vegetable oil

- May contain dairy from butter

- May contain peanuts from vegetable oil

- May contain soy from vegetable oil

Funghi all' Aglio e Olio (Mushrooms in Garlic and Olive Oil)
Mushrooms are a very popular Italian side dish, with this style being the most common in restaurants. Mushrooms such as cremini, porcini and portabella are sautéed in olive oil, garlic, salt and pepper. In Northern Italian restaurants, butter may be added along with various Italian herbs and bread crumbs. The dish is usually garnished with chopped parsley.

Gluten-Free Decision Factors:
- Ensure no wheat flour as ingredient

- Ensure no bread crumbs

Food Allergen Preparation Considerations:
- May contain corn from bread crumbs and vegetable oil

- May contain dairy from bread crumbs and butter

- May contain eggs from bread crumbs

- May contain peanuts from bread crumbs and vegetable oil

- May contain soy from bread crumbs and vegetable oil

- May contain tree nuts from bread crumbs

Melanzane alla Griglia (Grilled Eggplant)

Italian cuisine features eggplant more than most international cuisines, with grilled being one of the more common styles of preparation. Slices of eggplant are marinated in garlic, olive oil, salt and pepper, then scored and grilled over an open flame. In some cases, the eggplant may be dusted with wheat flour or coated with bread crumbs. Grilled eggplant is usually garnished with chopped parsley.

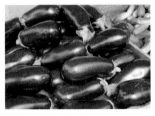

Melanzane (Eggplant)

Gluten-Free Decision Factors:

- Ensure eggplant is not dusted with wheat flour

- Ensure no bread crumbs

Food Allergen Preparation Considerations:

- May contain corn from bread crumbs and vegetable oil

- May contain dairy from bread crumbs

- May contain eggs from bread crumbs

- May contain peanuts from bread crumbs and vegetable oil

- May contain soy from bread crumbs and vegetable oil

- May contain tree nuts from bread crumbs

Polenta (Boiled Corn Meal)

Polenta has been a starch staple in Northern Italy for hundreds of years, far more so than pasta. The standard preparation involves boiling corn meal in water with salt. Once the water has been boiled out, the corn meal is malleable and can be formed into many different shapes. Depending on the restaurant, you may see *polenta* served on the side topped with butter and various Italian cheeses. It may also be cut into sticks or wedges and fried crisp in oil. Grilling is another popular preparation style. *Polenta* also serves as an excellent substitute for pasta when available and can be topped with any type of standard Italian sauce.

7

Gluten-Free Decision Factors:

- Ensure no wheat flour in sauce

- Ensure oil used for frying is designated for polenta only and is not used to fry other items that may be battered or dusted with wheat flour

Food Allergen Preparation Considerations:

- Contains corn from corn meal and possibly from vegetable oil

- May contain dairy from butter, cheese and sauce

- May contain peanuts from vegetable oil

- May contain soy from vegetable oil

- May contain tree nuts from sauce

Desserts
Frutti di Stagione (Fresh Fruit in Season)

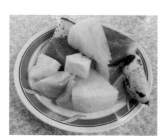

Italians love fresh fruit and generally only eat fruit when it is in season. Apples, berries, melons and oranges are usually available, but any combination of fruit can be offered. The fruit may be served plain or topped with whipped cream or *zabaglione,* an Italian custard.

Frutti di Stagione (Fresh Fruit in Season)

Gluten-Free Decision Factors:

- None

Food Allergen Preparation Considerations:

- May contain dairy from whipped cream

- May contain eggs from custard

Gelato (Italian Ice Cream or Sherbet)

Gelato is somewhere between ice cream and sherbet. There are many flavors including chocolate, custard, fruits and nuts. Many restaurants make it fresh in their kitchens, while others may opt to purchase pre-fabricated *gelato.* Puréed fruit or other natural flavors and sugar are mixed with heavy whipping cream and frozen, either in a freezer or in an ice cream machine. As is the case with most ice cream, ask your server to read the ingredients listed on the container if available and keep your flavor choices simple. Gelato may be served with a cookie.

Gluten-Free Decision Factors:
- Ensure no stabilizers which may contain gluten
- Request no cookie

Food Allergen Preparation Considerations:
- Contains dairy as an ingredient and possibly from cookie
- May contain corn from colors or flavors
- May contain eggs from cookie and colors or flavors
- May contain peanuts from cookie and various flavors
- May contain soy from cookie and colors or flavors
- May contain tree nuts from cookie and various flavors

7

Granita (Italian Ice)

It was known as *Ghiaccio Italiano* (Italian ice) in the immigrant neighborhoods of New York City, as well as in other cities on the east coast of the US for the first half of the 20th century. *Granita* is still found on the streets of Italy, as well as in restaurants. It is shaved ice with fruit syrup poured over the top, rather like a snow cone. What separates it from the standard snow cone in Italy is that the syrups are made fresh. Fruit is puréed and boiled with sugar and sometimes wine or liquor added to flavor the syrup.

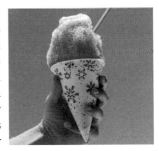

Granita (Italian Ice)

Gluten-Free Decision Factors:
- Ensure no malt or stabilizers which may contain gluten

Food Allergen Preparation Considerations:
- May contain corn from colors or flavors
- May contain soy from colors or flavors

Zabaglione (Italian Custard)

Unlike most custards, *zabaglione* is usually free of dairy products. It is made by whipping egg yolks and sugar together while cooking in a double boiler. Sweet *Marsala* wine is added toward the end of this process. When finished, it resembles a thick whipped cream with a yellow tint. *Zabaglione* is served warm or chilled, by itself or over fresh fruit. It may also be served on top of cake.

Gluten-Free Decision Factors:

- Ensure no cake

Food Allergen Preparation Considerations:

- Contains eggs from egg yolks and possibly from cake

- May contain dairy from cake

- May contain peanuts from cake

- May contain tree nuts from cake

7

7

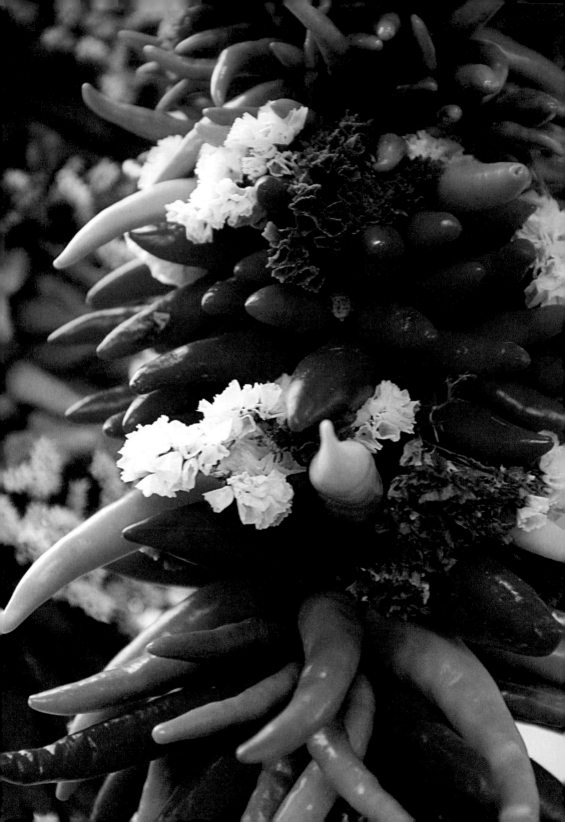

Conversation is food for the soul.
—Mexican proverb

Chapter 8
Let's Eat Mexican Cuisine

Cuisine Overview

With a landmass almost four times the size of Spain or three times the size of Texas, Mexico consists of 31 states, each of which has its own culinary traditions. The cultural identity of Mexico comes from a mixture of three distinct groups of people. The native Indians, the descendants of Spanish settlers and a mixture of the two groups known as Mestizos. Mexican food, like its history, is reflective of these three distinctive cultural influences.

Each region of Mexico is known for certain culinary specialties. The central plains, called the *Altiplano,* are credited with *antojos* (snacks) or *antojitos* (little snacks), which include foods such as tacos, tamales and enchiladas. The coastal state of Veracruz is known for its seafood dishes, whereas Puebla is famous for its complex mole sauce. Sauces in Yucatan are fruit-based and not as spicy as the chili fortified sauces you encounter in Sonora or Chihuahua. Restaurants in Mexico City serve bread with every meal, which is reminiscent of the French who ruled for a brief time. The state of Oaxaca is famous for its strong coffee and *mezcal,* a cousin of tequila made from the *agave* plant.

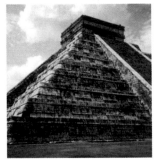
Chit'zen Itza

Mexican cuisine is based on fresh, seasonal produce. Chefs love to create dishes full of color and texture and typically present their plates in a simple fashion. Common culinary practices vary from state to state within Mexico. As you encounter restaurants outside the borders of Mexico, both authentic and derivative styles of Mexican cuisine maintain similar ingredients, while potentially incorporating different methods of preparation.

Traditional Ingredients

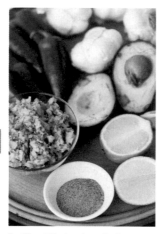

Traditional Mexican Ingredients

The traditional Mexican diet is rich in fresh vegetables, which are generally used only when in season. Various meats and seafood are balanced with vegetables. Cornmeal is the most common starch. Beans and rice are staples of every meal. The spices used in Mexican cooking are common to many cuisines, and yet, there are a number of seasonings that are unique to Mexican food. Desserts can range from simple tropical fruits to elaborate custards and cakes.

Called *verduras* in Spanish, vegetables are a part of the majority of Mexican meals, either as a side dish or in salads, soups and sauces. Onions, potatoes and tomatoes are common, with exotic fruits and vegetables such as avocado, *chayote* (gourd), *huitlacoche* (black mushrooms), jicama, prickly pear cactus and squash often featured. The most important spice used in Mexican cooking is also a vegetable in its fresh form: the chili pepper, spelled *chile* in Mexico.

Chile peppers are used as a dry spice as well as a fresh ingredient. There are many types, with the most common being ancho, habeñero, jalepeño, New Mexican green, New Mexican red, poblano and serrano. These peppers range from mild, like the poblano, to the extremely hot habenero. Other herbs and spices that flavor Mexican cuisine are anise, cilantro, cinnamon, clove, cumin, garlic, marjoram, Mexican oregano and thyme. *Azafran* (Mexican saffron) and the pungent *epazote* (wormseed) are popular indigenous spices. Contrary to popular belief, most Mexican cuisine is rather mild, yet there are certain regional specialties that are extraordinarily spicy.

Queso (cheese) is eaten on a daily basis in Mexico. There are many different types of Mexican cheese and they come in a variety of textures. The most common are queso añejo (a soft cheese), queso blanco (a fresh, white cheese) and queso Chihuahua (a semi-soft cheese). Most Mexican cheese is made from cow or goat's milk; however, some cheeses like queso fresco are a combination of the two.

Prior to the arrival of the Spanish, the Aztec and Mayan Indians survived on wild game and fowl such as rabbit, boar, venison, quail, turkey and pigeons. Today, wild game and fowl specialties are considered a delicacy. The Spanish introduced domesticated live-stock, which is the predominate meat currently served in Mexican restaurants. Beef, chicken and pork are most common and can be prepared every imaginable way in a Mexican kitchen including:

- Baked (*al horno*)

- Broiled (*asado*)

- Grilled (*a la parilla*)

- Fried (*frito*)

- Steamed (*al vapor*)

Salt water fish and shellfish are naturally popular in coastal areas, but you can also find fresh water fish on some menus.

Beer and tequila are the most popular alcoholic beverages in Mexico, with the popularity of wine gradu-ally gaining prominence. There is also a unique type of Mexican non-alcoholic beverage called *aguas frescas*. They are frappe-type drinks made with fresh fruit and puréed rice, melon seed or hibiscus flower. *Café de olla* is a popular form of Mexican coffee that is spiced with clove and cinnamon and is very high in caffeine.

Gluten Awareness

Although gluten is present in some areas of Mexican cuisine, we have outlined 30-plus items in our sample menu. There are six primary points that you need to consider when dining at a Mexican restaurant. To ensure a gluten-free experience, the areas of food preparation that you need to inquire about with your server or chef are listed below.

Sauces	Ensure sauces do not contain wheat flour
Stocks and Broths	Ensure all stocks and broths are made fresh and not from bouillon which may contain gluten
Cooking Oil	Ensure frying oil has not been used to fry battered foods that may contain gluten
Tortillas	Corn tortillas are typically used—ensure no wheat flour
Marinades	Although uncommon, ensure marinades do not contain soy sauce or wheat flour
Cross-Contamination	Ensure all utensils and cooking surfaces have been cleaned prior to the preparation of your meal

Sauces

Culinary practices vary in Mexican restaurants. Although it is uncommon, some sauces may have wheat flour added to them as a thickening agent. Tex-Mex and New Mexican style cuisines tend to add flour to sauces more frequently. Always be sure to confirm that flour is not added to any sauce. Below is a list of common Mexican sauces and their ingredients:

Green Chile	Green chile, garlic, onions with a cream or milk base
Red Chile	Puréed red chile, garlic, onions and water
Mole	Over 30 ingredients and spices, including chile, cinnamon, cardamom, garlic, chopped nuts, sesame seeds and chocolate
Pico de Gallo	A fresh salsa consisting of tomatoes, onions, garlic, jalapenos and cilantro
Salsa Picante	Puréed tomatoes, chile, garlic, onions and cilantro
Salsa Ranchero	A milder version of salsa picante with more tomato sauce

Stocks and Broths

Stocks and broths are used frequently in Mexican cuisines. They are present in sauces and soups, as well as in marinades for meats and vegetables. Ensure that stocks and broths are made fresh and not from bouillon, which may contain gluten.

Cooking Oil

Corn oil is typically used in Mexican restaurants; however other vegetable oils may be used from time to time. Oil is used to fry or sauté foods. When ordering food that is prepared by frying, ensure that there is a dedicated fryer in the kitchen for non-battered menu items. Since battered foods may contain wheat flour, this practice minimizes the potential of gluten cross-contamination from frying.

Tortillas

There are more than 160 different varieties of tortillas and nearly every Mexican meal will include at least one of them. Corn tortillas are the most common. The popularity of wheat flour tortillas has grown considerably during the last century in Northern Mexico and the United States. Cornmeal or wheat flour is combined with lard (animal fat) or vegetable oil/shortening to produce a thick dough. The dough is then made into thin circles and pre-cooked on a flat iron or griddle. Cross-contamination may occur during this process, as the cooking area and utensils might be used for both corn and flour tortillas. It is also important to ensure that a restaurant has a separate designated fryer for tortilla chips to avoid cross-contamination, as some establishments use only one. They may be served at room temperature, steamed, pan-fried or deep fried. Many restaurants make their own, while others prefer to purchase pre-made tortillas. Most dishes that use wheat flour tortillas can be easily modified by the substitution of corn tortillas.

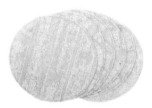

Nearly every Mexican meal will include tortillas.

Marinades

Marinades are used frequently in Mexican restaurants. In most cases they are citrus based; however, some restaurants may incorporate non-traditional ingredients in their marinades. If this is the case, ensure that the marinade does not include soy sauce, which contains wheat, or wheat flour.

Cross-Contamination

Cross-contamination occurs in two primary instances and should be considered at any restaurant you choose to dine in. One may occur when your meal is prepared in the same frying oil as foods containing other possible allergens. The second may occur when microbes or food particles are transferred from one food to another by using the same knife, cutting board, pots, pans or other utensils without washing the surfaces or tools in between uses. In the case of open flamed grills, the extreme temperature turns most food particles into carbon. Use of a wire brush designed for grill racks typically removes residual contaminants. To avoid cross-contamination, restaurants need to dedicate fryers for specific foods and wash all materials that may come in contact with food in hot, soapy water prior to preparing items for those with special dietary requirements. It is important to ensure that the restaurant follows these procedures for an allergen-free dining experience.

Other Allergy Considerations

If you have other food allergies or sensitivities, it is important to remain diligent in your approach to dining out. Because Mexican cuisine is complex, there are many common food allergens used on a regular basis. While in Mexico, be aware that corn oil is typically used to fry foods. Know that vegetable oil can always be substituted for any oil and may contain corn, peanuts or soy. If used, bouillon may contain Hydrolyzed Vegetable Protein (HVP) that can be derived from corn, soy or wheat. We have indicated the potential presence of bouillon and vegetable oil.

From the 30-plus items we have listed in our sample menu, we have identified each common allergen typically included in the dish as an ingredient. We have also indicated other potential allergens that may be present based upon non-traditional culinary practices. The chances of encountering common food allergens in items specific to our sample menu are outlined on the next page.

High likelihood   Corn, dairy, eggs, fish, and shellfish

Moderate likelihood Gluten, soy and wheat

Low likelihood   Peanuts and tree nuts

Dining Considerations

Mexican menu items are usually presented in Spanish. You may often find menu descriptions in the language of the country you are in following the name of the Mexican menu item. While traveling, be sure to familiarize yourself with the common Mexican culinary terms included in this chapter to assist you in your dining experience.

Native Mexicans generally eat four meals a day. The first meal of the day, *desayuno,* is taken early in the morning and consists of coffee, juice, fruit and hot cereal. At around 11 a.m., *almuerzo* is served and usually consists of eggs, beans and rice. *Comida* takes place between 2 p.m. and 5 p.m. and serves as the largest meal of the day. *Antojos* (snacks) or *antojitos* (little snacks) are featured in a *plato fuerte* (main dish) with rice and beans at this meal, along with *sopas* (soups). This usually tides over the appetite until 8 p.m. when *cena* is served, which is a light meal similar in size to *desayuno.* A more substantial evening meal, called *merienda,* is sometimes eaten in the evening depending upon how extensive the *comida* of the day was.

Like the Italians and French, Mexicans like to eat slowly and savor their food. The afternoon and evening meals are usually served in a modified course structure inspired by the French *service à la russe* and can last about two to three hours. This casual dining style means that the check, or *la cuenta*, is typically delivered when asked for. This relaxed style of service can often be confused with poor service. If you have time constraints, it is best to let your server know in advance so that they may expedite your meal appropriately.

Buen Provecho!

8

Sample Mexican Menu

Appetizers
Ceviche (Raw Fish Salad)
Chile con Queso (Chili Cheese Dip)
Guacamole (Avocado Dip)
Queso Fundido (Cheese Dip)
Tortillas y Salsa (Chips and Salsa)

Soups
Posole (Chili Corn Soup)
Sopa Azteca (Lime Chicken Soup)

Salads
Ensalada (House Salad)
Taco Salad

Egg Entrees
Huevos Mexicanos (Mexican Eggs)
Huevos Rancheros (Ranch Style Eggs)

Antojos (Mexican Specialties)
Enchiladas
Enfrijoladas
Tacos
Tamales (Stuffed Corn Meal)
Tostadas Compuestas (Filled Corn Tortillas)

Meat Entrees
Arracheras (Flank or Skirt Steak)
Bistek (Steak)
Carne Asada (Broiled Beef)
Carnitas (Simmered Pork)
Machaca (Shredded Beef)

8

Sample Mexican Menu

Chicken and Turkey Entrees
Mole
Pechuga de Pollo (Chicken Breast)
Pollo Asado (Broiled Chicken)

Seafood Entrees
Langosta (Lobster)
Paella Mariscos (Seafood and Rice)

Side Dishes
Arroz (Rice)
Frijoles (Beans)

Desserts
Arroz con Leche (Rice Pudding)
Flan (Custard)
Helados (Ice Cream, Sherbet or Sorbet)

8

We would like to thank Freddie Sanchez, owner and chef of Adobo Grill in Chicago, Illinois and the Crawley Family of El Sombrero Patio Cafe in Las Cruces, New Mexico for their valuable contributions in reviewing the following menu items.

Mexican Menu Item Descriptions

Appetizers
Ceviche (Raw Fish Salad)

Ceviche is a popular appetizer enjoyed worldwide, specifically in Latin America and Spain. In most cases, it is raw white fish with chopped jalepeños, cilantro and onions tossed in lime juice with salt. Ceviche may also include other *mariscos* (seafood) such as calamari, crab,

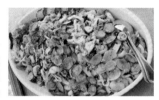
Ceviche (Raw Fish Salad)

lobster, octopus or shrimp; however, these ingredients are usually cooked. The dish may be served with corn tortilla chips.

Gluten-Free Decision Factors:

- Ensure that the oil used for frying is designated for corn tortilla chips only and is not used to fry other items that may be dusted with flour

- Request corn tortilla chips—ensure no wheat flour

Food Allergen Preparation Considerations:

- Contains fish

- May contain corn from tortilla chips and vegetable oil

- May contain shellfish

- May contain peanuts from vegetable oil

- May contain soy from tortilla chips and vegetable oil

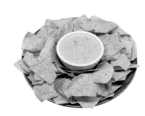

Chile con Queso (Chili Cheese Dip)

Chile con Queso (Chili Cheese Dip)

Traditional *Chile con Queso* is a blend of butter, cheese and chopped chile pepper. Any type of cheese or chile pepper can be used. It is usually served with corn tortilla chips or plain hot tortillas.

Gluten-Free Decision Factors:

- Ensure no wheat flour in sauce

- Ensure that the oil used for frying is designated for corn tortilla chips only and is not used to fry other items that may be battered or dusted with wheat flour

- Request corn tortillas—ensure no wheat flour

Food Allergen Preparation Considerations:

- Contains dairy from butter and cheese

- May contain corn from tortilla chips and vegetable oil

- May contain peanuts from vegetable oil

- May contain soy from tortilla chips and vegetable oil

Guacamole (Avocado Dip)

Guacamole is crushed avocado with garlic, lime juice, onions and tomatoes. Other ingredients may include diced chile pepper and cilantro. It is usually served with corn tortilla chips or plain hot tortillas.

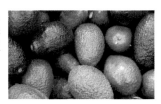

Guacamole is Crushed Avocado

Gluten-Free Decision Factors:

- Ensure that the oil used for frying is designated for corn tortilla chips only and is not used to fry other items that may be battered or dusted with wheat flour

- Request corn tortilla chips—ensure no wheat flour

Food Allergen Preparation Considerations:

- May contain corn from tortilla chips and vegetable oil

- May contain peanuts from vegetable oil

- May contain soy from tortilla chips and vegetable oil

Queso Fundido (Cheese Dip)

Queso Fundido is another variety of Mexican cheese dip. Cheese is melted together with butter and served in a hot ceramic dish. It may include sliced vegetables such as bell peppers, onions and tomatoes. Sometimes *chorizo* (Mexican pork sausage) may be added. It is usually served with corn tortilla chips or plain hot tortillas.

Gluten-Free Decision Factors:

- Ensure no wheat flour in sauce

- Ensure oil used for frying is designated for corn tortilla chips only and is not used to fry other items that may be battered or dusted with wheat flour

- Request corn tortillas—ensure no wheat flour

Food Allergen Preparation Considerations:
- Contains dairy from butter and cheese
- May contain corn from tortillas and vegetable oil
- May contain peanuts from vegetable oil
- May contain soy from tortillas and vegetable oil

Tortillas y Salsa (Chips and Salsa)

Tortillas y Salsa (Chips and Salsa)

Any Mexican meal would be incomplete without a bowl of chips and salsa. Corn tortilla chips are accompanied by any type of fresh salsa.

Gluten-Free Decision Factors:
- Ensure no wheat flour in salsa
- Ensure that the oil used for frying is designated for corn tortilla chips only and is not used to fry other items that may be battered or dusted with wheat flour
- Request corn tortilla chips—ensure no wheat flour

Food Allergen Preparation Considerations:
- May contain corn from salsa, tortilla chips and vegetable oil
- May contain peanuts from vegetable oil
- May contain soy from tortilla chips and vegetable oil

Soups
Posole (Chili Corn Soup)

Posole is a traditional, spicy Mexican soup. Although there are many recipes, most follow these guidelines: chunks of pork are simmered in fresh chicken stock with garlic, hominy, onions, chile peppers and tomato. With the exception of hominy, the other ingredients will likely be sautéed in oil prior to being added to the soup. It can be seasoned with *azafran* (Mexican saffron), chile powder, cilantro, Mexican oregano or any other Mexican herbs and spices. Both *Posole* and *Menudo* (a similar soup that features tripe) are considered excellent hangover remedies in Mexico.

Gluten-Free Decision Factors:
- Ensure stocks and broths are made fresh and not from bouillon which may contain gluten

- Ensure no wheat flour as thickening agent

Food Allergen Preparation Considerations:
- Contains corn from hominy and possibly from bouillon and vegetable oil

- May contain peanuts from vegetable oil

- May contain soy from bouillon and vegetable oil

Sopa Azteca (Lime Chicken Soup)

Sopa Azteca may also be called tortilla soup on some restaurant menus. There are many variations of this soup, but most are similar in preparation. Garlic, onions, sliced chicken and tomatoes are simmered in fresh chicken stock and lime juice. The soup is often topped with crunchy corn tortilla strips and grated cheese. Some recipes call for a greater variety of vegetables and may also include cream.

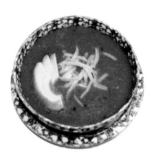

Sopa Azteca (Lime Chicken Soup)

Gluten-Free Decision Factors:
- Ensure no wheat flour tortillas—corn tortillas are typically used

- Ensure stocks and broths are made fresh and not from bouillon which may contain gluten

- Ensure no wheat flour as thickening agent

- Ensure oil used for frying is designated for corn tortilla chips only and is not used to fry other items that may be battered or dusted with wheat flour

Food Allergen Preparation Considerations:
- Contains dairy from cheese and possibly from cream

- May contain corn from bouillon, tortilla chips and vegetable oil

- May contain peanuts from vegetable oil

- May contain soy from bouillon, tortilla chips and vegetable oil

Salads
Ensalada (House Salad)

An *Ensalada* will usually be included with a *plato fuerte* or main dish. This salad usually consists of lettuce, onions and tomatoes. Salad dressings are uncommon; usually a wine vinegar and oil are available if needed.

Gluten-Free Decision Factors:
- None

Food Allergen Preparation Considerations:
- May contain corn from vegetable oil

- May contain peanuts from vegetable oil

- May contain soy from vegetable oil

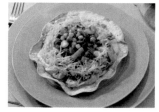

Taco Salad

Taco Salad

Taco salads are found on restaurant menus outside of Mexico. They can be served in a corn tortilla bowl, flour tortilla bowl or on a plate, topped with tortilla chips. The dish contains mixed greens, beans, grated cheese, onions and tomatoes. Your options usually include sliced marinated chicken, ground beef or steak. The salad is typically topped with fresh salsa and sour cream since salad dressings are uncommon.

Gluten-Free Decision Factors:
- Ensure no soy sauce or wheat flour in marinade

- Ensure no wheat flour in salsa

- Ensure no wheat flour in beans

- Ensure oil used for frying is designated for corn tortillas only and is not used to fry other items that may be battered or dusted with wheat flour

- Request corn tortilla bowl and chips—ensure no wheat flour

Food Allergen Preparation Considerations:
- Contains dairy from cheese and sour cream

- May contain corn from salsa, tortillas and vegetable oil

- May contain peanuts from vegetable oil

- May contain soy from soy sauce in marinade, tortillas and vegetable oil

Egg Entrees
Huevos Mexicanos (Mexican Eggs)
Huevos Mexicanos are scrambled eggs with chopped chile, onions and tomatoes. Eggs are usually cooked with vegetable oil or occasionally butter. They are often served with steamed tortillas and beans, which may be topped with cheese. Salsa picante (puréed tomatoes, chile, garlic, onions and cilantro) or pico de gallo (a fresh salsa consisting of tomatoes, onions, garlic, jalapenos and cilantro) may be offered on the side.

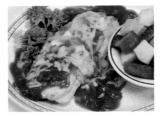

Huevos Mexicanos (Mexican Eggs)

8

Gluten-Free Decision Factors:
- Ensure no wheat flour in salsa

- Ensure no wheat flour in beans

- Request corn tortillas—ensure no wheat flour

- Ensure oil used for frying has not been used to fry other items which may be battered or dusted with wheat flour

Food Allergen Preparation Considerations:
- Contains eggs as ingredient

- May contain corn from salsa, tortillas and vegetable oil

- May contain dairy from butter and cheese

- May contain peanuts from vegetable oil

- May contain soy from tortillas and vegetable oil

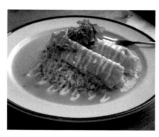

Huevos Rancheros (Ranch Style Eggs)

Huevos Rancheros (Ranch Style Eggs)

Huevos Rancheros consist of eggs fried in vegetable oil or occasionally butter. They are usually sunny side up, on top of a corn tortilla that has been lightly fried in vegetable oil. The eggs are topped with chile con carne (meat simmered in red or green chile) and cheese. Chopped lettuce, onions, tomatoes, beans and pico de gallo may also accompany the dish.

Gluten-Free Decision Factors:

- Ensure no wheat flour in salsa or sauce

- Ensure no wheat flour in beans

- Ensure oil used for frying is designated for corn tortillas only and is not used to fry other items that may be battered or dusted with wheat flour

- Request corn tortillas—ensure no wheat flour

Food Allergen Preparation Considerations:

- Contains dairy from cheese and possibly from butter

- Contains eggs as ingredient

- May contain corn from salsa, tortillas and vegetable oil

- May contain peanuts from vegetable oil

- May contain soy from tortillas and vegetable oil

Antojos (Mexican Specialties)
Enchiladas

Enchiladas are prepared two different ways: rolled and stuffed with ingredients or stacked like pancakes and layered with ingredients. When rolled, the tortillas are lightly fried in vegetable oil, stuffed with the ingredients of your choice and then topped with mole, red chile sauce or green chile sauce and cheese. The stacked variety is prepared a little differently. After the tortillas have been lightly fried, they are dipped in red or green chile and then layered with the ingredients of your choice. Standard *enchilada* ingredients include

Enchiladas with green chile sauce

cheese and onions, served plain or with your choice of beef, chicken or pork. However, there are hundreds of recipes, many of which can include any number of ingredients. Stacked *enchiladas* are often topped with a fried egg.

Gluten-Free Decision Factors:

- Ensure no wheat flour in sauce

- Ensure oil used for frying is designated for corn tortillas only and is not used to fry other items that may be battered or dusted with wheat flour

- Request corn tortillas—ensure no wheat flour

Food Allergen Preparation Considerations:

- Contains dairy from cheese and possibly from cream

- May contain corn from tortillas and vegetable oil

- May contain eggs as ingredient

- May contain peanuts from mole sauce and vegetable oil

- May contain soy from chocolate in mole sauce, tortillas and vegetable oil

- May contain tree nuts from mole sauce

Enfrijoladas

Enfrijoladas are like enchiladas, but feature beans as a major ingredient. Tortillas are lightly fried in oil then dipped in a crushed or puréed bean sauce with garlic. They can be rolled or stacked with cheese and onions and are typically topped with salsa and sour cream. Sometimes beef or chicken may be offered as fillings. Stacked *enfrijoladas* are often topped with a fried egg.

Gluten-Free Decision Factors:

- Ensure oil used for frying is designated for corn tortillas only and is not used to fry other items that may be battered or dusted with wheat flour

- Ensure no wheat flour in salsa or sauce

- Request corn tortillas—ensure no wheat flour

Food Allergen Preparation Considerations:
- Contains dairy from cheese and sour cream

- May contain corn from salsa, tortillas and vegetable oil

- May contain eggs as ingredient

- May contain peanuts from vegetable oil

- May contain soy from tortillas and vegetable oil

Tacos

Tacos al Carbon

Tacos are the Mexican version of a sandwich. They come in fried or steamed corn tortillas or in soft wheat flour tortillas. In most cases, they are folded; however, you may come across fried rolled tacos called *Flautas* or *Taquitos*. Ingredients vary widely depending on where you are and what type you decide to order. Some varieties include *al carbon* (grilled beef), *al dorado* (rolled and fried with shredded chicken or beef), *al pastor* (shaved marinated pork), *carnitas* (pork simmered with orange rind), *camarones* (shrimp), *machaca* (shredded beef), *pescado* (fish) and *pollo* (chicken). In addition to shredded lettuce and cheese, other garnishes may include sliced cucumbers, radishes, red and green salsas, sour cream, lime wedges and guacamole.

Gluten-Free Decision Factors:
- Ensure no wheat flour in salsa

- Ensure oil used for frying is designated for corn tortillas only and is not used to fry other items that may be battered or dusted with flour

- Request corn tortillas—ensure no wheat flour

Food Allergen Preparation Considerations:
- Contains dairy from cheese and sour cream

- May contain corn from salsa, tortillas and vegetable oil

- May contain fish if ordered

- May contain shellfish if ordered

- May contain peanuts from vegetable oil

- May contain soy from tortillas and vegetable oil

Tamales (Stuffed Corn Meal)

Tamales are made of *masa* (corn meal and vegetable oil or lard), which is stuffed with various ingredients, wrapped in a corn husk and steamed. There are a number of different types of tamale ingredients, the most common being shredded beef, chicken or pork that is simmered in red chile sauce.

Gluten-Free Decision Factors:
- Ensure no wheat flour in sauce

Food Allergen Preparation Considerations:
- Contains corn from *masa* and possibly from vegetable oil

- May contain peanuts from vegetable oil

- May contain soy from *masa* and from vegetable oil

Tostadas Compuestas (Filled Corn Tortillas)

Tostadas Compuestas are crisp fried corn tortillas, either flat or shaped in a bowl, which are topped or filled with various ingredients. The most common are red or green chile con carne, shredded cheese, lettuce and tomatoes. Some recipes may also call for beans, sliced marinated beef or chicken, pico de gallo and sour cream.

Gluten-Free Decision Factors:
- Ensure no wheat flour in salsa

- Ensure no wheat flour in beans

- Ensure no soy sauce or wheat flour in marinade

- Ensure oil used for frying is designated for corn tortillas only and is not used to fry other items that may be battered or dusted with wheat flour

- Request corn tortillas—ensure no wheat flour

Food Allergen Preparation Considerations:
- Contains dairy from cheese and possibly sour cream

- May contain corn from salsa, tortillas and vegetable oil

- May contain peanuts from vegetable oil

- May contain soy from soy sauce in marinade, tortillas and vegetable oil

Meat Entrees
Arracheras (Flank or Skirt Steak)

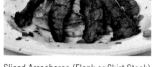

Sliced Arracheras (Flank or Skirt Steak)

Arracheras are thin cuts of meat and are used for making fajitas. The only real difference between the two is that fajitas are sliced into thinner strips. Flank or skirt steak is marinated in lime juice, garlic, salt, pepper and sometimes diced chile peppers. The beef is cooked over an open flame to temperature and served with steamed tortillas, shredded lettuce, tomatoes, beans and rice. The beans may be topped with cheese and salsa picante or pico de gallo.

Gluten-Free Decision Factors:
- Ensure no wheat flour in salsa

- Ensure no wheat flour in beans

- Ensure no soy sauce or wheat flour in marinade

- Request corn tortillas—ensure no wheat flour

Food Allergen Preparation Considerations:
- May contain corn from salsa, tortillas and vegetable oil in beans

- May contain dairy from cheese

- May contain peanuts from vegetable oil in beans

- May contain soy from soy sauce in marinade, tortillas and vegetable oil in beans

Bistek (Steak)

Steaks come in a variety of cuts, the most popular being filet, New York strip, porterhouse, and rib eye. The type of cut varies widely depending upon where you are eating and what is available at any given restaurant. Steaks are generally seasoned with salt and pepper and broiled or grilled. They may also be marinated in fresh lime juice, garlic and diced chile peppers. Beans (which may be topped with cheese) and rice are common side dishes. You may also encounter *papas fritas* (fried potatoes). Occasionally a menu will offer *Bistek Ranchero*, in which case the beef is smothered in salsa ranchero.

Gluten-Free Decision Factors:

- Ensure no wheat flour in salsa

- Ensure no wheat flour in beans

- Ensure no soy sauce or wheat flour in marinade

- Ensure oil used for frying is designated for potatoes only and is not used to fry other items that may be battered or dusted with wheat flour

Food Allergen Preparation Considerations:

- May contain corn from salsa, vegetable oil in beans and fried potatoes

- May contain dairy from cheese

- May contain peanuts from vegetable oil in beans

- May contain soy from soy sauce in marinade and vegetable oil in beans and fried potatoes

Carne Asada (Broiled Beef)

Carne Asada is marinated broiled beef and can be any of the smaller cuts of beef not considered bistek. These types include everything from butt steak to tri-tip. Mexican restaurants generally season *Carne Asada* with a marinade of lime juice, garlic, Mexican oregano, salt, pepper, and sometimes diced chile peppers. The dish is usually served with steamed tortillas, shredded lettuce, tomatoes, rice and beans, which may be topped with cheese. Salsa picante or pico de gallo may be offered on the side.

Gluten-Free Decision Factors:

- Ensure no wheat flour in salsa

- Ensure no wheat flour in beans

- Ensure no soy sauce or wheat flour in marinade

- Request corn tortillas—ensure no wheat flour

Food Allergen Preparation Considerations:

- May contain corn from salsa, tortillas and vegetable oil in beans

- May contain dairy from cheese

- May contain peanuts from vegetable oil

- May contain soy from soy sauce in marinade, tortillas and vegetable oil in beans

Carnitas (Simmered Pork)

Carnitas are a popular delicacy all over Mexico. Pork is slowly roasted and simmered in its own juices with orange rinds and any number of Mexican spices. In fact, purveyors of *Carnitas* in Mexico closely guard the specific spices they use; however, these secret recipes typically consist of dried Mexican chile powders and herbs such as cumin, *epazote* (wormseed), garlic, Mexican oregano, salt and pepper. The dish is usually served with steamed tortillas, shredded lettuce, tomatoes, rice and beans, which may be topped with cheese. Salsa picante or pico de gallo may be offered on the side.

Gluten-Free Decision Factors:

- Ensure no wheat flour in salsa

- Ensure no wheat flour in beans

- Request corn tortillas—ensure no wheat flour

Food Allergen Preparation Considerations:

- May contain corn from salsa, tortillas and

vegetable oil in beans

- May contain dairy from cheese

- May contain peanuts from vegetable oil in beans

- May contain soy from tortillas and vegetable oil in beans

Machaca (Shredded Beef)

Machaca is a Northern Mexican specialty. Beef shoulder or chuck roast is simmered for hours in water, oil and spices (usually chile powder, cumin, garlic, salt and pepper). Once all the fat has been cooked out of the beef, it is pulled apart or shredded. The dish is usually served with steamed tortillas, shredded lettuce, tomatoes, rice and beans, which may be topped with cheese. Salsa picante or pico de gallo may be offered on the side.

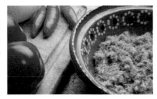
Machaca (Shredded Beef)

8

Gluten-Free Decision Factors:

- Ensure no wheat flour in salsa

- Ensure no wheat flour in beans

- Request corn tortillas—ensure no wheat flour

Food Allergen Preparation Considerations:

- May contain corn from salsa, tortillas and vegetable oil

- May contain dairy from cheese

- May contain peanuts from vegetable oil

- May contain soy from tortillas and vegetable oil

Chicken and Turkey Entrees
Mole

Mole is a specialty from the states of Puebla and Oaxaca. It is a thick brown sauce, usually served over chicken or turkey. Although there are hundreds, if not thousands, of recipes for *Mole*, the sauce is typically made from a lengthy list of ingredients that include unsweetened chocolate, chile peppers, cinnamon, cloves, coriander, cumin, garlic, peanuts, sesame seeds, and tree nuts. The dish is usually served with steamed tortillas, shredded lettuce, tomatoes, rice and beans, which may be topped with cheese. Salsa picante or pico de gallo may be offered on the side.

Gluten-Free Decision Factors:
- Ensure no wheat flour in sauce

- Ensure no wheat flour in beans

- Request corn tortillas—ensure no wheat flour

Food Allergen Preparation Considerations:
- May contain corn from tortillas and vegetable oil in beans

- May contain dairy from cheese

- May contain peanuts from sauce and vegetable oil in beans

- May contain soy from chocolate, tortillas and vegetable oil in beans

- May contain tree nuts from sauce

Pechuga de Pollo (Chicken Breast)
Chicken breasts are usually marinated in lime juice, garlic, Mexican oregano, salt, pepper and sometimes diced chile peppers. They are cooked *asado* (broiled) or *a la parilla* (grilled). The dish is usually served with steamed tortillas, shredded lettuce, tomatoes, rice and beans, which may be topped with cheese. Salsa picante or pico de gallo may be offered on the side.

Gluten-Free Decision Factors:
- Ensure no wheat flour in salsa

- Ensure no wheat flour in beans

- Ensure no soy sauce or wheat flour in marinade

- Request corn tortillas—ensure no wheat flour

Food Allergen Preparation Considerations:
- May contain corn from salsa, tortillas and

vegetable oil in beans

- May contain dairy from cheese

- May contain peanuts from vegetable oil in beans

- May contain soy from soy sauce in marinade, tortillas and vegetable oil in beans

Pollo Asado (Broiled Chicken)

Pollo Asado is a whole chicken, usually marinated in lime juice, garlic, Mexican oregano, salt, pepper and sometimes diced chile peppers. It is then broiled or charbroiled so that the skin is very crispy. The standard serving is half of a chicken on the bone. The dish is usually served with steamed tortillas, shredded lettuce, tomatoes, rice and beans, which may be topped with cheese. Salsa picante or pico de gallo may be offered on the side.

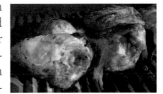

Pollo Asado (Broiled Chicken)

8

Gluten-Free Decision Factors:

- Ensure no wheat flour in salsa

- Ensure no wheat flour in beans

- Ensure no soy sauce or wheat flour in marinade

- Request corn tortillas—ensure no wheat flour

Food Allergen Preparation Considerations:

- May contain corn from salsa, tortillas and vegetable oil in beans

- May contain dairy from cheese

- May contain peanuts from vegetable oil in beans

- May contain soy from soy sauce in marinade, tortillas and vegetable oil in beans

Seafood Entrees

Langosta (Lobster)

Mexican restaurants generally offer the clawless spiny lobsters available in the Caribbean or off the coast of the Baja peninsula. Whole lobster or just the tails may be featured on the menu. Lobster tails are usually broiled or grilled, whereas whole lobsters are traditionally boiled in water, fish stock or seafood stock. Most lobster is served with drawn butter (melted butter and vegetable oil), lime wedges and steamed tortillas. Salsa picante or pico de gallo may be offered on the side.

Gluten-Free Decision Factors:

- Ensure no wheat flour in salsa

- Ensure stocks and broths are made fresh and not from bouillon which may contain gluten

- Request corn tortillas—ensure no wheat flour

Food Allergen Preparation Considerations:

- Contains shellfish from lobster and possibly from seafood stock

- May contain corn from bouillon, salsa, tortillas and vegetable oil in drawn butter

- May contain dairy from drawn butter

- May contain fish from seafood stock

- May contain peanuts from vegetable oil in drawn butter

- May contain soy from bouillon, tortillas and vegetable oil in drawn butter

Paella Mariscos (Seafood and Rice)

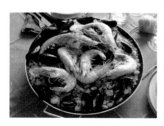
Paella Mariscos (Seafood and Rice)

Paella is a popular Spanish rice dish that is enjoyed all over the Latin world including Mexican restaurants. Rice is boiled in fresh chicken or fish stock. Clams, calamari, fish, mussels, scallops and shrimp that have been sautéed in vegetable oil, herbs and spices are then added. These herbs and spices usually include *azafran* (Mexican saffron), chile powder, garlic, salt and pepper. The dish usually includes bell peppers, sliced chile peppers, onions and tomatoes.

Gluten-Free Decision Factors:
- Ensure stocks and broths are made fresh and not from bouillon which may contain gluten

Food Allergen Preparation Considerations:
- Contains fish

- Contains shellfish

- May contain corn from bouillon and vegetable oil

- May contain peanuts from vegetable oil

- May contain soy from bouillon and vegetable oil

Side Dishes
Arroz (Rice)
Most rice served in Mexican restaurants is similar in preparation and may be referred to as Spanish rice. After the rice has been boiled, usually in water or fresh chicken stock, crushed tomatoes or tomato sauce and sliced onions are added. Sometimes the tomatoes and onions may be sautéed in vegetable oil prior to being added. The rice is seasoned with salt and may also be seasoned with *azafran*.

Gluten-Free Decision Factors:
- Ensure stocks and broths are made fresh and not from bouillon which may contain gluten

Food Allergen Preparation Considerations:
- May contain corn from bouillon and vegetable oil

- May contain peanuts from vegetable oil

- May contain soy from bouillon and vegetable oil

Frijoles (Beans)
Pinto beans are the most popular variety in Northern Mexico, while black beans are mostly enjoyed in southern Mexico. Dried beans are boiled until soft, then mashed and fried with lard or oil to make *Frijoles*. This preparation style is called *Frijoles Refritos* or

"refried beans" and is typically topped with cheese. Beans can also be served whole in their own broth and may be flavored with salted pork.

Gluten-Free Decision Factors:
- Ensure no wheat flour in beans

Food Allergen Preparation Considerations:
- May contain corn from vegetable oil
- May contain dairy from cheese
- May contain peanuts from vegetable oil
- May contain soy from vegetable oil

Desserts

Arroz con Leche (Rice Pudding)

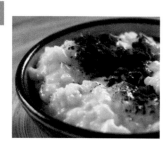

Arroz con Leche (Rice Pudding)

Mexican rice pudding is a great dessert choice. Rice is boiled with cinnamon until soft. Milk or cream, raisins, sugar and vanilla beans or extract are then added. This is heated for a few minutes, then eggs and more cinnamon are added. This dessert can be served chilled or warm.

Gluten-Free Decision Factors:
- None

Food Allergen Preparation Considerations:
- Contains dairy from milk or cream
- Contains eggs as ingredient
- May contain corn from vanilla extract

Flan (Custard)

Flan is the national dessert of Spain and itt is a common dessert in most Latin cuisines. Its ingredients are simple: cream, eggs, sugar and vanilla beans or extract. You may see it on the menu as *"Flan con Dulce de Leche,"* which means it is topped with caramel sauce.

Gluten-Free Decision Factors:
- Ensure no wheat flour

Food Allergen Preparation Considerations:
- Contains dairy from cream

- Contains eggs as ingredient

- May contain corn from caramel sauce and vanilla extract

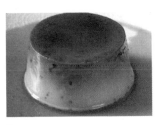

Flan

Helados (Ice Cream, Sherbet or Sorbet)

Helados are usually available in Mexican restaurants. Many establishments make these items in-house, yet others prefer to offer pre-fabricated *Helados*. It is generally best to keep your flavor choices simple. In either case, inquire about the ingredients.

Gluten-Free Decision Factors:
- Ensure no malt or wheat as ingredients

- Ensure no stabilizers which may contain gluten

- Request no cookie

Food Allergen Preparation Considerations:
- May contain corn from caramel, colors or flavors

- May contain dairy as ingredient, from cookie and possibly from chocolate

- May contain eggs from cookie

- May contain peanuts from various flavors and from cookie

- May contain soy from chocolate, colors or flavors

- May contain tree nuts from cookie and various flavors

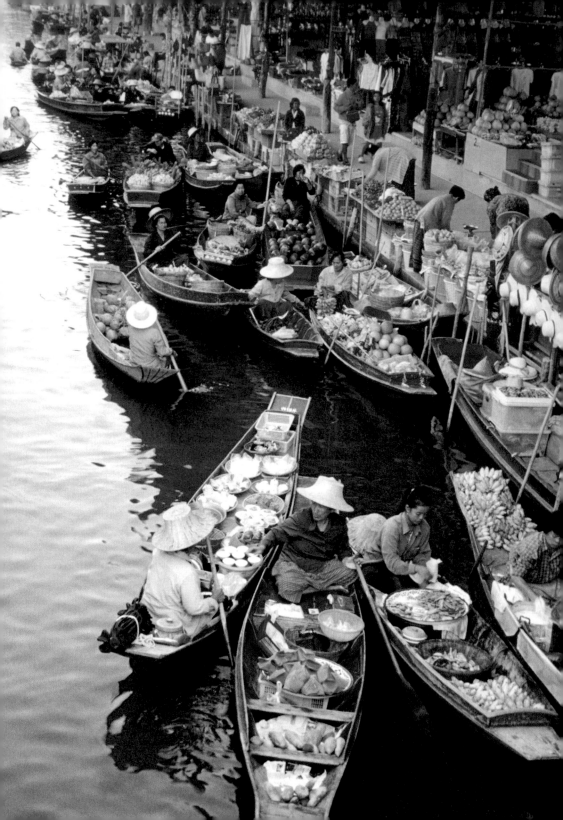

If you knew what I know about the power of giving,
you would not let a single meal pass without
sharing it in some way.
—Buddha

Chapter 9
Let's Eat Thai Cuisine

Cuisine Overview

Thailand lies in the heart of Southeast Asia and encompasses a land mass slightly larger than Spain or Italy and two times the size of Wyoming. The country has 76 provinces and almost 65 million inhabitants, 95% of which are Buddhist. A unified Thai kingdom was established in the mid-14th century and was known as Siam until 1939 when a bloodless coup instituted a constitutional monarchy and the name The Kingdom of Thailand. Thailand is the only Southeast Asian country never to have been conquered by a European power.

Thai food is unique among the cuisines of Southeast Asia. Its colorful and aromatic nature is uncommon in both appearance and flavor. It is a distinct cuisine in its own right; largely due to the ability of the Thai people to absorb outside influences or culinary practices and develop them into something uniquely their own. The skill of blending the five flavors—sweet, sour, salty, bitter and hot—is the hallmark of this cuisine. Thai food has the texture of Chinese food, minus the complicated sauces, and the spiciness of Indian food without the use of dairy products. Although gluten is often found in other

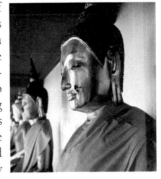
Line of Golden Buddhas

Asian noodle dishes and hidden in soy sauce, Thai food differs in this respect. Most noodle dishes have rice flour-based noodles and soy sauce is rarely used. Regardless of the dish, the influence of Buddhism on Thai cuisine requires a harmony of tastes and textures, both within a dish and throughout the meal.

Like most Asian cuisines, chefs in Thai restaurants use Chinese cooking techniques. These techniques of preparing food grew out of an economic need rather than an aesthetic aspiration, as there were periods in history of famine and fuel shortage. Stir frying eliminated food waste and reduced the amount of fuel necessary to prepare a meal, which ultimately solved two problems at the same time. Cooking foods for a short time at a high temperature also allows vegetables to remain crisp, thereby retaining a greater amount of their raw nutritional value.

9

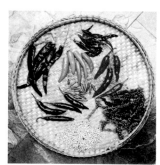

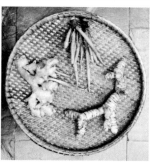

Chili Peppers (top); Galangal, Ginger and Lemongrass (bottom)

Traditional Ingredients

Thailand's culinary palate is similar to other Asian cuisines in its use of vegetables, proteins and starch. Protein and vegetable dishes are balanced with noodle and rice dishes at every meal. Soups are also an important source of daily nutrition.

Vegetables used in Thai cooking are similar to those used in most cuisines in Southeast Asia. Bamboo shoots, bean sprouts, broccoli, celery, eggplant, mushrooms, onions and shallots are common, along with fruits such as coconut, lime and pineapple. Thai cooking's use of fresh aromatic herbs and spices is unique and includes basil, chili pepper, coriander, cumin, garlic, galangal, ginger, lemongrass and turmeric.

There are many different types of protein featured in Thai cuisine. Meats such as beef, chicken, duck and pork are commonly used. Other sources of protein include bean curd, eggs, fish, nuts and shellfish.

Rice is the main form of starch. In addition to eating the whole grain, rice is also converted into flour used to make noodles, rice paper and dumpling skins. The influence of China has also brought wheat flour-based noodles into many Thai kitchens; however, most still prefer to use traditional rice noodles.

Beverages in Thailand are quite interesting. In addition to tropical fruit juices, thick Thai style iced coffee and tea are very popular. Both are prepared in a similar fashion with lots of sugar and topped with sweet condensed milk. Beers such as Singha malt beverage are very common and are not gluten-free.

Gluten Awareness

Since gluten can be found in some areas of Thai cuisine, we have outlined 20-plus items in our sample menu. There are eight primary points that you need to consider when dining at a Thai restaurant. To ensure a gluten-free experience, the areas of food preparation that you need to inquire about with your server or chef are listed below.

Fish Sauce	Ensure no wheat as ingredient
Soy Sauce	Although an unusual additive in Thai food, ensure no soy sauce
Flour Dusting	Tapioca, potato or corn starch is typically used—ensure no wheat flour
Stocks and Broths	Ensure all stocks and broths are made fresh and not from bouillon which may contain gluten
Cooking Oil	Ensure frying oil has not been used to fry battered foods that may contain gluten
Noodles and Dumplings	Rice flour is typically used—ensure no wheat flour
Battering	Request plain-cooked food—ensure no batter
Cross-Contamination	Ensure all utensils and cooking surfaces have been cleaned prior to the preparation of your meal

Fish Sauce

Fish sauce, rather than soy sauce, is used in Thai cuisine to add the flavor of salt to a dish. Called "*nam pla*" in Thai, or literally, "fish water," genuine fish sauce is the juice in the flesh of fish and is extracted via prolonged salting and fermentation. It is made from small saltwater or freshwater fish that would otherwise have

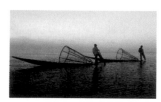

Thai Fishermen

little value for consumption. Today, most fish sauce is made from saltwater fish, as pollution and dams have drastically reduced the once plentiful supply of freshwater fish in the heartlands of Southeast Asia. Top quality fish sauce is naturally gluten-free. Tra Chang™, Golden Boy®, King Crab™ and Squid™ are the most common gluten-free fish sauce brands used in restaurants worldwide.

How does one tell which fish sauce brands are good? Respected Thai cooking guru and author Kasma Loha-unchit (http://www.thaifoodandtravel.com) suggests the following guidelines to choose the right fish sauce:

- "Check the labels, though unfortunately, the certification of quality is not always clearly translated into English. Nutritional analyses cannot be relied upon, as they are outside the scopes of many manufacturers..."

- "...look for fish sauce with a clear, reddish brown color, like the color of good whisky or sherry, without any sediment. If the color is a dark or muddy brown, the sauce is likely to be either a lower grade or one that is not properly or naturally fermented..."

- "It also appears suspicious [if] the label states that the fish sauce is a product of Thailand but is 'processed in Hong Kong,' further indicating that it is more highly processed than naturally fermented fish sauce."

- "Good fish sauce also has a pleasant aroma of the sea, not an overwhelming, smelly fishiness, and should not be overly salty."

When you are planning to go to a Thai restaurant, you may want to call in advance to inquire about the fish sauce. If you are at a restaurant and have not called in advance, ask your waiter what brand they use and request to see the bottle. Again, in most cases Tra Chang™, Golden Boy®, King Crab™ and Squid™ will be used. If the restaurant presents you with a bottle of fish sauce, for easy reference, the following guidelines will help you discern whether it is gluten-free:

9

- As previously noted, fish sauce should have a clear, reddish brown color similar to a good whiskey or sherry

- The bottle should not state that it is processed in Hong Kong

- Make sure the ingredients list is free of wheat—fish, salt, sugar and water should be the only ingredients listed

Soy Sauce

Although it is uncommon, soy sauce may be used in some Thai restaurants. Soy sauce has a stronger flavor than fish sauce, so some chefs incorporate it into vegetarian dishes. Occasionally, it may also be used in a marinade for *Gai Yang* (roasted chicken). Black sauce (*siew dam*) is a thick sweet sauce made by fermenting soy beans with molasses. It may be present in noodle dishes; however, most brands produced in Thailand do not contain wheat. If used, request to see the bottle to verify the ingredients. Since most establishments prepare dishes made to order, soy sauce can easily be omitted from the few dishes where it is possibly present.

Flour Dusting

Flour dusting is common in Thai cuisine. Most restaurants prefer to dust meat or fish with tapioca, potato or corn starch—rather than wheat flour—for texture prior to pan-frying, allowing a sauce to be evenly distributed. Ensure that wheat flour is not used to dust meat or fish in the preparation of your meal.

Stocks and Broths

Stocks and broths are used frequently in Thai cuisines and are present in sauces and soups. Ensure that stocks and broths are made fresh and not from bouillon, which may contain gluten.

Cooking Oil

Canola oil is typically used in Thai restaurants; however peanut oil and other vegetable oils may be used from time to time. Oil is used to fry or sauté foods.

9

When ordering food that is prepared by frying, ensure that there is a dedicated fryer in the kitchen for non-battered menu items. Since battered foods may contain wheat flour, this practice minimizes the potential of gluten cross-contamination from frying.

Noodles and Dumplings

Rice flour is used for most dumpling skins and noodles. Although it is uncommon for Thai restaurants to serve wheat flour-based noodles and dumpling skins, lack of availability or non-traditional culinary practices may cause these ingredients to be present in some establishments. It is important to ensure with your server or chef that only rice flour is used.

Battering

Battering of meats is uncommon in Thai cuisine. Some restaurants use tempura battering for a few dishes, so it important to ensure that the oil used for frying is fresh and has not been used to fry other foods whose batter may contain gluten.

Cross-Contamination

Cross-contamination occurs in two primary instances and should be considered at any restaurant you choose to dine in. One may occur when your meal is prepared in the same frying oil as foods containing other possible allergens. The second may occur when microbes or food particles are transferred from one food to another by using the same knife, cutting board, pots, pans or other utensils without washing the surfaces or tools in between uses. In the case of open flamed grills, the extreme temperature turns most food particles into carbon. Use of a wire brush designed for grill racks typically removes residual contaminants. To avoid cross-contamination, restaurants need to dedicate fryers for specific foods and wash all materials that may come in contact with food in hot, soapy water prior to preparing items for those with special dietary requirements. It is important to ensure that the restaurant follows these procedures for an allergen-free dining experience.

9

Other Allergy Considerations

If you have other food allergies or sensitivities, it is important to remain diligent in your approach to dining out. Because Thai cuisine is complex, there are many common food allergens used on a regular basis. As previously noted, canola oil is typically used in Thai restaurants; however, corn, peanut and vegetable oil (which may contain corn, peanuts or soy) can also be used. If used, bouillon may contain Hydrolyzed Vegetable Protein (HVP) that can be derived from corn, soy or wheat. We have indicated the potential presence of bouillon and oils.

From the 20-plus items we have listed in our sample menu, we have identified each common allergen typically included in the dish as an ingredient. We have also indicated other potential allergens that may be present based upon varied culinary practices. The chances of encountering common food allergens in items specific to our sample menu are outlined below.

High Likelihood   Fish, peanuts, shellfish and tree nuts

Moderate Likelihood Corn, eggs and soy

Low Likelihood   Dairy, gluten and wheat

In addition, your sensitivity to spice levels can be an important concern. If you see the words *"prik"* or *"kra prow,"* you can be sure that the dish is going to be spiced with chili peppers or curry powder. The term *"pet mak"* indicates that a dish is made especially spicy. You can have almost any Thai dish made spicier by requesting that it be prepared in one of these styles. If you are especially sensitive, it is important to discuss these concerns with your server or chef.

Dining Considerations

Menus in Thai restaurants tend to be presented in the language that you're dining in. Since the Thai language has a different alphabet than the English language, menus may have the name of a dish spelled phonetically in English. With this in mind, you will soon realize that there are many different ways to phonetically spell a Thai dish. *Pad Thai,* whether it

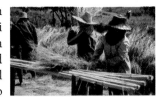
Rice Harvest in Thailand

is spelled *Phad Thai, Phat Thai* or *Pat Thai*, are all the same delicious rice noodle dish.

As is the case with most Asian cuisines, Thai food is designed to be enjoyed family style. Most food is brought to the table at one time in Thailand and they do not follow a course structure. Restaurants outside of Thailand allow you to eat your meal in a Western fashion. Finding a balance between dishes and sharing them with your table is a very important part of the Thai gastronomic experience. Due to the influences of Buddhism, Hinduism and Taoism on Thai culture, it is customary to order a combination of dishes that compliment each other, balancing noodle and rice dishes with meat and vegetable dishes.

Gkin Kao!
(Bon Appetit in Thai,
literally means "Eat Rice!")

Sample Thai Menu

Appetizers
Kanom Jeeb (Shrimp Dumplings)
Satay (Skewered Beef, Chicken or Shrimp)
Som Tam (Papaya Salad)
Summer Rolls

Soups
Tom Kha Gai (Chicken and Coconut Soup)
Tom Yum Groong (Spicy Shrimp Soup)

Noodles and Rice
Kaw Pad (Thai Fried Rice)
Pad See Yu
Pad Thai
Sticky Rice

Curries (Kang)
Kang Dang or Malay (Red Curry)
Kang Khiao Wan (Green Curry)
Kang Massaman (Tamarind Curry)
Kang Panang (Peanut Curry)

Beef Entrees
Braised Beef Short Ribs

Chicken Entrees
Gai Yang (Thai Barbeque Chicken)

Seafood Entrees
Pla Rad Prik (Crispy Whole Fish)

Desserts
Fresh Tropical Fruits
Sweet Sticky Rice
Tropical Fruit Sorbets

9

We would like to thank Chef Pam Panyasiri of Pam Real Thai in New York, New York for her valuable contribution in reviewing the following menu items.

Thai Menu Item Descriptions

Appetizers
Kanom Jeeb (Shrimp Dumplings)

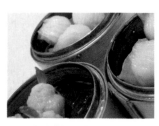

Kanom Jeeb (Shrimp Dumplings)

Dumplings are a regular appetizer at Asian restaurants. *Kanom Jeeb* differ from other Southeast Asian dumplings in that rice flour skins made of rice flour and eggs are almost always used. The dumplings are usually steamed; however, you can get them pan fried in oil if you prefer the texture and flavor. Inside the dumpling skin is a combination of ground shrimp, garlic, ginger and chives, with a little fish sauce for seasoning. A touch of egg is usually used to seal the dumpling. The accompanying dipping sauce, *nam pla prik*, is made from fish sauce, garlic and chili peppers.

Gluten-Free Decision Factors:

- Ensure no wheat in fish sauce

- Ensure no soy sauce in dumplings

- Ensure no soy sauce in dipping sauce

- Ensure no wheat flour—rice flour is typically used

Food Allergen Preparation Considerations:

- Contains fish from fish sauce

- Contains shellfish from shrimp

- May contain corn from vegetable oil

- May contain eggs from dumpling skin and seal

- May contain peanuts from vegetable oil

- May contain soy from soy sauce and vegetable oil

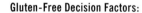

9

Satay (Skewered Beef, Chicken or Shrimp)

Satay is an appetizer that you will find in virtually every Thai restaurant. There are three basic types of *satay*: beef, chicken and shrimp. *Chicken Satay* is prepared by marinating slices of chicken breast in coconut milk, yellow curry, coriander, cumin, turmeric and, possibly, fish sauce for seasoning. The marinade for *Beef* and *Shrimp Satay* is fish sauce, rice vinegar, garlic and onions. The beef, chicken or shrimp is then skewered and grilled. *Satays* are served with a peanut dipping sauce that is made from puréed peanuts and tamarind juice. Sometimes chili is added to give the sauce a little kick. *Satays* are usually garnished with a side of cucumber and onion salad with rice wine vinegar.

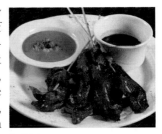
Beef Satay

Gluten-Free Decision Factors:
- Ensure no wheat in fish sauce
- Ensure no soy sauce or wheat flour in marinade
- Ensure no soy sauce in dipping sauce

Food Allergen Preparation Considerations:
- Contains fish from fish sauce
- Contains peanuts from dipping sauce
- May contain shellfish from shrimp if ordered
- May contain soy from soy sauce in dipping sauce and marinade

Som Tam (Papaya Salad)

This salad is made from either unripened green papaya or ripe papaya. It contains chili, green beans, tomatoes, garlic, onions and peanuts. It is then tossed in fish sauce, tamarind juice and lime. Some restaurants may include dried shrimp to add a saltier flavor and crunchy texture. Sometimes there is a garnish of ground nuts that may contain tree nuts in addition to peanuts. The flavor profile of *som tam* is sweet, tangy and spicy.

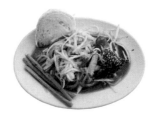
Som Tam (Papaya Salad)

9

Gluten-Free Decision Factors:

- Ensure no wheat in fish sauce

- Ensure no soy sauce as ingredient

Food Allergen Preparation Considerations:

- Contains fish from fish sauce

- Contains peanuts as ingredient

- May contain shellfish from shrimp

- May contain soy from soy sauce

- May contain tree nuts from garnish

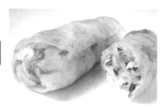

Summer Rolls

Summer Rolls

A cold appetizer, summer rolls are a light choice to begin your Thai meal. Julienned carrots, cucumber, onions, scallions and ginger are wrapped in a thin layer of rice paper. Fish sauce may be used for seasoning. The vegetables can either be steamed or boiled in fresh chicken stock prior to wrapping. Sometimes the vegetables are left raw, giving a nice, crunchy texture. The dipping sauce is usually a plum sauce and may be mild or spicy. Its ingredients are puréed plums, ginger and sometimes chili pepper. Although most restaurants will make fresh plum sauce, some may opt for the prefabricated variety. If the restaurant cannot verify the nature of the plum sauce, *nam pla prik* or peanut sauce may be substituted.

Gluten-Free Decision Factors:

- Ensure no wheat in fish sauce

- Ensure no soy sauce as seasoning

- Ensure no soy sauce in dipping sauce

- Ensure no wheat flour—rice flour paper is typically used

- Ensure stocks and broths are made fresh and not from bouillon which may contain gluten

- Ensure plum sauce is made fresh and not prefabricated which may contain gluten

Food Allergen Preparation Considerations:
- May contain corn from bouillon

- May contain fish from fish sauce

- May contain peanuts from peanut sauce

- May contain soy from bouillon, soy sauce as seasoning and in dipping sauce

Soups
Tom Kha Gai (Chicken and Coconut Soup)

Tom Kha Gai is a very popular Thai soup. At first glance, it appears to be a dairy-based soup but in reality, coconut milk gives *Tom Kha Gai* its look and texture. The broth is made with fresh chicken stock, coconut milk, lime juice and possibly fish sauce. Slices of chicken breast, fresh mushrooms, bamboo shoots, lemon grass and galangal root provide the bulk of the soup. *Tom Kha Gai* is usually garnished with a kaffir lime leaf or coriander leaf (cilantro) and sliced Thai chili peppers. It may also be garnished with crushed peanuts or tree nuts. This soup is moderately spicy, but you can most likely have it made mild because Thai soups are almost always made to order.

Gluten-Free Decision Factors:
- Ensure no wheat in fish sauce

- Ensure no soy sauce as ingredient

- Ensure stocks and broths are made fresh and not from bouillon which may contain gluten

Food Allergen Preparation Considerations:
- May contain corn from bouillon

- May contain fish from fish sauce

- May contain peanuts from garnish

- May contain soy from bouillon and soy sauce

- May contain tree nuts from garnish

9

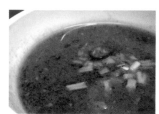

Tom Yum Groong (Spicy Shrimp Soup)

Tom Yum Groong (Spicy Shrimp Soup)

Tom Yum Groong is another common soup found on most Thai menus. It is similar to hot and sour soup found in Chinese restaurants. Shrimp, straw mushrooms, lemon grass, galangal root, Thai chili peppers, coriander and garlic are simmered in fresh chicken broth with lime juice and a touch of fish sauce. *Tom Yum Groong* is usually garnished with a kaffir lime leaf or coriander leaf and sliced Thai chili peppers. It may also be garnished with crushed peanuts or tree nuts. This soup can be very spicy, but since Thai soups are usually made to order, you will likely have the opportunity to request it mild, if you prefer.

Gluten-Free Decision Factors:

- Ensure no wheat in fish sauce

- Ensure no soy sauce as ingredient

- Ensure stocks and broths are made fresh and not from bouillon which may contain gluten

Food Allergen Preparation Considerations:

- Contains fish from fish sauce

- Contains shellfish from shrimp

- May contain corn from bouillon

- May contain peanuts from garnish

- May contain soy from bouillon and soy sauce

- May contain tree nuts from garnish

Noodle and Rice Dishes
Kaw Pad (Thai Fried Rice)

Kaw Pad (Thai Fried Rice)

There are literally hundreds of recipes for *Kaw Pad*. Luckily, they are all variations on one theme so you may be fairly certain of the ingredients. Whether you want chicken, beef, pork, shrimp, vegetarian or even pineapple *Kaw Pad*, the base of all of these dishes is the same. Steamed jasmine, white or brown rice—preferably a day old—is tossed in a wok with fish sauce, garlic, scallions, eggs and tomatoes. Bean curd is also typically included in this dish. Fresh basil is added to give it that authentic Southeast Asian flavor and the dish is garnished with kaffir lime wedges and bean sprouts. Occasionally, ground peanuts or tree nuts are also used as a garnish. If you see the words *"prik"* or *"kra prow"* after *Kaw Pad,* you can be sure that the rice is going to be spiced with chili pepper or red curry powder.

Gluten-Free Decision Factors:
- Ensure no wheat in fish sauce

- Ensure no soy sauce as ingredient

Food Allergen Preparation Considerations:
- Contains eggs as ingredient

- Contains fish from fish sauce

- Contains soy from bean curd and possibly from soy sauce and vegetable oil

- May contain corn from vegetable oil

- May contain peanuts from garnish, peanut oil and vegetable oil

- May contain shellfish from shrimp

- May contain tree nuts from garnish

9

Pad See Yu

Pad See Yu is very prevalent in Thai restaurants. At the center of this simple stir-fried dish are broad rice noodles, similar to *chow fun* noodles found in Chinese restaurants. *Pad See Yu* comes with sliced chicken or beef and contains Chinese broccoli, onions and egg. The sauce is made from canola oil, fish sauce, garlic and palm sugar. Black sauce (*siew dam*) may also be used as a substitution for fish sauce and palm sugar. It is usually garnished with kaffir lime wedges and basil, and may additionally be garnished with chopped peanuts or tree nuts. Though Thai noodle dishes are generally lighter than most Asian noodle dishes, *Pad*

See Yu is definitely a hearty meal. It is easily shared as an accompaniment to other menu items when eating family style.

Gluten-Free Decision Factors:

- Ensure no wheat in fish sauce

- Ensure no soy sauce as ingredient

- Ensure black sauce *(siew dam)* does not list wheat as ingredient

- Ensure no wheat flour—rice flour noodles are typically used

Food Allergen Preparation Considerations:

- Contains eggs as ingredient and possibly from noodles

- Contains fish from fish sauce

- May contain corn from vegetable oil

- May contain peanuts from garnish, peanut oil and vegetable oil

- May contain soy from black sauce *(siew dam)*, soy sauce and vegetable oil

- May contain tree nuts from garnish

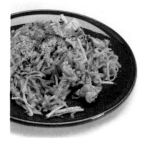

Pad Thai

Pad Thai

Pad Thai is by far the most popular Thai noodle dish worldwide. It is difficult to find a Thai menu that does not include this classic. *Pad Thai* is typically made of bean curd, bean sprouts, cabbage, carrots, chicken, chili powder, fish sauce, garlic, ground peanuts, lime, onions, palm sugar, pickled radish, rice vinegar, canola oil and narrow rice noodles. Black sauce *(siew dam)* may also be used as a substitution for fish sauce and palm sugar. Depending on the restaurant, shrimp may also be included. The chef sautés garlic and onions with oil, adds eggs, then the other ingredients. The contents of the dish are then tossed in the wok and plated. *Pad Thai* is garnished with chopped peanuts or tree nuts, bean sprouts, cabbage, carrots and sliced lime. Due to the nature of its preparation, *Pad Thai* is always made to order. With this in mind, it is easy to omit any ingredients.

Gluten-Free Decision Factors:
- Ensure no wheat in fish sauce

- Ensure no soy sauce as ingredient

- Ensure black sauce *(siew dam)* does not list wheat as ingredient

- Ensure no wheat flour—rice flour noodles are typically used

Food Allergen Preparation Considerations:
- Contains eggs as ingredient and possibly from noodles

- Contains fish from fish sauce

- Contains peanuts from garnish and possibly from peanut oil and vegetable oil

- Contains soy from bean curd and possibly from black sauce *(siew dam)*, soy sauce and vegetable oil

- May contain corn from vegetable oil

- May contain shellfish from shrimp

- May contain tree nuts from garnish

Sticky Rice

Sticky rice is a fun, hands-on experience. It is prepared by first letting the rice sit in water for a day or so. This process allows the starch of the rice to expand through the shell of the grain. As a result, the rice sticks together when steamed and can be formed into any shape desired. The Thai use sticky rice to soak up the sauces or curries in their meals. This custom is sure to lighten the atmosphere of any Thai dining experience, especially when eating family style.

9

Gluten-Free Decision Factors:
- None

Food Allergen Preparation Considerations:
- None

Curries (Kang)
Kang Dang or Malay (Red Curry)
Shrimp is the most common protein item in *Kang Dang*, but you can also have sliced chicken, pork or beef. The sauce is made of red curry paste and coconut milk. Thai long beans, bamboo shoots and fresh basil are usually present, as are onions, pineapple, tomato, sliced chili peppers and possibly fish sauce for seasoning. Because coconut milk is at the base of this curry, it will look like a bowl of soup. It is meant to be spooned over steamed rice, but diners often dip chunks of sticky rice straight into the bowl. The garnish is usually basil and sliced chili peppers, but crushed peanuts and tree nuts may also be used.

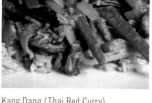

Kang Dang (Thai Red Curry)

9

Gluten-Free Decision Factors:
- Ensure no wheat in fish sauce
- Ensure no soy sauce as ingredient
- Ensure chicken is not battered or dusted with wheat flour

Food Allergen Preparation Considerations:
- May contain corn from vegetable oil
- May contain eggs from batter
- May contain fish from fish sauce
- May contain peanuts from garnish, peanut oil and vegetable oil
- May contain shellfish from shrimp if ordered
- May contain soy from soy sauce and vegetable oil
- May contain tree nuts from garnish

Kang Khiao Wan (Green Curry)

Like all Thai curries, *Kang Khiao Wan* can be made with your choice of chicken, pork, beef or shrimp; however, chicken is usually the meat of choice. Be sure to request plain, sliced chicken because of the tendency to tempura-fry chicken in curry dishes. The sauce for this dish is made up of green curry paste, coconut milk and possibly fish sauce for seasoning. Bamboo shoots and fresh basil are staple ingredients, and some-

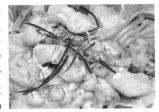

Kang Khiao Wan Gai (Thai Green Curry with Chicken)

times Japanese eggplant and sliced chili peppers are included. *Kang Khiao Wan* is a little milder than kang dang, but it is still spicy. It is difficult to adjust the level of spiciness in curry dishes, but some chefs suggest adding pineapple to even out the flavor profile. The garnish is usually Thai basil and sliced chili peppers, but crushed peanuts and tree nuts may also be used.

Gluten-Free Decision Factors:

- Ensure no wheat in fish sauce

- Ensure no soy sauce as ingredient

- Ensure chicken is not battered or dusted with wheat flour

Food Allergen Preparation Considerations:

- May contain corn from vegetable oil

- May contain eggs from batter

- May contain fish from fish sauce

- May contain peanuts from garnish, peanut oil and vegetable oil

- May contain shellfish from shrimp if ordered

- May contain soy from soy sauce and vegetable oil

- May contain tree nuts from garnish

9

Kang Massaman (Tamarind Curry)

Kang Massaman is a delicacy, combining almost all the spices featured in Thai cuisine. This complex, brown curry is moderately spicy to very spicy, depending on the restaurant, and resembles a stew. The usual ingre-

Kang Massaman (Tamarind Curry)

dients are cardamom, coconut milk, coriander, cumin, curry powder, galangal root, garlic, lemon grass, lime zest, palm sugar, peanuts and tamarind juice. Fish sauce may be added for seasoning. Whole shallots, potatoes and cherry tomatoes round out the bulk of the dish. Although chicken or beef is commonly ordered, duck is preferred by some since the richness of the sauce is considered the perfect complement to its bold flavor. Shrimp may also be ordered if available. The garnish is usually basil, though crushed peanuts and tree nuts may also be used.

Gluten-Free Decision Factors:
- Ensure no wheat in fish sauce

- Ensure no soy sauce as ingredient

- Ensure chicken is not battered or dusted with wheat flour

Food Allergen Preparation Considerations:
- Contains peanuts as ingredient and possibly from peanut oil and vegetable oil

- May contain corn from vegetable oil

- May contain eggs from batter

- May contain fish from fish sauce

- May contain shellfish from shrimp if ordered

- May contain soy from soy sauce and vegetable oil

- May contain tree nuts from garnish

Kang Panang (Peanut Curry)

This mild curry contains chopped peanuts, so it is often referred to as peanut curry. It is brownish green in color and more like a thick sauce, as opposed to a soupy curry. Beef is the meat of choice for this dish; however, chicken, duck, pork or shrimp can also be ordered. Thin slices of beef are tossed in the peanut curry with one or two vegetables, usually Chinese broccoli and onions. Sometimes pineapple is added to balance out the flavor and fish sauce may be added

9

for seasoning. The garnish is usually basil, though crushed peanuts and tree nuts may also be used. If your stomach is sensitive to spicy foods, the relatively mild *Kang Panang* curry is your best bet.

Gluten-Free Decision Factors:

- Ensure no wheat in fish sauce

- Ensure no soy sauce as ingredient

- Ensure chicken is not battered or dusted with wheat flour

Food Allergen Preparation Considerations:

- Contains peanuts as ingredient and possibly from peanut oil and vegetable oil

- May contain corn from vegetable oil

- May contain eggs from batter

- May contain fish from fish sauce

- May contain shellfish from shrimp if ordered

- May contain soy from soy sauce and vegetable oil

- May contain tree nuts from garnish

9

Beef Entrees

Braised Beef Short Ribs

Braised beef short ribs are a delicacy served at many upscale Thai restaurants and can be prepared a number of different ways. The most common is with traditional green curry. First, the short ribs are removed from the bone and pan seared. They are then marinated in green curry and coconut milk for six to 24 hours. After this, the ribs are braised in a wok with green curry and served with vegetables, usually Thai eggplant (which resembles a green tomato), onions and tomatoes. The dish is usually garnished with a large sprig of basil and sometimes crushed peanuts or tree nuts. Additional ingredients may include cardamom, coriander, cumin, fish sauce, galangal root, garlic, lemon grass and sliced Thai chili pepper. The result of this process is beef so tender and savory, a fork slices through it with ease.

Gluten-Free Decision Factors:

- Ensure no wheat in fish sauce

- Ensure no soy sauce as ingredient

- Ensure no soy sauce or wheat flour in marinade

Food Allergen Preparation Considerations:

- May contain fish from fish sauce

- May contain peanuts from garnish

- May contain soy from soy sauce

- May contain tree nuts from garnish

Chicken Entrees
Gai Yang (Thai Barbeque Chicken)

Gai Yang can be prepared in many different ways, due to the fact that there are hundreds of recipes for the marinade. The most common style is usually some variation of the following recipe. Half a chicken is marinated in a combination of coconut milk, rice vinegar and fish sauce for two to twenty-four hours. It is seasoned with cilantro, curry powder, garlic, palm sugar, chili pepper and turmeric. The chicken is then removed from the marinade and cooked on the grill. The garnish for this dish is usually basil or coriander leaf. The most common dipping sauces provided are a sweet chili dipping sauce made with fish sauce, vinegar, palm sugar, garlic and chili pepper; or a garlic and rice vinegar sauce with sliced chili peppers and shallots.

Gluten-Free Decision Factors:

- Ensure no wheat in fish sauce

- Ensure no soy sauce in dipping sauce

- Ensure no soy sauce or wheat flour in marinade

Food Allergen Preparation Considerations:

- Contains fish from fish sauce

- May contain soy from soy sauce in dipping sauce and marinade

Seafood Entrees
Pla Rad Prik (Crispy Whole Fish)

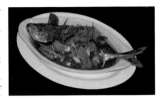

Pla Rad Prik (Crispy Whole Fish)

Having a cooked whole fish staring at you during your dinner may be a bit hard for some to handle. Even though this type of presentation is, at the very least, "foreign" to many in the Western world, *Pla Rad Prik* is an amazing treat. Although a two to three pound red snapper is usually the fish of choice, any fish of similar size can be used. The fish is deeply scored at an angle on both sides and then dredged in corn, potato or tapioca starch with salt and pepper. The fish is then, typically, pan fried in canola oil until golden brown. An accompanying spicy, tangy tamarind sauce combines chopped garlic, shallots and chili peppers with tamarind juice, fish sauce and palm sugar. It is reduced in a hot wok to the consistency of maple syrup. The sauce is then poured over the whole fried fish and garnished with basil or coriander leaves. The texture and flavor of the fish combined with the sweet, sour and spicy flavor of the sauce is heaven to Thai food aficionados.

9

Gluten-Free Decision Factors:
- Ensure no wheat in fish sauce
- Ensure no soy sauce as ingredient
- Ensure fish is not dusted with wheat flour

Food Allergen Preparation Considerations:
- Contains fish
- May contain corn from corn starch and vegetable oil
- May contain peanuts from peanut oil and vegetable oil
- May contain soy from soy sauce and vegetable oil

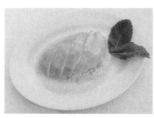
Sweet Sticky Rice served with a mango

Desserts
Fresh Tropical Fruits

Fresh tropical fruit makes a light choice for dessert. Bite-sized chunks of pineapple, guava, papaya and banana are the most common fruits served. Some restaurants serve "fruit sushi," which is sweet sticky rice topped with slices of tropical fruit and drizzled with liquid palm sugar.

Gluten-Free Decision Factors:
- None

Food Allergen Preparation Considerations:
- None

9

Sweet Sticky Rice

Sweet sticky rice is prepared like regular sticky rice except that palm sugar is added to the rice during the soaking process. It can be served plain or rolled into balls and served with coconut milk.

Gluten-Free Decision Factors:
- None

Food Allergen Preparation Considerations:
- None

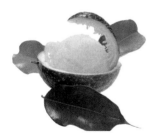
Tropical Fruit Sorbets

Tropical Fruit Sorbets

Sorbet is great for cleansing the palate after a Thai dining experience. If the restaurant offers sorbets, tropical flavors such as mango, guava and banana will usually be available. Raspberry, lemon and lime sorbets are also common.

Gluten-Free Decision Factors:
- Ensure no flavors containing gluten
- Ensure no stabilizers which may contain gluten
- Request no cookie

Food Allergen Preparation Considerations:
- May contain corn from colors or flavors

- May contain dairy from cookie and colors or flavors

- May contain eggs from cookie and colors or flavors

- May contain peanuts from cookie

- May contain soy from cookie and colors or flavors

- May contain tree nuts from cookie

9

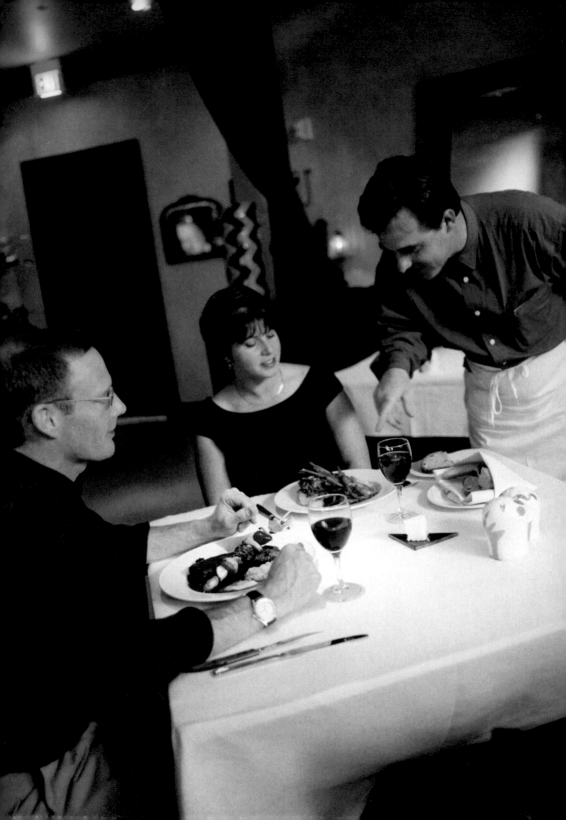

*You are never given a wish
or a dream without also being given
the power to make it come true.*
—Richard Bach

Chapter 10
Cuisine Quick Reference Guides

Chapter Overview

The quick reference guides represent each of the seven international cuisines detailed in this book including:

- American Steak and Seafood

- Chinese

- French

- Indian

- Italian

- Mexican

- Thai

The guides have been designed to assist you in simplifying the ordering process. They allow you to walk into any restaurant that serves these cuisines, scan the menu and quickly spot the safest choices based upon your specific food allergies. These are intended to refresh your memory, providing you with quick and easy access to the detailed information outlined in each of the cuisine chapters.

Quick Reference Guide Descriptions

Color Key for the Quick Reference Guides

Corn–dark brown
Soy–light brown
Dairy–light yellow
Gluten/wheat–dark yellow
Fish–dark blue
Shellfish–light blue
Peanuts–dark green
Tree Nuts–light green
Eggs–pink

The guides reflect where you may potentially encounter 10 common allergens by each sample menu item. These allergens are color-coded based on allergen type in an easy-to-follow format and include:

- Brown for corn and soy

- Yellow for dairy and gluten/wheat

- Blue for fish and shellfish

- Green for peanuts and tree nuts

- Pink for eggs

The *Quick Reference Guides* identify the specific allergen by menu item indicated by an ● for "typically contains allergen" or an ○ for "may contain allergen" recommending that you check with your server about this allergen.

The guide is designed to provide you with a level of comfort while dining out. With key information at your finger tips necessary to guide your decisions, you can effectively communicate your needs, ensure hidden allergens are addressed and concentrate on enjoying your experience.

10

American Steak and Seafood Cuisine:
Quick Reference Guide
(Appetizers – Chicken Entrees)

	Corn	Dairy	Eggs	Fish	Gluten/Wheat	Peanuts	Shellfish	Soy	Tree Nuts
Appetizers									
Oysters on the Half Shell	O	O	O	O	O		●	O	
Shrimp Cocktail	O		O	O	O		●	O	
Soups									
Bisque (Cream Soup)	O	●	O	O	O	O	O	O	O
Salads									
Buffalo Mozzarella and Tomato Salad	O	●				O		O	
Chopped Salad	O	O	O	O	O	O		O	
Cobb Salad	O	●	●	O	O	O		O	
Hearts of Palm Salad	O		O			O		O	
Mixed Green Salad	O	O	O	O	O	O		O	
Meat Entrees									
Hamburgers	O	O	O		O	O		O	O
Pork Chops*	O	O			O	O		O	
Lamb Chops	O	O	O		O	O		O	O
Steaks	O	O	O		O	O		O	
Chicken Entrees									
Grilled Chicken Breast*	O	O			O	O		O	
Roasted Chicken*	O	O			O	O		O	

10

Always ensure no cross-contamination in food preparation
● Typically contains allergen   O May contain allergen
* Food allergens may vary depending upon type of accompaniment

American Steak and Seafood Cuisine:
Quick Reference Guide
(Seafood Entrees – Desserts)

	Corn	Dairy	Eggs	Fish	Gluten/Wheat	Peanuts	Shellfish	Soy	Tree Nuts
Seafood Entrees									
Crab	O	O	O	O	O	O	●	O	O
Fish Filet	O	O		●	O	O		O	
Lobster	O	O	O	O	O	O	●	O	O
Side Dishes									
Asparagus	O	O	O		O	O		O	
Baked Potato	O	O			O			O	
Broccoli	O	O			O	O		O	
French Fried Potatoes	O	O			O	O		O	
Green Beans	O	O	O		O	O		O	O
Hash Browns	O	O			O	O		O	
Mashed Potatoes	O	O			O			O	
Potatoes Lyonnaise	O	O			O	O		O	
Spinach	O	O			O	O		O	
Desserts									
Chocolate Mousse	O	●	●		O	O		O	O
Crème Brulée (Baked Custard)	O	●	●		O			O	O
Flourless Chocolate Torte	O	●	●		O	O		O	O
Fresh Berries with Whipped Cream		●							
Ice Cream	O	●	O		O	O		O	O
Sorbet	O	O	O		O	O		O	O

Always ensure no cross-contamination in food preparation

● Typically contains allergen   O May contain allergen

10

Chinese Cuisine:
Quick Reference Guide
(Soup – Desserts)

	Corn	Dairy	Eggs	Fish	Gluten/Wheat	Peanuts	Shellfish	Soy	Tree Nuts
Soup									
Egg Drop Soup	O		●		O	O		O	
Sizzling Rice Soup	O		O		O	O	O	O	
Chicken Entrees									
Lemon Chicken	O		O		O	O		O	
Steamed Chicken and Broccoli					O			O	
Seafood Entrees									
Steamed Fish				●	O			O	
Vegetarian Entrees									
Buddha's Feast	O				O	O		O	
Noodle and Rice Dishes									
Steamed Rice									
Desserts									
Fresh Tropical Fruit									

10

Always ensure no cross-contamination in food preparation

● Typically contains allergen   O May contain allergen

French Cuisine:
Quick Reference Guide
(Appetizers – Beef Entrees)

	Corn	Dairy	Eggs	Fish	Gluten/Wheat	Peanuts	Shellfish	Soy	Tree Nuts
Appetizers									
Crevette Cocktail (Shrimp Cocktail)	O		O	O	O		●	O	
Escargot (Snails)	O	●	O		O	O	●	O	O
Foies Gras (Fat Liver)	O	O	O		O	O		O	O
Les Huîtres (Oysters on the Half Shell)	O	O	O	O	O		●	O	
Steak Tartare (Beef Tartar)	O		O	O		O		O	
Tartare de Saumon (Salmon Tartar)	O		O	●		O		O	
Soups									
Bisque (Cream Soup)	O	●	O	O	O	O	O	O	O
Vichyssoise (Potato Leek Soup)	O	●			O			O	
Salads									
Artichauts à la Vinaigrette (Artichoke Salad)	O					O		O	
Asperge à la Vinaigrette (Asparagus Salad)	O		O			O		O	
Mesclun de Salade (Mixed Green Salad)	O					O		O	O
Salade Niçoise (Nice Style Salad)	O		●	●		O		O	
Egg Entrees									
Les Oeufs (Fried Eggs)	O	O	●		O	O		O	
Les Omelettes (Omelets)	O	O	●		O	O		O	
Beef Entrees									
Filet de Boeuf (Beef Filet)	O	O	O		O	O		O	
Fondue Bourguignon (Beef Fondue)	O	O	O		O	O		O	
Steak au Poivre (Peppered Steak)	O	●			O	O		O	
Steak Frites (Steak and French Fried Potatoes)	O	O	O		O	O		O	

Always ensure no cross-contamination in food preparation
● Typically contains allergen O May contain allergen

French Cuisine:
Quick Reference Guide
(Chicken Entrees – Desserts)

	Corn	Dairy	Eggs	Fish	Gluten/Wheat	Peanuts	Shellfish	Soy	Tree Nuts
Chicken Entrees									
Poulet Provençal (Roasted Chicken with Herbs)	○			○				○	○
Seafood Entrees									
Bouillabaise (Seafood Stew)	○	○	○	●	○		●	○	○
Moules Frites (Mussels and French Fried Potatoes)	○	●	○	○	○	○	●	○	○
Saumon en Papillote (Baked Salmon)	○	○	○	●	○	○		○	
Side Dishes									
Gratin Dauphinois (Creamed Potatoes)	○	●	○		○	○		○	○
Haricots Verts (French Green Beans)	○	○	○		○	○		○	○
Pommes Frites (French Fried Potatoes)	○	○	○		○	○		○	
Ratatouille (Vegetable Stew)	○	○			○	○		○	
Desserts									
Assiette de Fromage (Cheese Plate)	○	●	○		○	○		○	○
Crème Brulée (Baked Custard)	○	●	●		○			○	○
Fruits à la Crème (Fresh Fruit with Cream)		●							
Mousse au Chocolat (Chocolate Mousse)	○	●	●		○	○		○	○
Les Sorbets (Sorbet)	○	○	○		○	○		○	○

10

Always ensure no cross-contamination in food preparation

● Typically contains allergen   ○ May contain allergen

Indian Cuisine:
Quick Reference Guide
(Appetizers – Curry Entrees)

	Corn	Dairy	Eggs	Fish	Gluten/Wheat	Peanuts	Shellfish	Soy	Tree Nuts
Appetizers									
Aloo Tikki (Potato Patty)	O	O			O	O		O	
Kabobs (Skewered Meat)	O	●		O	O	O	O	O	
Pakoras (Vegetable Fritters)	O	O			O	O		O	
Papadam (Spicy Crackers)	O	O			O	O		O	
Soups									
Curried Coconut Soup		●	O		O				O
Mulligatawny (Chicken and Vegetable Soup)	O	O			O	O		O	O
Sambar (Lentil and Vegetable Stew)	O	O			O	O		O	
Salads									
Kachumber (Chopped Salad)	O					O		O	
Curry Entrees									
Channa Masala (Chickpeas in Tomato Curry)	O	O			O	O		O	
Gosht Vindaloo (Spicy Lamb Curry)	O	O			O	O		O	
Jhinga Masala (Shrimp in Coconut Curry)	O	O			O	O	●	O	
Malai Kofta (Vegetarian Croquettes in Mild Curry)	O	●			O	O		O	●
Murg Korma (Chicken in Cream Curry)	O	●			O	O		O	O
Murg Tikki Masala (Chicken in Tomato Curry)	O	●			O	O		O	O
Rogan Josh (Mild Lamb Curry)	O	●			O	O		O	
Saag Paneer (Indian Cheese and Spinach Curry)	O	●			O	O		O	

Always ensure no cross-contamination in food preparation

● Typically contains allergen   O May contain allergen

Indian Cuisine:
Quick Reference Guide
(Tandoor Specialties – Desserts)

	Corn	Dairy	Eggs	Fish	Gluten/Wheat	Peanuts	Shellfish	Soy	Tree Nuts
Tandoor Specialties									
Boti Kabob (Skewered Lamb)	○	●			○	○		○	
Murg Tandoori (Tandoori Barbeque Chicken)	○	●			○	○		○	
Murg Tikka (Yogurt Marinated Chicken)	○	●			○	○		○	
Seekh Kabob (Skewered Minced Lamb)	○	○	●		○			○	●
Dosas (South Indian Specialties)									
Masala Dosa (Spicy Vegetable Filled Crepe)	○	○			○	○		○	
Sada Dosa (Lentil and Rice Crepe)	○	○			○	○		○	
Uthappam (Lentil and Rice Pancake)	○	○			○	○		○	●
Desserts									
Kheer (Rice Pudding)		●			○				●
Kulfi (Indian Ice Cream)		●			○				○
Rasmalai (Cheese Balls in Sweet Cream)	○	●							●

10

Always ensure no cross-contamination in food preparation

● Typically contains allergen   ○ May contain allergen

Italian Cuisine:
Quick Reference Guide
(Appetizers, Soups and Salads)

	Corn	Dairy	Eggs	Fish	Gluten/Wheat	Peanuts	Shellfish	Soy	Tree Nuts
Appetizers									
Calamari alla Griglia (Grilled Calamari)	○	○	○		○	○	●	○	○
Carpaccio di Manzo (Beef Carpaccio)	○	●				○		○	
Carpaccio di Salmone (Salmon Carpaccio)	○			●	○	○		○	
Cocktail di Gamberi (Shrimp Cocktail)	○		○	○	○		●	○	
Cozze al Vapore (Steamed Mussels)	○	●	○	○	○	○	●	○	○
Prosciutto e Melone (Cured Ham and Melon)		○							
Soups									
Gazpaccio	○		○		○				
Salads									
Insalata Caprese (Mozzarella Tomato Salad)	○	●				○		○	
Insalata Mista (Mixed Green Salad)	○		○	○	○	○		○	

Always ensure no cross-contamination in food preparation

● Typically contains allergen   ○ May contain allergen

10

Italian Cuisine:
Quick Reference Guide
(Italian Specialties and Meat Entrees)

	Corn	Dairy	Eggs	Fish	Gluten/Wheat	Peanuts	Shellfish	Soy	Tree Nuts
Italian Specialties									
Risotto ai Frutti di Mare (Arborio Rice and Seafood Dish)	O	●		●	O	O	●	O	
Risotto ai Funghi (Arborio Rice and Mushroom Dish)	O	●			O	O		O	
Risotto al Pollo (Arborio Rice and Chicken Dish)	O	●			O	O		O	
Risotto ai Quattro Formaggi (Arborio Rice and Cheese Dish)	O	●			O	O		O	
Meat Entrees									
Costatella D'Agnello (Rack of Lamb)*	O	O	O		O	O		O	O
Fileto di Manzo (Filet Mignon)*	O	O	O		O	O		O	
Medalione di Manzo (Beef Tenderloin Medallions)*	O	O	O		O	O		O	O
Vitello (Veal)*	O	O	O		O	O		O	O

Always ensure no cross-contamination in food preparation

● Typically contains allergen   O May contain allergen

* Food allergens may vary in side dishes and accompaniments

10

Italian Cuisine:
Quick Reference Guide
(Chicken Entrees, Seafood Entrees and Side Dishes)

	Corn	Dairy	Eggs	Fish	Gluten/Wheat	Peanuts	Shellfish	Soy	Tree Nuts
Chicken Entrees									
Petti di Pollo (Chicken Breast)*	O	O	O		O	O		O	O
Pollo Arrosto Rosmarino (Rosemary Roasted Chicken)*	O	O	O		O	O		O	O
Seafood Entrees									
Salmone alla Griglia (Grilled Salmon)*	O	O	O	●	O	O		O	O
Scampi (Prawns)	O	O	O		O	O	●	O	O
Side Dishes									
Broccoli Rabe (Broccoli Florets)	O	O			O			O	
Funghi all' Aglio e Olio (Mushrooms in Garlic and Olive Oil)	O	O	O		O	O		O	O
Melanzane alla Griglia (Grilled Eggplant)	O	O	O		O	O		O	O
Polenta (Boiled Corn Meal)	●	O			O	O		O	O

Always ensure no cross-contamination in food preparation
● Typically contains allergen   O May contain allergen
* Food allergens may vary in side dishes and accompaniments

10

Italian Cuisine:
Quick Reference Guide
(Desserts)

Desserts	Corn	Dairy	Eggs	Fish	Gluten/Wheat	Peanuts	Shellfish	Soy	Tree Nuts
Frutti di Stagione (Fresh Fruit in Season)		O	O						
Gelato (Italian Ice Cream or Sherbert)	O	●	O		O	O		O	O
Granita (Italian Ice)	O				O			O	
Zabaglione (Italian Custard)		O	●		O	O		O	O

Always ensure no cross-contamination in food preparation

● Typically contains allergen   O May contain allergen

10

Mexican Cuisine: Quick Reference Guide
(Appetizers – Antojos)

	Corn	Dairy	Eggs	Fish	Gluten/Wheat	Peanuts	Shellfish	Soy	Tree Nuts
Appetizers									
Ceviche (Raw Fish Salad)	O			●	O	O	O	O	
Chile con Queso (Chili Cheese Dip)	O	●			O	O		O	
Guacamole (Avocado Dip)	O				O	O		O	
Queso Fundido (Cheese Dip)	O	●			O	O		O	
Tortillas y Salsa (Chips and Salsa)	O				O	O		O	
Soups									
Posole (Chili Corn Soup)	●				O	O		O	
Sopa Azteca (Lime Chicken Soup)	O	●			O	O		O	
Salads									
Ensalada (House Salad)	O					O		O	
Taco Salad	O	●			O	O		O	
Egg Entrees									
Huevos Mexicanos (Mexican Eggs)	O	O	●			O		O	
Huevos Rancheros (Ranch Style Eggs)	O	●	●			O		O	
Antojos (Mexican Specialties)									
Enchiladas	O	●	O		O	O		O	O
Enfrijoladas	O	●	O		O	O		O	
Tacos	O	●		O	O	O	O	O	
Tamales (Stuffed Corn Meal)	●				O	O		O	
Tostadas Compuestas (Filled Corn Tortillas)	O	●			O	O		O	

Always ensure no cross-contamination in food preparation
● Typically contains allergen   O May contain allergen

Mexican Cuisine:
Quick Reference Guide
(Meat Entrees – Desserts)

	Corn	Dairy	Eggs	Fish	Gluten/Wheat	Peanuts	Shellfish	Soy	Tree Nuts
Meat Entrees									
Arracheras (Flank or Skirt Steak)	○	○			○	○		○	
Bistek (Steak)	○	○			○	○		○	
Carne Asada (Broiled Beef)	○	○			○	○		○	
Carnitas (Simmered Pork)	○	○			○	○		○	
Machaca (Shredded Beef)	○	○			○	○		○	
Chicken and Turkey Entrees									
Mole	○	○			○	○		○	○
Pechuga de Pollo (Chicken Breast)	○	○			○	○		○	
Pollo Asado (Broiled Chicken)	○	○			○	○		○	
Seafood Entrees									
Langosta (Lobster)	○	○		○	○	○	●	○	
Paella Mariscos (Seafood and Rice)	○		●		○	○	●	○	
Side Dishes									
Arroz (Rice)	○				○	○		○	
Frijoles (Beans)	○	○			○	○		○	
Desserts									
Arroz con Leche (Rice Pudding)	○	●	●						
Flan (Custard)	○	●	●		○				
Helados (Ice Cream, Sherbet or Sorbet)	○	○	○		○	○		○	○

Always ensure no cross-contamination in food preparation

● Typically contains allergen   ○ May contain allergen

10

Thai Cuisine:
Quick Reference Guide
(Appetizers – Curries)

	Corn	Dairy	Eggs	Fish	Gluten/Wheat	Peanuts	Shellfish	Soy	Tree Nuts
Appetizers									
Kanom Jeeb (Shrimp Dumplings)	○		○	●	○	○	●	○	
Satay (Skewered Beef, Chicken or Shrimp)				●	○	●	○	○	
Som Tam (Papaya Salad)				●	○	●	○	○	○
Summer Rolls				○	○	○		○	
Soups									
Tom Kha Gai (Chicken and Coconut Soup)				○	○	○		○	○
Tom Yum Groong (Spicy Shrimp Soup)				●	○	○	●	○	○
Noodles and Rice									
Kaw Pad (Thai Fried Rice)	○		●	●	○	○	○	●	○
Pad See Yu	○		●	●	○	○		○	○
Pad Thai	○		●	●	○	●	○	●	○
Sticky Rice									
Curries (Kang)									
Kang Dang or Malay (Red Curry)	○		○	○	○	○	○	○	○
Kang Khiao Wan (Green Curry)	○		○	○	○	○	○	○	○
Kang Massaman (Tamarind Curry)	○		○	○	○	●	○	○	○
Kang Panang (Peanut Curry)	○		○	○	○	●	○	○	○

Always ensure no cross-contamination in food preparation

●   Typically contains allergen   ○   May contain allergen

Thai Cuisine:
Quick Reference Guide
(Beef Entrees – Desserts)

	Corn	Dairy	Eggs	Fish	Gluten/Wheat	Peanuts	Shellfish	Soy	Tree Nuts
Beef Entrees									
Braised Beef Short Ribs				O	O	O		O	O
Chicken Entrees									
Gai Yang (Thai Barbeque Chicken)				●	O			O	
Seafood Entrees									
Pla Rad Prik (Crispy Whole Fish)	O			●	O	O		O	
Desserts									
Fresh Tropical Fruits									
Sweet Sticky Rice									
Tropical Fruit Sorbets	O	O	O		O	O		O	O

10

Always ensure no cross-contamination in food preparation
● Typically contains allergen   O May contain allergen

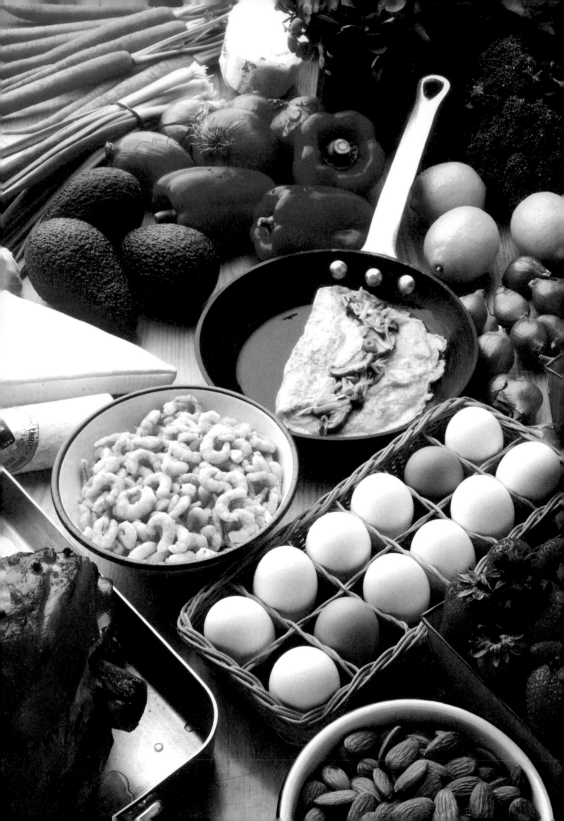

"When you wake up in the morning, Pooh," said Piglet at last,
"what's the first thing you say to yourself?"
"What's for breakfast?" said Pooh. "What do you say, Piglet?"
"I say, I wonder what's going to happen exciting today?" said Piglet
Pooh nodded thoughtfully. "It's the same thing," he said.
—Benjamin Hoff

Chapter 11

Breakfast Meal Suggestions

Chapter Overview

The suggestions for breakfast meals represent a variety of guidelines to help you eat your first meal of the day away from home. These suggestions provide you with the opportunity to enjoy breakfast in a restaurant or in your hotel room with room service and include:

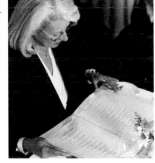

11

- Breakfast meal and side dish overview

- Sample breakfast menu

- Breakfast quick reference guide

Breakfast Meal and Side Dish Overview

The breakfast suggestions have been developed based upon research, personal global travel experience and proven choices, after asking the right questions, for eating breakfast outside your home.

To facilitate an easy-to-use format while ordering, the breakfast meals and side dishes are grouped into 12 categories for your reference as follows:

- Egg dishes

- Eggs—made to order

- Egg preparation

- Omelets and potential ingredients

- Cheese and yogurts

- Meat side dishes

- From the sea side dishes

- Potato and salad side dishes

- Fruits

- Spreads, jams, and jellies

- Bakery products

- Breakfast specialties

11

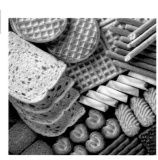

Restaurants are starting to offer gluten and wheat-free bakery products to their guests.

The list of breakfast specialties and bakery products included in these suggestions typically contain gluten and wheat. For those of you who are concerned about allergens other than gluten and wheat, these are acceptable alternatives to the breakfast suggestions.

For those of you allergic to gluten and wheat, more restaurants are starting to offer gluten and wheat-free products to their guests. To assist you, a list of gluten and wheat-free grains/flours is included which may be available at a restaurant or hotel depending upon your location by country. It is recommended that you ask the restaurant management and staff if any gluten and wheat-free products are available. If these products are available—great, then enjoy them as part of your breakfast. If not, you need to refer to the other sample breakfast menu items for potential gluten and wheat-free alternatives.

Sample Breakfast Menu

The following menu details 125-plus breakfast suggestions
listed by category.

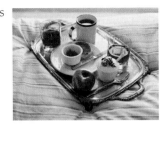

Egg Dishes
eggs benedict
huevos mexicanos
huevos rancheros
skillets–american style

Eggs—Made to Order
eggs (white and yolk)
egg beaters
egg whites
egg yolks

Egg Preparation
boiled
fried in butter
fried in oil
hard boiled
poached
scrambled with milk and
   cooked in butter
scrambled plain or with
   water and cooked in oil
soft boiled
sunny side up
yolk broken

Omelets and Potential Ingredients
plain
asparagus
avocado
bacon
broccoli
cheese
chicken
chiles
chives
chorizo
garlic

Omelets and Potential Ingredients, continued
green beans
green peppers
ham
herbs
jalapeños
mushrooms
olives
onions
potatoes
red peppers
sausage–chicken
sausage–pork
sausage–turkey
spinach
tomatoes

Cheese and Yogurts
cheese
cottage cheese
fruit yogurt
natural yogurt
plain yogurt
soy yogurt
soy fruit yogurt
yogurt drink

Fruits
apple
apricots
banana
berries
blueberries
blackberries
boysenberries
cantaloupe
cherries
clementines

11

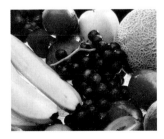

Fruits, continued
cranberries
grapes
grapefruit
honey dew
kumquats
loganberries
melon
nectarine
orange
papaya
peach
pear
plantain
pineapple
plum
prunes
raisins
raspberries
strawberries
tangerine

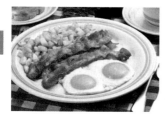

Meat Side Dishes
bacon
canadian bacon
chorizo
corned beef hash
ham
sausage–chicken
sausage–pork
sausage–turkey
steak
turkey

From the Sea Side Dishes
lox or smoked salmon
sardines
shrimp
tuna
white fish

Potato & Salad Side Dishes
french fries
hash browns
sautéed potatoes
fruit salad
mixed green salad

Spreads, Jams and Jellies
butter
confiture
cream cheese
honey
jams
jellies
margarine
marmalades
peanut butter
preserves

Breakfast Specialties
blintzes
cereal–cold
cereal–hot
crepes
french toast
pancakes
toast
waffles

Bakery Products
bagels
biscuits
breads
buns
coffee cake
crackers
croissant
donuts
muffin
rolls
rice cakes
scones

11

Acceptable Gluten-Free Grains/Flours

amaranth	potato
arrowroot	quinoa
buckwheat	rice
chickpea	sorghum (milo)
corn	soy
manioc (tapioca)	teff
millet	

Breakfast Quick Reference Guide

Similar to the international cuisine quick reference guides, this guide has been designed to help simplify the ordering process for your breakfast meals. It allows you to walk into any restaurant that serves breakfast or call room service, scan the menu or view the breakfast buffet options and quickly spot the safest choices based upon your specific food allergies.

The *Breakfast Quick Reference Guide* reflects where you may potentially encounter 10 common allergens by each sample breakfast item found on the menu or on the buffet. These allergens are color-coded based on allergen type in an easy-to-follow format and include:

- Brown for corn and soy

- Yellow for dairy and gluten/wheat

- Blue for fish and shellfish

- Green for peanuts and tree nuts

- Pink for eggs

It identifies the specific allergen by menu item indicated by an ● for "typically contains allergen" or an o for "may contain allergen" recommending that you check with your server about this allergen.

**Color Key for the
Quick Reference Guides**

Corn–dark brown
Soy–light brown
Dairy–light yellow
Gluten/wheat–dark yellow
Fish–dark blue
Shellfish–light blue
Peanuts–dark green
Tree Nuts light green
Eggs–pink

11

Breakfast:
Quick Reference Guide
(Egg Dishes, Eggs—Made to Order and Egg Preparation)

	Corn	Dairy	Eggs	Fish	Gluten/Wheat	Peanuts	Shellfish	Soy	Tree Nuts
Egg Dishes									
Eggs Benedict	○	●	●		○	○		○	
Huevos Mexicanos	○	○	●		○	○		○	
Huevos Rancheros	○	○	●		○	○		○	
Skillets- American Style	○	○	●		○	○		○	
Eggs—Made to Order									
Eggs (White and Yolk)	○	○	●			○		○	
Egg Beaters	○	○	●			○		○	
Egg Whites	○	○	●			○		○	
Egg Yolks	○	○	●			○		○	
Egg Preparation									
Boiled			●						
Fried in Butter		●	●						
Fried in Oil	○		●			○		○	
Hard Boiled			●						
Poached			●						
Scrambled with milk and cooked in butter		●	●		○				
Scrambled plain or with water and cooked in oil	○		●		○	○		○	
Soft Boiled			●						
Sunny Side Up	○	●	●			○		○	
Yolk Broken	○	●	●			○		○	

11

Always ensure no cross-contamination in food preparation

● Typically contains allergen   ○ May contain allergen

Breakfast:
Quick Reference Guide
(Omelet Preparation and Potential Omelet Ingredients)

	Corn	Dairy	Eggs	Fish	Gluten/Wheat	Peanuts	Shellfish	Soy	Tree Nuts
Omelet Preparation									
Plain–cooked in butter		●	●		○				
Plain– cooked in oil	○	○	●		○	○		○	
With ingredients–cooked in butter		●	●		○				
With ingredients–cooked in oil	○	○	●		○	○		○	
Potential Omelet Ingredients									
Asparagus									
Avocado									
Bacon	○				○	○		○	
Broccoli									
Cheese	○	●			○			○	
Chicken					○			○	
Chiles									
Chives									
Chorizo	○				○	○		○	
Garlic									
Green Beans									
Green Peppers									
Ham	○	○			○	○		○	○
Herbs									
Jalapeños									

Always ensure no cross-contamination in food preparation

● Typically contains allergen   ○ May contain allergen

Breakfast:
Quick Reference Guide
(Potential Omelet Ingredients, Cheese & Yogurts)

	Corn	Dairy	Eggs	Fish	Gluten/Wheat	Peanuts	Shellfish	Soy	Tree Nuts
Potential Omelet Ingredients									
Mushrooms									
Olives									
Onions									
Potatoes	O				O			O	
Red Peppers									
Sausage–Chicken	O				O	O		O	
Sausage–Pork	O				O	O		O	
Sausage–Turkey	O				O	O		O	
Spinach									
Tomatoes									
Cheese & Yogurts									
Cheese		●			O				
Cheese (American)	O	●			O			O	
Cottage Cheese		●							
Fruit Yogurt	O	●			O			O	
Natural Yogurt		●							
Plain Yogurt		●							
Soy Yogurt								●	
Soy Fruit Yogurt	O				O			●	
Yogurt Drink	O	●			O			O	

Always ensure no cross-contamination in food preparation
● Typically contains allergen   O May contain allergen

Breakfast:
Quick Reference Guide
(Fresh Fruits, Meat Side Dishes and From the Sea Side Dishes)

	Corn	Dairy	Eggs	Fish	Gluten/Wheat	Peanuts	Shellfish	Soy	Tree Nuts
Fresh Fruits									
All Fresh Fruits									
Meat Side Dishes									
Bacon	O				O	O		O	
Canadian Bacon	O				O	O		O	
Chorizo	O				O	O		O	
Corned Beef Hash	O	O				O		O	
Ham	O	O			O	O		O	
Sausage–Chicken	O				O	O		O	
Sausage–Pork	O				O	O		O	
Sausage–Turkey	O				O	O		O	
Steak	O	O			O	O		O	
Turkey	O				O			O	
From the Sea Side Dishes									
Lox or Smoked Salmon				●					
Sardines	O			●			O	O	
Shrimp					O		●		
Tuna	O			●			O	O	
White Fish				●					

Always ensure no cross-contamination in food preparation

● Typically contains allergen   O May contain allergen

11

Breakfast:
Quick Reference Guide
(Potato & Salad Side Dishes, Spreads and Breakfast Specialties)

	Corn	Dairy	Eggs	Fish	Gluten/Wheat	Peanuts	Shellfish	Soy	Tree Nuts
Potato & Salad Side Dishes									
French Fries	O				O	O		O	
Hash Browns	O	O			O	O		O	
Sautéed Potatoes	O	O			O	O		O	
Fruit Salad									
Mixed Green Salad	O	O	O		O	O		O	
Spreads, Jams, and Jellies									
Butter		●							
Confiture/Jams/Jellies/Preserves	O				O			O	
Cream Cheese	O	●			O			O	
Honey									
Margarine	O					O		O	
Marmelades	O				O			O	
Peanut Butter					O	●			
Breakfast Specialties									
Blintzes	O	O	O		O	O		O	O
Cereal–Cold	O	O			O	O		O	O
Cereal–Hot	O	O			O	O		O	O
Crêpes	O	O	O		O	O		O	O
French Toast	O	O	O		O	O		O	O
Pancakes/Waffles	O	O	O		O	O		O	O
Toast	O	O	O		O	O		O	O

Always ensure no cross-contamination in food preparation

● Typically contains allergen   O May contain allergen

Breakfast:
Quick Reference Guide
(Bakery Products)

Bakery Products	Corn	Dairy	Eggs	Fish	Gluten/ Wheat	Peanuts	Shellfish	Soy	Tree Nuts
Bagels	O	O	O		O	O		O	O
Biscuits	O	O	O		O	O		O	O
Breads/Buns/Rolls	O	O	O		O	O		O	O
Coffee Cake	O	O	O		O	O		O	O
Crackers	O	O	O		O			O	O
Croissant	O	O	O		O	O		O	O
Donuts/Muffins	O	O	O		O	O		O	O
Rice Cakes	O	O			O			O	
Scones	O	O	O		O	O		O	O

Always ensure no cross-contamination in food preparation

O   May contain allergen

11

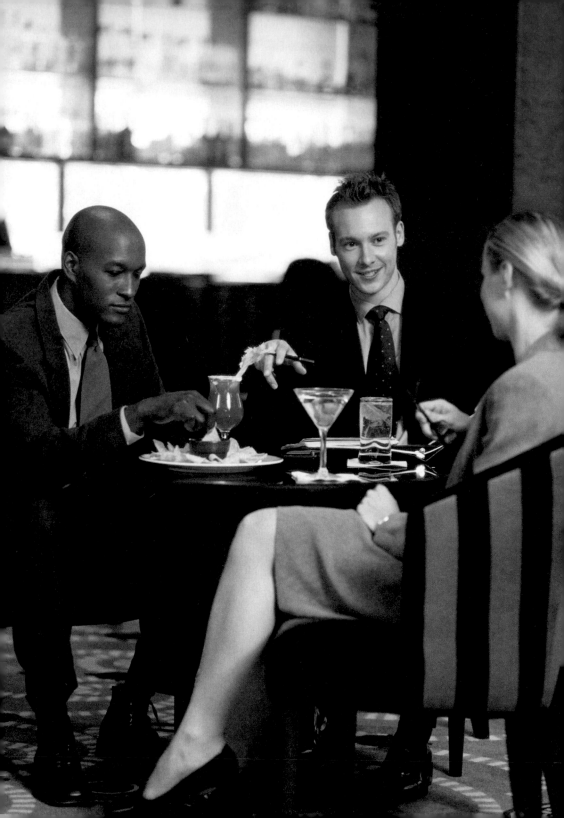

Okay, so it has sophisticated assertiveness,
presumptuous breeding, crisp authority, complex
balance, elegant power and respected finesse:
What's it taste like?
—Anonymous

Chapter 12
Allergy-Free Beverage Suggestions

Chapter Overview

The suggestions for non-alcoholic and alcoholic beverages represent a variety of guidelines to help you in choosing beverages throughout the day. These suggestions can assist you in curbing your thirst safely —whether it's in your car, at a café or at the airport— anywhere you may be, even in your own home. The beverage guidelines include:

- Allergy awareness with beverages

- Non-alcoholic beverage suggestions

- Non-alcoholic beverage quick reference guide

- Alcoholic beverage suggestions

- Alcoholic beverage quick reference guide

12

Allergy Awareness in Beverages

There are a variety of choices when it comes to allergy-free non-alcoholic and alcoholic beverages. At the

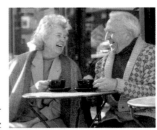

same time, it is extremely important to ensure that there are no hidden allergens or ingredients used in the manufacturing process that you may have a reaction to. Non-alcoholic beverages label the specific ingredients found in their products, so it is necessary to read these labels carefully. By contrast, alcohol manufacturers in Europe and North America are not required by law to list their ingredients. Some alcoholic products list what ingredients they are distilled from and some do not.

Below is a list of common ingredients that contain hidden allergens in non-alcoholic and alcoholic beverages. Actual contents of some ingredients may vary based upon your location. If you find any of these ingredients listed on a beverage label or you think it is included in the alcoholic beverage, you may want to choose another beverage option.

- Colors or flavors (may contain corn, gluten/wheat, soy, peanuts or treenuts)

- Brown rice syrup (frequently made with barley/gluten)

- Caramel color (may contain corn, gluten/wheat or soy)

- Corn syrup (contains corn)

- Dextrin (made from corn or wheat)

- High fructose corn syrup (contains corn)

- Vegetable protein, hydrolyzed vegetable protein (HVP), hydrolyzed plant protein (HPP), or textured vegetable protein (TVP) (may contain corn, gluten/wheat or soy)

- Hydrolyzed corn protein (contains corn)

- Hydrolyzed soy protein (contains soy)

- Hydrolyzed wheat protein (contains gluten/ wheat)

- Malt or malt flavoring (made from barley/gluten or corn)

- Modified food starch or modified starch (made from corn or gluten/wheat)

12

Non-Alcoholic Beverage Suggestions

These beverage suggestions have been developed based upon personal global travel experience, research and product label reviews. The following reflects two categories of non-alcoholic beverages to order around the corner or around the world:

- Hot beverages
- Cold beverages

Hot Beverage Suggestions

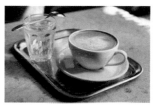

Coffee
Suggestions: café au lait, cappuccino, coffee syrup, decaffeinated, espresso, flavored, instant, instant espresso, latte, powdered, regular

Tea
Suggestions: decaffeinated, flavored, herbal, regular

Gluten-Free Hot Ciders and Cocoas
Suggestions: apple cider, hot chocolate

12

Cold Beverage Suggestions

Gluten-Free Iced Coffee and Iced Teas
Suggestions: decaffeinated, flavored, herbal, iced cappuccino, iced coffee, iced tea, regular

Fruit Juice
Suggestions: apple, banana, cherry, cranberry, grape, grapefruit, orange, peach, pear, pineapple, plum, prune

Vegetable Juice
Suggestions: carrot, celery, aloe vera, tomato, vegetable

Mineral Water
Suggestions: Most still and sparkling waters—some flavored waters may contain colors or flavors

Gluten-Free Carbonated Soft Drinks

Suggestions: cola, ginger ale, grape, orange, root beer, soda water, tonic water

Gluten-Free Non-Carbonated Beverages

Suggestions: fruit drink, fruit punch, lemonade, sports drinks, powdered drinks

Gluten-Free Dairy and Soy Drinks

Suggestions: milk, protein drinks, smoothie, soy drinks, yogurt drinks

Non-Alcoholic Beverage Quick Reference Guide

Color Key for the Quick Reference Guides

Corn–dark brown
Soy–light brown
Dairy–light yellow
Gluten/wheat–dark yellow
Fish–dark blue
Shellfish–light blue
Peanuts–dark green
Tree Nuts–light green
Eggs–pink

Based on these hot and cold beverages, the *Non-Alcoholic Beverage Quick Reference Guide* reflects where you may potentially encounter 10 common allergens. These allergens are color-coded based on allergen type in an easy-to-follow format and include:

- Brown for corn and soy
- Yellow for dairy and gluten/wheat
- Blue for fish and shellfish
- Green for peanuts and tree nuts
- Pink for eggs

The Quick Reference Guide identifies the specific allergen by suggestion type indicated by an o for "may contain allergen" recommending that you need to carefully check each label when possible to ensure the absence of your specific food allergens.

This guide is designed to provide you with a level of comfort. With key information at your finger tips necessary to guide your decisions, you can effectively ensure hidden allergens are addressed and concentrate on enjoying your experience.

12

Non-Alcoholic Beverages:
Quick Reference Guide

	Corn	Dairy	Eggs	Fish	Gluten/Wheat	Peanuts	Shellfish	Soy	Tree Nuts
Hot Beverages									
Coffee	O	O			O			O	O
Tea	O				O			O	O
Ciders and Cocoas	O	O			O			O	
Cold Beverages									
Iced Coffee and Teas	O				O			O	O
Fruit Juices	O				O			O	
Vegetable Juices	O				O			O	
Mineral Water	O				O			O	
Carbonated Soft Drinks	O				O			O	
Non-Carbonated Beverages	O				O			O	
Dairy and Soy Drinks	O	O	O		O			O	O

O   May contain allergen

12

Alcoholic Beverage Suggestions

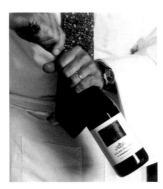

In your allergy-free journeys, you may have discovered a broad spectrum of opinions on alcoholic beverages. Some sources of information advise you to stay away from alcohol all together, while others provide listings of products that may be allergy-free.

The distillation process removes all proteins from alcohol; thereby eliminating the substance in food that the body reacts to in an allergic response. We have noted the source of distilled alcohol for all products listed in our *Alcoholic Beverage Quick Reference Guide* for your reference.

You need to consider whether colors or flavors are used in the production of the product. Colors and flavors may contain corn, dairy, eggs, gluten/wheat, peanuts, soy or treenuts. In addition, some alcoholic beverages may be fortified with grain alcohol. Grain alcohol may be distilled from corn or wheat. Finally, some alcoholic beverages may contain malt which is derived from barley/gluten or corn.

As discussed earlier, manufacturers of alcoholic beverages are not required by law to list their ingredients on product labels. Although efforts were made with manufacturers to confirm their ingredients, we were unable to obtain information. Therefore, these beverage suggestions have been based upon personal global travel experience and research.

The following reflect 10 categories of alcoholic beverages that you may want to consider ordering around the corner or around the world:

- Vodkas

- Rums

- Tequilas and mezcals

- Gins and jenevers

- Whiskeys

- Beers, ciders and sake

- Wine and wine beverages

- Brandys

12

- Liqueurs

- Beverage mixes

The vodkas have been categorized by the following six suggestion types:

- Vodka from corn

- Vodka from grains

- Vodka from grapes

- Vodka from potatoes

- Vodka from soy

- Flavored vodka

The rums have been categorized by the following five suggestion types:

- Añejo rum

- Blanco (clear) rum

- Dark rum

- Flavored rum

- Spiced rum

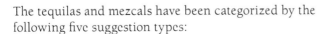

12

The tequilas and mezcals have been categorized by the following five suggestion types:

- Añejo tequila

- Blanco (clear) tequila

- Gold tequila

- Mezcal

- Reposado

The gins have been categorized by the following four suggestion types:

- Gin (London Dry and Plymouth styles)

- Flavored gin

- Jenever (Dutch and European styles)

- Flavored jenever

The whiskeys have been categorized by the following four suggestion types:

- American (bourbon, sour mash, rye)

- Canadian (rye)

- Irish

- Scotch

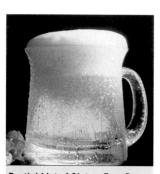

The beers, ciders and sakes have been categorized by the following five suggestion types:

- Gluten-free beer

- Beer (ale, lager, pilsner, porter, stout, wheat-beer)

- Non-alcoholic beer

- Hard cider

- Sake

Partial List of Gluten-Free Beer Manufacturers

Canada – Baluchon
http://www.baluchon.com/microbrewery
Phone: (819) 268-5500

UK – Green's
http://www.glutenfreebeers.co.uk
Phone: 44 0113 2502 036

US – Bard's Tale
http://www.bardsbeer.com
Phone: (816) 896-2273

US – Ramapo Valley
http://www.ramapovalleybrewery.com
Phone: (845) 369-7827

12

The wine and wine beverages have been categorized by the following five suggestion types:

- Champagne and sparkling wine

- Red, white and blush wine

- Fortified wine and port (Madeira, port, sherry)

- Vermouth (French dry and Italian sweet styles)

- Wine Coolers

Brandy has been categorized by the following nine suggestion types:

- Brandy

- Flavored brandy

- Armagnac

- Calvados

- Cognac

- Flavored cognac

- Eaux de Vie

- Grappa

- Kirshwasser

The liqueurs have been categorized by the following eight suggestion types:

- Anise-flavored liqueur (anisette, absinthe, ouzo, pastis, sambucca)

- Coffee liqueurs

- Cream-based liqueur

- Fruit flavored liqueur

- Melon flavored liqueur

- Nut flavored liqueur

- Orange flavored liqueur

- Schnapps

The beverage mixers have been categorized by the following five suggestion types:

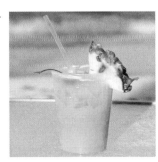

- Bloody Mary mixers

- Colada mixers

- Daiquiri mixers

- Margarita mixers

- Pre-mixed alcoholic cocktails

12

Alcoholic Beverage Quick Reference Guide

Color Key for the Quick Reference Guides

Corn–dark brown
Soy–light brown
Dairy–light yellow
Gluten/wheat–dark yellow
Fish–dark blue
Shellfish–light blue
Peanuts–dark green
Tree Nuts–light green
Eggs–pink

Based on these 10 categories and associated 50-plus suggestion types, the *Alcoholic Beverage Quick Reference Guide* reflects where you may potentially encounter 10 common allergens. These suggestion types identify the source of distilled alcohol and other alcohol that may be included in the beverage. Please note that alcohol, which may be distilled from a potential allergen, is not listed as containing the allergen in the reference guides based upon the standards of the Codex Alimentarius.

These allergens are color-coded based on allergen type for an easy-to-use format and include:

- Brown for corn and soy

- Yellow for dairy and gluten/wheat

- Blue for fish and shellfish

- Green for peanuts and tree nuts

- Pink for eggs

The Quick Reference Guide identifies the specific allergen by alcoholic beverage indicated by an ● for "typically contains allergen" or an ○ for "may contain allergen".

This guide is designed to provide you with a level of comfort. With key information at your finger tips necessary to guide your decisions, you can effectively communicate your needs, ensure hidden allergens are addressed and concentrate on enjoying your experience. You need to carefully order your alcoholic beverages and ensure that you are served your respective choices. Be sure to consume alcoholic beverages sensibly and remember to drink moderately as a rule for healthy living.

Alcoholic Beverages:
Quick Reference Guide
(Vodkas, Rums, Tequilas & Mezcals)

Vodkas	Distilled/ Made from	Corn	Dairy	Eggs	Fish	Gluten/Wheat	Peanuts	Shellfish	Soy	Tree Nuts
Vodka from Corn (e.g. Rain)	Corn									
Vodka from Grapes (e.g. Ciroc)	Grapes									
Vodka from Grain	Grains									
Vodka from Potato (e.g.Chopin, Glacier Teton, Luksusowa, Monopolowa, Jarzebiak, Bison, and Viking Fjord)	Potato									
Vodka from Soy (e.g. 3)	Soy									
Flavored Vodkas	Grains or Corn	O				O			O	O
Rums										
Añejo Rum	Sugar Cane									
Blanco (Clear) Rums (e.g. Bacardi Silver)	Sugar Cane									
Dark Rum	Sugar Cane	O				O			O	
Flavored Rum	Sugar Cane	O				O			O	
Spiced Rum	Sugar Cane	O				O			O	
Tequilas & Mezcals										
Añejo Tequila (Aged at least one year)*	Agave									
Blanco (Clear) Tequila (Aged no more than two months)*	Agave									
Gold Tequila (Aged no more than two months)*	Agave	O				O			O	
Mezcal*	Agave									
Reposado (Aged at least six months)*	Agave									

O   May contain allergen

*   Unless stated 100%, may be mixed with grain
     alcohol distilled from corn or sugar cane

Alcoholic Beverages:
Quick Reference Guide
(Gins & Jenever, Whiskeys, Beers, Ciders & Sake)

Gins & Jenever	Distilled/ Made from	Corn	Dairy	Eggs	Fish	Gluten/Wheat	Peanuts	Shellfish	Soy	Tree Nuts
Gin (London Dry & Plymouth Styles)	Grains									
Flavored Gin	Grains	O				O			O	
Jenever (Dutch & European Styles)	Grains									
Flavored Jenever	Grains	O				O			O	
Whiskeys										
American (Bourbon, Sour Mash, Rye)	Grains	O				O			O	
Canadian (Rye)	Grains	O				O			O	
Irish	Grains	O				O			O	
Scotch	Grains	O				O			O	
Beers, Ciders & Sake										
Gluten-free Beer (e.g. Baluchon-Canada, Greens- UK, Bard's Tale-US, Ramapo Valley-US)	Gluten-Free Grains	O								
Beer (Ale, Lager, Pilsner, Porter, Stout, Wheat-Beer)	Hops, Barley, Malt & Wheat	O				●				
Non-Alcoholic Beer	Hops, Barley, Malt & Wheat	O				●				
Hard Cider	Apples and possibly Barley	O				O			O	
Sake (Known as rice wine, but fermented and brewed like beer)	Rice and Koji Enzymes grown on Miso (typically made from barley)					O				

● Typically contains allergen   O May contain allergen

12

Alcoholic Beverages:
Quick Reference Guide
(Wine, Wine Beverages and Brandy)

Wine & Wine Beverages	Distilled/ Made from	Corn	Dairy	Eggs	Fish	Gluten/Wheat	Peanuts	Shellfish	Soy	Tree Nuts
Champagne and Sparkling Wine	Grapes									
Red, White and Blush Wines	Grapes									
Fortified Wine and Port (Madeira, Port, Sherry)*	Grapes									
Vermouth (French dry & Italian sweet styles- e.g. Cinzano, Dubonnet, Lillet)*	Grapes	O				O			O	
Wine Coolers	Grapes	O				O			O	
Brandy										
Brandy	Grapes									
Flavored Brandy	Grapes	O				O			O	
Armagnac	Grapes									
Calvados	Apples									
Cognac	Grapes									
Flavored Cognac	Grapes	O				O			O	
Eaux de Vie	Fruit									
Grappa	Grapes or Fruit									
Kirschwasser	Cherries									

O   May contain allergen
*   May be mixed with alcohol distilled from corn or grain

12

Alcoholic Beverages:
Quick Reference Guide
(Liqueurs and Beverage Mixes)

Liqueurs	Distilled/ Made from	Corn	Dairy	Eggs	Fish	Gluten/Wheat	Peanuts	Shellfish	Soy	Tree Nuts
Anise-Flavored Liqueur (e.g. Anisette, Absinthe, Ouzo, Pastis, Sambucca)		O				O			O	
Coffee Liqueur*	Coffee	O				O			O	
Cream-Based Liqueur*	Cream	O	●			O			O	
Fruit Flavored Liqueur*	Fruit	O				O			O	
Melon Liqueur*	Melon	O				O			O	
Nut Flavored Liqueur*	Melon	O				O	O		O	O
Orange Flavored Liqueur*	Orange	O				O			O	
Schnapps*	Fruit and Herbs	O				O			O	O
Beverage Mixes										
Bloody Mary Mixers	Tomato-based mixture	O				O		O	O	
Colada Mixers	Coconut-based mixture	O	O	O		O			O	
Daiquiri Mixers	Fruit-based mixture	O				O			O	
Margarita Mixers	Lime-based mixture	O				O			O	
Pre-mixed Alcoholic Cocktails	Ingredients vary	O	O	O		O	O		O	O

● Typically contains allergen   O May contain allergen
* May be mixed with alcohol distilled from corn or grain

12

12

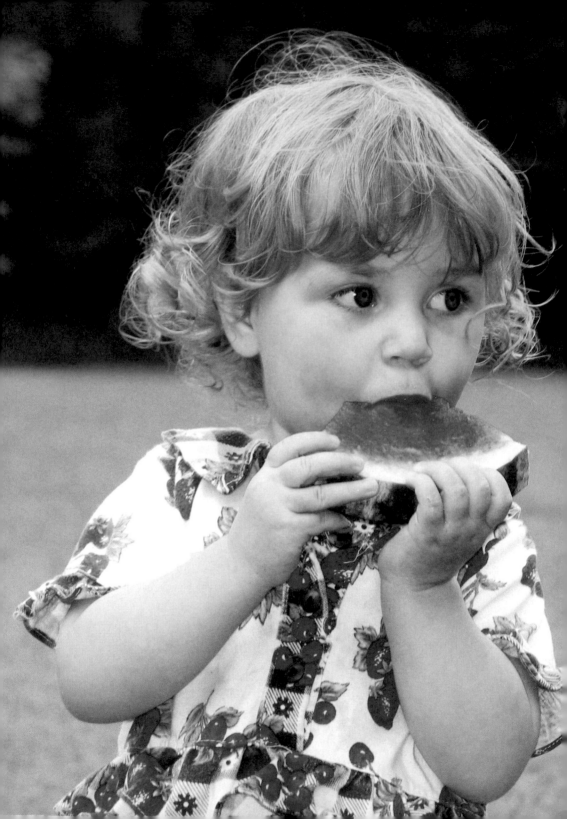

Every now and then,
bite off more than you can chew.
—Kobi Yamada

Chapter 13
On The Go Snacks And Light Meal Suggestions

Chapter Overview

The suggestions for snacks and light meals represent a variety of guidelines to help you in choosing snacks away from home. These can help to curb your hunger throughout the day—if it's at the office, at school, at the airport—anywhere you may be, even in your own home. The snack and light meal guidelines include:

- Snack and light meal overview

- Snack and light meal shopping checklists

- Snack and light meal Quick Reference Guide

Snack and Light Meal Overview

The snack and light meal suggestions have been developed based upon personal global travel experience, research and product label reviews. It is assumed that microwaves, ovens, stoves, toasters, toaster ovens and freezers are not available for your use.

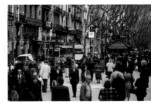

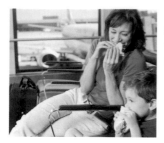

The following reflect three categories of snacks and light meals that you may want to consider bringing while outside the comforts of your home—either on the go or on the road around the globe requiring:

- No preparation

- Hot water preparation

- Cooler required

To facilitate an easy-to-use format, we have further detailed each of these categories by snack and light meal types. The 12 types of suggestions requiring no preparation include:

- Fresh Fruits

- Canned/Packaged Fruits

- Dried Fruits

- Fresh Vegetables

- Cereals

- Biscuits, Breads, Crackers and Rice Cakes

- Cakes, Cookies and Sweet Biscuits

- Canned and Pre-Packed Meats & Fish

- Nuts and Trail Mixes

- Candy and Confectionery

- Energy Bars

- Chips and Crisps

The three types of snack and light meal suggestions requiring hot water preparation include:

- Hot Cereals

- Instant Soups and Meals

- Rice Noodle Dishes

The six types of snack and light meal suggestions requiring a cooler include:

13

- Fresh Fruits

- Fresh Vegetables and Salads

- Cheese and Yogurts

- Deli/Packaged Meats and Seafood

- Condiments, Dips and Spreads

- Desserts and Other Packaged Snacks

In addition, some of the following items may be helpful to carry along with you for eating your snacks and light meals: aluminum foil, cold pack, individual packets of condiments, packaged wet napkins, paper napkins, paper plates, plastic cups, plastic containers, plastic silverware, pocket knife, re-sealable plastic bags and small cutting board.

No Preparation Suggestions: Sample Shopping Checklist

These snacks and light meal suggestions can be carried with you in your backpack, purse, briefcase or kept in your office, school locker, automobile—anywhere you may find yourself hungry. Be sure to read product labels and review country-specific regulations.

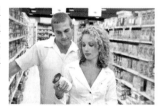

13

Fresh Fruits	Canned/Packaged Fruits
apples	apples
apricots	apple sauce
bananas	apricots
cherries	cherries
clementines	fruit cocktail
grapes	mandarin oranges
nectarines	peaches
oranges	pears
peaches	pineapples
pears	
pineapples	
plums	
tangerines	

Dried Fruits
apples
apricots
banana chips
cherries
cranberries
currants
dates
figs
ginger
mango
papaya
peaches
pineapples
plantains
raisins
strawberries

Fresh Vegetables
broccoli
carrots
cauliflower
celery
cherry tomatoes
green beans
soy beans

Gluten-Free Cereals
amaranth
buckwheat flakes
corn flakes
corn puffs
granola- no oats
millet
muesli
quinoa
rice bran/crisps
rice flakes/puffs
soy flakes
teff

Gluten-Free Biscuits, Breads, Crackers & Rice Cakes
baguettes
biscuits
breads
breadsticks
corn cakes
crispbreads
crackers
rice cakes
toast

Gluten-Free Cakes, Cookies and Sweet Biscuits
biscotti
brownies
cake bars
cookies
digestives
macaroons
magdalenas
mini cheesecakes
muffins
wafers

Gluten-Free Canned/Packaged Meats & Fish
anchovies
beef jerky
canned chicken
pepperoni
salmon
sardines
sausage
spreadables
tofu jerky
canned/packaged tuna
canned turkey
turkey jerky
white fish

13

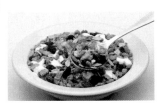

Gluten-Free Nuts and Trail Mixes
almonds
brazil nuts
cashews
flax seed
filberts
hemp nuts
macadamia nuts
nut butter
peanuts
peanut butter
pecans
pinenuts
pistachios
pumpkin seeds
sesame seeds
soynuts
sunflower seeds
walnuts
yogurt covered nuts

Gluten-Free Candy and Confectionery
bars
chewing gums
chocolates
cremes
diabetic
drops
fudges
fruit snacks
gummi candies
hard candies

Gluten-Free Candy and Confectionery, continued
jellies
lollipops
marshmallows
mints
pastilles
soothers
tablets
toffee
yogurt covered fruits

Gluten-Free Energy Bars
fruit and nut bars
fruit filled bars
protein bars
rice bars
sesame seed bars
vegan bars

Gluten-Free Chips and Crisps
caramel corn
corn chips
corn tortilla chips
cheese snacks
packaged popcorn
potato chips
potato sticks
gluten-free pretzels
rice chips
rice sticks
soy crisps
veggie chips

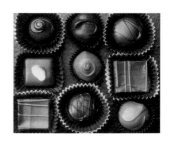

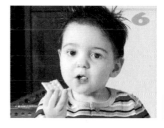

13

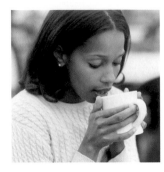

Hot Water Preparation Suggestions: Sample Shopping Checklist

These snack and light meal suggestions can also be carried with you for when you may find yourself hungry. You just need to ask for hot water in a container wherever you may be. Hot water is available in many locations including: convenience stores, restaurants, coffee shops, bars, petrol stations, airplanes, airports, etc. Be sure to read product labels and review country-specific regulations.

Hot Cereals
buckwheat
corn cereal
corn grits
corn meal
rice cereal
porridge flakes
rice porridge
quinoa

Gluten-Free Rice Noodle Dishes
instant rice noodles
instant rice lunch cups

Instant Soups and Meals
beans
beef and vegetable
broccoli
chicken
chili
miso
mushroom
onion
split pea
potato
rice
shrimp
stroganoff
vegetable

13

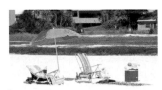

Cooler Required Suggestions: Sample Shopping Checklist

The following snacks and light meal suggestions that require cooling may be refrigerated in a small portable cooler, insulated mug, and small refrigerator in your hotel room or office. Be sure to read product labels and review country-specific regulations.

Fresh Fruits
blueberries
blackberries
cantaloupe
grapefruit
honey dew

melon
mango
papaya
raspberries
strawberries

Fresh Vegetables and Salads

cucumbers
hearts of palm
lettuce
peppers
tomatoes
gluten-free salad dressings

Gluten-Free Cheese and Yogurts

cheese
cheese spreads
cottage cheese
cream cheese
string cheese
soy yogurt
yogurt

Gluten-Free Deli/Packaged Meats and Seafood

bologna
caviar
chicken
corned beef
ham
liverwurst
mortadella
pancetta
pepperoni
prosciutto
roast beef
salami
salmon (lox)
shrimp
summer sausage
turkey

Gluten-Free Condiments, Dips and Spreads

baba gannouj
bean dip
butter
chutney
dressing
guacamole
hummus
ketchup
mayonnaise
mustard
pâtés
preserves
salsa
tapenade
tzatziki

Gluten-Free Desserts and Other Packaged Snacks

eggs-hard boiled
falafel
flan
gelatin
mousse
olives
pickles
pudding
whipped topping

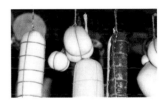

13

Snack and Light Meal Quick Reference Guide

Color Key for the Quick Reference Guides

Corn–dark brown
Soy–light brown
Dairy–light yellow
Gluten/wheat–dark yellow
Fish–dark blue
Shellfish–light blue
Peanuts–dark green
Tree Nuts–light green
Eggs–pink

Based on these three categories, the *Quick Reference Guide* reflects where you may typically encounter the 10 common allergens by each sample snack and light meal category and suggestion type. These allergens are color-coded based on allergen type for an easy-to-use format and include:

- Brown for corn and soy
- Yellow for dairy and gluten/wheat
- Blue for fish and shellfish
- Green for peanuts and tree nuts
- Pink for eggs

These 20-plus suggested types identify the ingredients which may be found in these products indicated by an ● for "typically contains allergen" or an ○ for "may contain allergen" recommending that you need to carefully check each label to ensure the absence of your specific food allergens.

13

Snacks and Light Meals Suggestions:
Quick Reference Guide

	Corn	Dairy	Eggs	Fish	Gluten/Wheat	Peanuts	Shellfish	Soy	Tree Nuts
No Preparation Suggestions									
Fresh Fruits									
Canned/Packaged Fruits	○				○			○	
Dried Fruits					○			○	
Fresh Vegetables									
Cereals	○	○	○		○	○		○	○
Biscuits, Breads, Crackers and Rice Cakes	○	○	○		○	○		○	○
Cakes, Cookies and Sweet Biscuits	○	○	○		○	○		○	○
Nuts and Trail Mixes					○	●		○	●
Canned/Pre-packed Meats & Fish	○	○	○	○	○			○	
Candy and Confectionery	○	○			○	○		○	○
Energy Bars	○	○			○	○		○	○
Chips and Crisps	○	○			○	○	○	○	
Hot Water Preparation Suggestions									
Hot Cereals	○	○			○			○	
Instant Soups and Meals		○			○		○	○	
Rice Noodle Dishes					○	○		○	○
Cooler Required Suggestions									
Fresh Fruits									
Fresh Vegetables and Salads	○	○			○			○	
Cheese and Yogurts		○			○			○	
Deli/Packaged Meats and Seafood				○	○		○	○	
Condiments, Dips and Spreads	○	○			○			○	
Desserts and Other Packaged Snacks		○	○		○			○	

● Typically contains allergen
○ May contain allergen; refer to package labeling

13

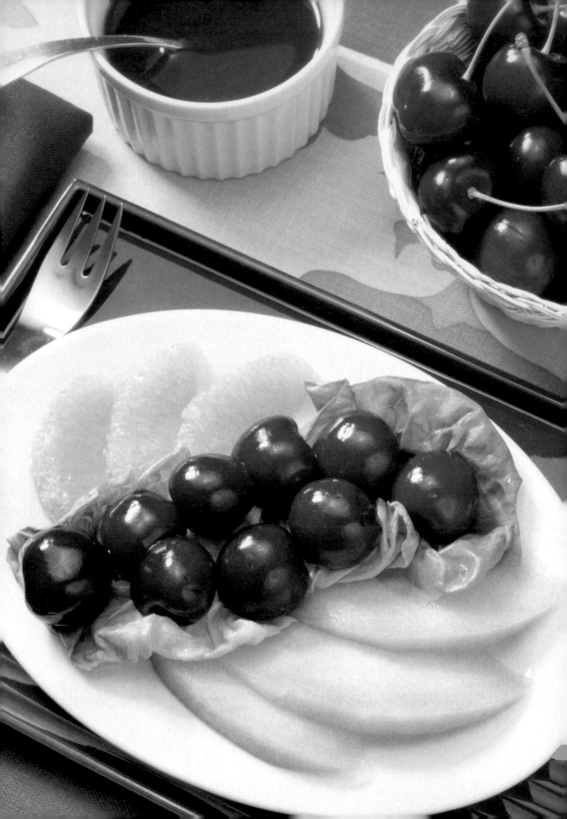

*Twenty years from now you will be
more disappointed by the things you didn't do
than by the ones you did. So throw off the bowlines.
Sail away from the safe harbor. Catch the trade
winds in your sails. Explore. Dream. Discover.*
—Unknown

Chapter 14
Airline Meal Suggestions

Chapter Overview

The airline suggestions represent a variety of guidelines to help you order and obtain special meals while traveling by air. These suggestions may assist you in choosing your airline carrier based upon your special dietary considerations and include:

- Airline meal guidelines overview

- Airline special meal descriptions and notification policy

- Special meal availability by global airlines

- Global airline contact listings

14

Airline Meal Guidelines Overview

If the carrier you are flying offers special meals, it is necessary to make airline personnel aware of your needs in advance. In most instances, you can communicate your special meal needs and make these arrangements at the time of your booking. Airlines that offer special meals typically need advance notification anywhere between 24 to 96 hours to ensure that your special meal is ready at the time of your departure. It

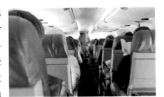

is advised to confirm your meal request directly with the airline or with your travel agent prior to your departure.

Based upon your dietary requirements, you may be required to fly on an airline carrier that does not offer the special meal you need or prefer. In this case, refer to Chapter 12, Snack and Light Meal Suggestions, for on-the-go options to take with you to make your flight a more comfortable experience. Even if you have ordered a special meal, it is advised that you pack snacks as a precautionary measure, just in case your flight is delayed, plans change or a mistake happens.

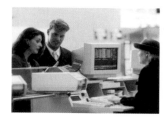

Airline Special Meal Descriptions and Notification Policy

Many global airlines are aware of and cater to those who need special meals when traveling by air. The selection and quality of these meals varies significantly from airline to airline. There are different types of special meals that are offered by specific airlines based on flight duration, destination and meal availability. These meals are categorized as follows:

- Medically prescribed lifestyles

- Recommended lifestyles

- Age considerations

- Religious considerations

- Health preferences

The airline industry has 25-plus standard codes for the various types of special meals. These codes, their definitions and associated descriptions are listed on the following page. The recommended special meal notification policy as of June 2005 is also outlined for your reference.

14

Meal Descriptions for Medically Prescribed & Recommended Lifestyles

Code	Definition	Description
GFML	Gluten-Free Meal	No wheat, rye, barley, or oats or their derivatives
NLML	Non-Lactose Meal	No milk, cheese, dairy products or their derivatives
PFML	Peanut-Free Meal	No peanuts or its derivatives
DBML	Diabetic Meal	No refined sugars, syrups, jams, cakes or chocolates, etc.
LFML	Low-Fat/Cholesterol Meal	Limited amount of fat (particularly saturated fat)
PRML	Low-Purine Meal	No anchovies, crab, herring, liver, offal or shrimp
LPML	Low-Protein Meal	Limited amount of protein
LSML	Low-Sodium/Salt Meal	Little salt, Monosodium Glutamate (MSG) or baking soda/powder used

Meal Descriptions based on Age Considerations

BBML	Baby Meal	Soft and/or liquid foods, usually canned baby food or formula for infants under 2 years old
CHML	Child Meal	A combination of familiar foods and fun food for children 2 – 12 years old

Meal Descriptions based on Religious Considerations

HNML	Hindu Meal	No beef, veal, pork or their derivatives
JNML	Jain Meal	No root vegetables, onion or garlic
KSML	Kosher Meal	Prepared to comply with Jewish dietary laws
MOML	Muslim Meal	No pork, by-products of pork, shellfish or foodstuffs containing alcohol—all meat is Halal

Meal Descriptions based on Health Preferences

HFML	High-Fiber Meal	Unrefined flours are used over white flour products
LCML	Low-Calorie Meal	Limited amounts of fat, sugar and protein
AVML	Asian-Vegetarian Meal	No fish, shellfish, meat, poultry or eggs—typically spicy in content
VGML	Vegan Meal	No meat, fish, seafood, eggs, honey, dairy products or their derivatives
RVML	Raw-Vegetarian Meal	Combination of raw vegetables and fruit (ie salad)
VLML	Lacto-Ovo Vegetarian Meal	No meat, fish, or seafood—may contain dairy products such as milk, butter, cheese and eggs
ORML	Oriental Meal	Cooked in oriental or Chinese style—it avoids meat, fish, milk, dairy products and root vegetables
FPML	Fruit Plate Meal	Contains a variety of fresh fruits and possibly a bakery item
SFML	Seafood Meal	Contains only seafood
BLML	Bland Meal	No spicy or acidic ingredients

14

Global Airline Notification Policy
(Aer Lingus – Far Eastern Air Transport)

Airline Name	Country	Notification Policy
Aer Lingus	Ireland	24 hours
Aeroflot	Russia	72 hours
Aerolineas	Argentina	When booking
AeroMexico	Mexico	48 hours
Air Canada	Canada	24 hours
Air France	France	24 hours and 48 hours for Kosher
Air India	India	When booking
Air Malta	Malta	72 hours
Air New Zealand	New Zealand	48 hours
Air Pacific	Fiji	When booking
Air Tahiti Nui	Tahiti	When booking
Air Transat	Canada	72 hours
Alitalia	Italy	When booking
American Airlines	USA	8 – 24 hours
America West	USA	Offered in 1st class only - 48 hours
Asiana Airlines	South Korea	When booking
Austrian Airlines	Austria	24 hours
Britannia Airways	UK	3 days
British Airways	UK	24 hours and 48 hours for Kosher
British Midland	UK	24 hours and 48 hours for Kosher
Cathay Pacific	Hong Kong	24 hours
China Airlines	China	24 hours
Continental Airlines	USA	24 hours
CSA Czech Airlines	Czech Republic	When booking
Delta Airlines	USA	12 hours
El Al	Israel	24 hours
Emirates	United Arab Emirates	24 hours
Estonian Air	Estonia	When booking
Eurowings	Germany	When booking
Eva Airways	Taiwan	When booking
Far Eastern Air Transport	Taiwan	When booking

14

Global Airline Notification Policy
(Finnair – Virgin Atlantic)

Airline Name	Country	Notification Policy
Finnair	Finland	24 hours
Gulf Air	Bahrain	24 hours
Iberia	Spain	When booking
IcelandAir	Iceland	24 hours
Japan Airlines	Japan	24 - 72 hours
Kenya Airways	Kenya	24 hours and 48 hours for Kosher
KLM/Northwest	Netherlands / USA	36 hours
Korean Air	Korea	When booking
LAN Airlines	Chile	When booking
Lithuanian Airlines	Lithuania	24 hours
Lufthansa	Germany	When booking
Luxair	Luxembourg	When booking
Malev	Hungary	When booking
Olympic Airlines	Greece	When booking
Qantas	Australia	48 hours
SAS	Sweden	24 hours
SATA	Portugal	When booking
Saudi Arabian Airlines	Saudi Arabia	When booking
Singapore Airlines	Singapore	24 hours
South African Airlines	South Africa	72 hours
Swiss Int'l Airlines	Switzerland	72 hours
TAM Airlines	Brazil	When booking
TAP Air Portugal	Portugal	48 hours
Thai Airlines	Thailand	48 hours
Turkish Airlines	Turkey	When booking
United Airlines	USA	24 hours
US Air	USA	24 hours
Varig	Brazil	24 hours
Vietnam Airlines	Vietnam	24 hours
Virgin Atlantic	UK	72 hours

14

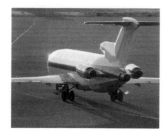

Special Meal Availability by Global Airlines

The following list outlines 50-plus international airline carriers by name, country of origin and different types of special meals offered to travelers. These meals are grouped by:

- Medically prescribed and recommended lifestyles
- Age or religious considerations
- Health preferences

These materials have been compiled based upon research and information provided by airline professionals as of June 2005. Availability of airline meals and notification policies change frequently so it is recommended that you use this as a guide and contact your specific airline for the most up-to-date information.

Special Meal Availability:
Medically Prescribed and Recommended Lifestyles
(Aer Lingus – Air Pacific)

Airline Name	Gluten-Free GFML	Non-Lactose NLML	Peanut-Free PFML	Diabetic DBML	Low-Fat/Chol LFML	Low-Purine PRML	Low-Protein LPML	Low-Sodium LSML
Aer Lingus	●	●		●	●	●	●	
Aeroflot	●	●		●	●	●	●	●
Aerolineas	●	●		●	●	●	●	●
AeroMexico				●	●			●
Air Canada	●	●		●	●			●
Air France	●			●				●
Air India	●	●		●	●	●	●	●
Air Malta	●			●	●			●
Air New Zealand	●	●		●	●	●	●	●
Air Pacific	●			●				

14

Special Meal Availability:
Medically Prescribed and Recommended Lifestyles
(Air Tahiti Nui – IcelandAir)

Airline Name	Gluten-Free GFML	Non-Lactose NLML	Peanut-Free PFML	Diabetic DBML	Low-Fat/Chol LFML	Low-Purine PRML	Low-Protein LPML	Low-Sodium LSML
Air Tahiti Nui	●			●			●	●
Air Transat	●	●		●	●			●
Alitalia								
American Airlines	●	●		●	●			●
America West				●	●			●
Asiana Airlines		●		●	●	●	●	●
Austrian Airlines	●	●		●	●	●	●	●
Britannia Airways	●		●	●				
British Airways	●	●		●	●	●	●	●
British Midland	●	●		●	●		●	●
Cathay Pacific	●	●						●
China Airlines	●	●		●		●	●	●
Continental Airlines	●			●	●			●
CSA Czech Airlines	●	●		●	●	●		●
Delta Airlines	●			●	●			●
El Al	●	●		●	●			●
Emirates	●	●	●	●	●	●	●	●
Estonian Air		●			●			
Eurowings	●	●		●				●
Eva Airways	●	●	●	●	●	●	●	●
Far Eastern Air Transport	●	●		●	●	●	●	●
Finnair	●	●		●	●	●	●	●
Gulf Air	●	●		●	●		●	●
Iberia	●			●	●		●	●
IcelandAir					●			●

14

Special Meal Availability:
Medically Prescribed and Recommended Lifestyles
(Japan Airlines – Virgin Atlantic)

Airline Name	Medically Prescribed and Recommended Lifestyles							
	Gluten-Free GFML	Non-Lactose NLML	Peanut-Free PFML	Diabetic DBML	Low-Fat/Chol LFML	Low-Purine PRML	Low-Protein LPML	Low-Sodium LSML
Japan Airlines	●	●		●	●	●	●	●
Kenya Airways	●	●		●	●	●	●	●
KLM/Northwest	●	●		●	●			●
Korean Air	●	●		●	●	●	●	●
LAN Airlines	●	●		●	●			●
Lithuanian Airlines				●	●			
Lufthansa	●	●		●	●	●	●	●
Luxair	●	●		●	●			
Malev		●		●				
Olympic Airlines	●	●		●	●		●	●
Qantas	●	●		●	●			●
SAS	●				●			●
SATA	●	●		●	●		●	●
Saudi Arabian Airlines	●			●	●			●
Singapore Airlines	●	●		●	●	●	●	●
South African Airlines	●	●		●	●	●	●	●
Swiss Int'l Airlines	●	●		●	●	●	●	●
TAM Airlines	●			●	●			●
TAP Air Portugal	●	●		●	●	●	●	●
Thai Airlines	●			●	●			●
Turkish Airlines	●	●		●	●	●	●	●
United Airlines	●			●	●	●	●	●
US Air	●	●	●	●	●			●
Varig	●	●		●	●		●	●
Vietnam Airlines	●	●		●	●	●	●	●
Virgin Atlantic	●		●	●	●			●

14

Special Meal Availability:
Age Considerations, Religious Considerations & Health Preferences
(Aer Lingus – Delta Airlines)

Airline Name	Age Considerations		Religious Considerations				Health Preferences	
	Baby BBML	Child CHML	Hindu HNML	Jain JNML	Kosher KSML	Muslim MOML	High-Fiber HFML	Low-Calorie LCML
Aer Lingus			●		●	●	●	
Aeroflot	●	●	●		●	●	●	●
Aerolineas	●	●	●			●	●	●
AeroMexico	●	●			●			
Air Canada	●	●	●		●	●		●
Air France	●	●	●		●	●		
Air India	●	●	●	●	●	●	●	●
Air Malta	●							
Air New Zealand	●	●	●		●	●		●
Air Pacific	●	●			●			
Air Tahiti Nui			●		●	●	●	●
Air Transat		●	●		●	●	●	●
Alitalia	●	●			●	●		
American Airlines			●		●	●		●
America West					●			●
Asiana Airlines			●		●	●		●
Austrian Airlines	●	●	●		●	●	●	●
Britannia Airways								
British Airways	●	●	●		●	●	●	●
British Midland		●	●		●	●	●	●
Cathay Pacific			●		●	●	●	●
China Airlines		●	●			●		●
Continental Airlines	●	●	●		●	●		
CSA Czech Airlines	●	●	●		●	●	●	
Delta Airlines	●	●	●		●	●		●

14

Special Meal Availability:
Age Considerations, Religious Considerations & Health Preferences
(El Al – Singapore Airlines)

Airline Name	Age Considerations		Religious Considerations				Health Preferences	
	Baby BBML	Child CHML	Hindu HNML	Jain JNML	Kosher KSML	Muslim MOML	High-Fiber HFML	Low-Calorie LCML
El Al					●			●
Emirates	●	●	●	●		●	●	●
Estonian Air		●				●		
Eurowings								
Eva Airways	●	●	●		●	●	●	●
Far Eastern Air Transport	●	●	●		●	●	●	
Finnair		●	●		●	●	●	●
Gulf Air	●	●	●			●	●	●
Iberia		●	●		●	●		
IcelandAir		●			●	●		●
Japan Airlines	●	●	●		●	●	●	●
Kenya Airways	●	●	●		●	●	●	●
KLM/Northwest	●	●	●		●	●		
Korean Air			●	●	●	●	●	●
LAN Airlines					●			●
Lithuanian Airlines	●	●						●
Lufthansa	●	●	●		●	●		●
Luxair	●	●			●	●		●
Malev		●			●			
Olympic Airlines	●	●	●		●	●	●	●
Qantas		●			●	●		●
SAS	●	●	●		●			
SATA	●	●	●		●	●	●	●
Saudi Arabian Airlines	●	●						
Singapore Airlines	●	●	●		●	●	●	●

14

Special Meal Availability:
Age Considerations, Religious Considerations & Health Preferences
(South African Airlines – Virgin Atlantic)

Airline Name	Age Considerations		Religious Considerations				Health Preferences	
	Baby BBML	Child CHML	Hindu HNML	Jain JNML	Kosher KSML	Muslim MOML	High-Fiber HFML	Low-Calorie LCML
South African Airlines	●	●	●		●	●	●	●
Swiss International Airlines	●	●	●		●	●	●	●
TAM Airlines	●	●	●		●		●	●
TAP Air Portugal	●	●	●		●	●	●	●
Thai Airlines	●	●	●		●	●	●	●
Turkish Airlines	●	●	●		●	●	●	●
United Airlines	●	●	●		●	●	●	●
US Air	●	●	●		●	●		●
Varig	●	●	●		●	●		●
Vietnam Airlines	●	●	●		●	●	●	
Virgin Atlantic			●	●	●	●		

14

Special Meal Availability:
Health Preferences, continued
(Aer Lingus – Delta Airlines)

Airline Name	Health Preferences							
	Asian-Veg AVML	Vegan VGML	Raw-Veg RVML	Lacto-Ovo Veg VLML	Oriental ORML	Fruit Plate FPML	Seafood SFML	Bland SPML
Aer Lingus	●	●	●		●			●
Aeroflot	●	●	●	●	●	●	●	●
Aerolineas	●	●		●	●	●	●	●
AeroMexico		●		●				
Air Canada	●	●		●	●	●		●
Air France		●		●			●	●
Air India	●	●	●	●	●		●	●
Air Malta				●				
Air New Zealand	●	●	●	●	●	●	●	●
Air Pacific		●		●		●		
Air Tahiti Nui	●	●		●		●	●	
Air Transat	●	●		●				
Alitalia	●			●				
American Airlines		●		●				●
America West		●				●		
Asiana Airlines					●		●	
Austrian Airlines	●	●	●	●		●	●	●
Britannia Airways		●		●				
British Airways	●	●		●		●	●	●
British Midland	●	●		●			●	●
Cathay Pacific		●		●	●	●		●
China Airlines	●	●	●	●	●			●
Continental Airlines		●				●	●	
CSA Czech Airlines	●	●	●	●	●		●	●
Delta Airlines		●		●		●	●	●

14

Special Meal Availability:
Health Preferences, continued
(El Al – Singapore Airlines)

Airline Name	Asian-Veg AVML	Vegan VGML	Raw-Veg RVML	Lacto-Ovo Veg VLML	Oriental ORML	Fruit Plate FPML	Seafood SFML	Bland SPML
El Al								●
Emirates	●	●	●	●	●	●	●	●
Estonian Air		●		●				
Eurowings				●				
Eva Airways	●			●		●	●	●
Far Eastern Air Transport	●	●	●	●		●	●	●
Finnair	●	●	●	●	●	●	●	●
Gulf Air	●	●	●	●	●	●	●	●
Iberia	●			●			●	●
IcelandAir	●			●				
Japan Airlines	●	●		●			●	●
Kenya Airways	●	●	●	●			●	●
KLM/Northwest	●	●	●	●		●		
Korean Air		●	●	●		●	●	●
LAN Airlines	●			●				
Lithuanian Airlines				●			●	
Lufthansa	●	●		●		●	●	●
Luxair		●		●		●	●	
Malev				●	●			
Olympic Airlines	●		●		●	●	●	●
Qantas	●	●		●		●		
SAS	●	●		●				
SATA	●	●		●	●	●	●	
Saudi Arabian Airlines	●			●			●	●
Singapore Airlines	●	●	●	●	●	●	●	●

14

Special Meal Availability:
Health Preferences, continued
(South African Airlines – Virgin Atlantic)

Airline Name	Asian-Veg AVML	Vegan VGML	Raw-Veg RVML	Lacto-Ovo Veg VLML	Oriental ORML	Fruit Plate FPML	Seafood SFML	Bland SPML
South African Airlines	●	●	●		●		●	
Swiss International Airlines	●	●		●				●
TAM Airlines	●							
TAP Air Portugal	●		●	●	●	●	●	●
Thai Airlines	●	●		●	●			●
Turkish Airlines	●	●	●	●	●		●	●
United Airlines	●	●	●	●				
US Air	●	●		●				●
Varig	●	●		●	●			●
Vietnam Airlines	●	●	●	●	●	●	●	●
Virgin Atlantic		●		●				

Health Preferences

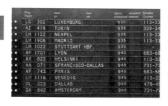

Global Airline Contact Listings

The following listing reflects 50-plus airlines on a worldwide basis that provide special meals. This listing gives you various contact methods for each airline either electronically or via telephone and includes the following information:

- Airline name

- Home country

- Website address

- Telephone numbers

These materials have been compiled based upon research and information provided by airline professionals as of June 2005. Airline contact information changes frequently so it is recommended that you use this as a guide and refer to the respective website for the most up-to-date information.

Please note: Multiple telephone numbers have been provided to assist you in contacting the respective airline personnel. In-country telephone numbers are included for each airline's home country e.g. Paris telephone number for Air France. Additional telephone numbers are included when in English-speaking countries such as Australia, Canada, Ireland, New Zealand, the United Kingdom and the United States.

Global Airline Contact Listings:
(Aer Lingus – Air Canada)

Airline	Country	Website	Phone Numbers
Aer Lingus	Ireland	http://www.aerlingus.com	in country- 0 1886 8844 UK- 0845 084 4444 Canada/US- 1 800 474 7424
Aeroflot	Russia	http://www.aeroflot.org	in country- 155 5045 UK- (44) 71 4911764 Ireland- 01 679 453 Australia- (61) 2 233 7911 Canada- 1 514 288 2125 US- 1 206 522 5995
Aerolineas	Argentina	http://www.aerolineas.com	in country- 0810 222 86527 UK- 020 7290 7887 Australia- 61 2 9234 9000 New Zealand- 64 9 379 3675 Canada/US- 1 800 333 0276
AeroMexico	Mexico	http://www.aeromexico.com	in country- 01 800 021 4050 UK- 020 7801 6234 Australia- 0 29 959 3922 New Zealand- 0 9 623 4294 Canada/US- 1 800 237 6639
Air Canada	Canada	http://www.aircanada.com	in country- 1 514 350 1086 UK- 0871 220 1111 Ireland- 0 1679 3958 Australia- 0 2 8248 5757 New Zealand- 0 9 969 7470 Canada/US- 1 888 247 2262

14

Global Airline Contact Listings:
(Air France – America West)

Airline	Country	Website	Phone Numbers
Air France	France	http://www.airfrance.com	in country- 0 820 820 820 UK- 0870 142 4343 Ireland- 01 605 0383 Australia- 1 300 361 400 Canada- 1 800 667 2747 US- 1 800 237 2747
Air India	India	http://www.airindia.com	in country- 22 22 79 6666 UK- 020 8745 1000 Australia- 02 928 34020 New Zealand- 09 303 1301 Canada/US- 1 800 223 7776
Air Malta	Malta	http://www.airmalta.com	in country- 0 2169 0890 UK- 020 8785 3199 Australia- 02 9244 2011; 1 800 756 2582 Canada- 1 877 23 MALTA US- 1 866 357 4155
Air New Zealand	New Zealand	http://www.airnewzealand.com	in country- 0 800 737 000 UK- 0 800 028 4149 Australia 13 24 76 Canada/US- 1 800 262 1234
Air Pacific	Fiji	http://www.airpacific.com	in country- (679) 6720888 UK- 0845 774 7767 Australia- 1 800 230 150 New Zealand- 0 800 800 178 Canada/US- 1 800 227 4446
Air Tahiti Nui	Tahiti	http://www.airtahitinui.com	in country- (689) 46 03 03 UK-(44) 1 239 59 6627 Australia- (61) 2 9244 2799 New Zealand- (64) 9 308 3360 Canada/US- 1 877 824 4846
Air Transat	Canada	http://www.airtransat.com	in country- 514 636 3630 UK- 0 800 283 87 673 US- 1 877 872 6728
Alitalia	Italy	http://www.alitalia.com	in country- Rome: 06 65 642 outside Rome: 84 88 65 642 UK- 0870 544 8259 Ireland- 01 677 5171 or 01 844 6035 Australia- 02 9244 2400 Canada/US 1 800 223 5730
America West	United States	http://www.americawest.com	North America- 1 800 235 9292 UK- 01483 440 490 Australia- 1 300 364 757

14

Global Airline Contact Listings:
(American Airlines – Continental Airlines)

Airline	Country	Website	Phone Numbers
American Airlines	United States	http://www.aa.com	North America- 1 800 433 7300 UK- 01293 555 400 Ireland- 01 602 0550 Australia- 1 300 650 747 New Zealand- 0 800 887 997
Asiana Airlines	South Korea	http://us.flyasiana.com	in country- 1588 8000 UK- 020 7514 0200 Australia- 1 300 767 234 New Zealand- 09 308 3359 Canada/US- 1 800 227 4262
Austrian Airlines	Austria	http://www.aua.com	in country- (43) (0) 5 1789 UK- 020 7766 0300 Ireland- 1 800 509 142 Australia- 800 642 438 Canada- 888 817 4444 US- 800 843 0002
Britannia Airways	United Kingdom	http://www.britanniaairways.com	in country- 0870 6076 0757
British Airways	United Kingdom	http://www.britishairways.com	in country- 0870 850 9850 Ireland- 1 890 626 747 Australia- 1 300 134 001 New Zealand- 09 966 9777 Canada/US- 1 800 247 9297
British Midland	United Kingdom	http://www.flybmi.com	in country- 01332 854000 Ireland- 0 1407 3036 Australia- 02 9922 3230 Canada/US- 1 800 788 0555
Cathay Pacific	Hong Kong	http://www.cathaypacific.com	in country- (852) 2747 1888 UK- 020 8834 8800 Australia- 131 747 New Zealand- 0 800 800 454 Canada/US- 1 800 233 2742
China Air	China	http://www.china-airlines.com	in country- 02 2715 1212 UK- 020 7436 9001 Australia- 1 300 668 052 Canada/US- 1 800 227 5118
Continental Airlines	United States	http://www.continental.com	North America- 1 800 523 3273 UK- 0845 607 6760 Ireland- 1890 925 252 Australia- 08 9229 9211

14

Global Airline Contact Listings:
(CSA Czech Airlines – Gulf Air)

Airline	Country	Website	Phone Numbers
CSA Czech Airlines	Czech Republic	http://www.csa.cz	in country- (420) 239 007 007 UK- 0870 444 3747 Ireland- 01 814 4626 Australia- 02 9247 7706 New Zealand- 31 20 62 00 719 Canada- Montreal: 1 514 844 4200 Toronto: 1 416 363 3174 US- 1 800 223 2365
Delta Airlines	United States	http://www.delta.com	North America- 1 800 241 4141 UK- 0 800 414 767 Ireland- 800 768 080 Australia- 1 300 302 849 New Zealand- 09 977 2232
El Al	Israel	http://www.elal.co.il	in country- 3 972 23 33 UK- 020 7957 4100 Ireland- 01 6704 731 Canada/US- 1 800 223 6700
Emirates	United Arab Emirates	http://www.emirates.com	in country- 2144 444 UK- 0870 243 2222 Australia- 1 300 303 777 New Zealand- 09 968 2200 Canada/US- 1 800 777 3999
Estonian Air	Estonia	http://www.estonian-air.com	in country- (372) 6401 163 UK- 020 7333 0196 Ireland- 01 844 4907 Canada 905 677 4295 US- 1 800 397 1354
Eurowings	Germany	http://www.eurowings.com	in country- 0231 92450
Eva Airways	Taiwan	http://www.evaair.com	incountry- 0 800 098 666 UK- 020 7380 8300 Australia- 02 9221 7055 New Zealand- 09 358 8300 Canada/US- 1 800 695 1188
Far Eastern Air Transport	Taiwan	http://www.fat.com.tw	in country- (886) 2 339 35388
Finnair	Finland	http://www.finnair.com	in country- (358) 9 818 7702 UK- 020 7629 4349 Ireland- 01 844 6565 Australia- 02 9244 2299 Canada/US- 1 800 950 5000
Gulf Air	Bahrain	http://www.gulfairco.com	in country- 17 335 777 UK- 0870 777 1717 Australia- 13 12 23 Canada/US- 1 888 359 4853

14

Global Airline Contact Listings:
(Iberia – Lufthansa)

Airline	Country	Website	Phone Numbers
Iberia	Spain	http://www.iberia.com	in country- 902 400 500; UK- 0845 850 9000; Ireland- 01 407 3017; Australia- 02 9244 2793; New Zealand- 09 630 7335; Canada/US- 1 800 772 4642
IcelandAir	Iceland	http://www.icelandair.com	in country- (354) 50 50 100 UK- 020 7874 1000; Australia- 02 9087 0244; Canada/US-1 800 223 5500
Japan Airlines	Japan	http://www.jal.com	in country- 0 120 25 59 31 UK- 0845 7747 700 Ireland- 0 1661 0749 Australia- 1 800 634 435 New Zealand- 09 379 3202 Canada/US- 1 800 525 3663
Kenya Airways	Kenya	http://www.kenya-airways.com	in country- (254) 2 327 4747 UK- 01784 888222 Canada/US- 1 866 536 9224
KLM/Northwest	Netherlands	http://www.klm.com	Netherlands- 020 474 7747 UK- 0870 507 4074 Australia- 300 303 747 New Zealand-09 309 1782 Canada/US- 1 800 374 7747
Korean Air	South Korea	http://www.korcanair.com	in country- 1588 2001 UK 0 800 41 3000 Ireland- 01 799 799 Australia- 02 9262 2009 New Zealand- 09 914 2000 Canada/US- 1 800 438 5000
LAN Airlines	Chile	http://www.lan.com	in country- 600 526 2000 UK- 0800 917 0572 Australia- 1 300 361 400 New Zealand- 09 977 2233 Canada/US- 1 866 435 9526
Lithuanian Airlines	Lithuania	http://www.lal.lt/en	in country- 8 800 25252 UK- 01293 579900 Canada/US- 1 877 454 8482
Lufthansa	Germany	http://www.lufthansa.com	in country- 0180 5 83 84 26 UK- 0845 773 7747 Ireland- 01 844 5544 Australia- 02 9367 3888 New Zealand- 0 800 945 220 Canada/US- 1 800 399 LUFT (5838)

14

Global Airline Contact Listings:
(Luxair – Swiss Int'l Airlines)

Airline	Country	Website	Phone Numbers
Luxair	Luxembourg	http://www.luxair.lu	in country- (352) 2456 4242 UK- 0800 38 99 443 Ireland 800 38 99 443
Malev	Hungary	http://www.malev.com	in country- 06 40 212121 UK- 0870 9090 577 Ireland- 01 844 4303 Canada/US- 1 800 262 5380
Olympic Airlines	Greece	http://www.olympicairlines.com	in country- 80 111 444 444 UK- 0870 6060 460 Australia- 02 9251 1048 Canada- 514 878 3891 US- 1 800 223 1226
Qantas	Australia	http://www.qantas.com	in country- 13 13 13 UK- 0845 7 747 767 Ireland- 01 407 3278 New Zealand- 0800 808 767 Canada/US- 1 800 227 4500
SAS	Sweden	http://www.scandinavian.net	in country- 0770 727 727 UK- 0870 60 727 727 Ireland- 01 844 5440 Australia-1 300 727 707 New Zealand- 09 977 2214 Canada/US- 1 800 221 2350
SATA	Portugal	http://www.sata.pt	in country- (351) 707 22 72 82 UK- 0870 6066 664 Canada- 1 800 387 0365 US-1 800 762 9995
Saudi Arabian Airlines	Saudi Arabia	http://www.saudiairlines.com	in country- 802 22222 UK- 020 7798 9890 Canada/US- 1 800 472 8342
Singapore Airlines	Singapore	http://www.singaporeair.com	in country- (65) 6223 8888 UK- 0870 608 8886 Ireland- 01 6710 722 Australia- 13 10 11 New Zealand- 04 499 0271 Canada/US- 1 800 742 3333
South African Airlines	South Africa	http://www.flysaa.com	in country- 0861 359 722 UK- 020 7312 5005 Australia- 13 12 23 New Zealand- 09 977 2237 Canada/US- 1 800 722 9675
Swiss Int'l Airlines	Switzerland	http://www.swiss.com	in country- 0848 85 2000 UK- 0845 601 0956 Ireland- 1 890 200 515 New Zealand- 09 977 2238 Canada/US- 1 877 359 7947

14

Global Airline Contact Listings:
(TAM Airlines – Virgin Atlantic)

Airline	Country	Website	Phone Numbers
TAM Airlines	Brazil	http://www.tamairlines.com	in country- 3123 1000/ 0 300 123 1000 UK- 0118 903 4003 Australia- 02 9232 5866 New Zealand- 09 308 5206 Canada/US- 1 888 235 9826
TAP Air Portugal	Portugal (UK)	http://www.tap-airportugal.com	in country- 707 205 700 UK- 0845 601 0932 Australia- 02 9244 2344 Canada/US- 1 800 221 7370
Thai Airways	Thailand	http://www.thaiair.com	in country- (66-2) 545 3690 92 UK- 0870 606 0911 Australia- 1 300 651 960 New Zealand- 09 377 3886 Canada/US- 1 800 426 5204
Turkish Airlines	Turkey	http://www.thy.com	in country- (90) 212 444 0 849 UK 020 7766 9300 Australia- 02 9299 8400 Canada/US- 1 800 874 8875
United Airlines	United States	http://www.unlted.com	North America- 1 800 241 6522 UK- 0845 8444 777 Ireland- 01 819 1761 Australia- 13 17 77 New Zealand- 0800 508 648
US Air	United States	http://www.usairways.com	North America- 1 800 428 4322 UK- 020 7484 2100 Ireland- 1 890 925 065 Australia- 02 9959 3922
Varig	Brazil	http://www.varigbrasil.com	in country- 0300 788 7000 UK- 0870 1203 020 Ireland- 01 819 1089 Australia- 02 9244 2179 Canada/US- 1 800 468 2744
Vietnam Airlines	Vietnam	http://www.vietnamairlines.com	in country- (84) 4 8320 320 UK- 0870 2240 211 Australia- 1 300 888 028 Canada- 1 416 599 6555 US- 1 415 677 0888
Virgin Atlantic	United Kingdom	http://www.virgin-atlantic.com	in country- 0870 5747 747 Ireland- 01 435 0055 Australia- 1 300 727 340 Canada/US- 1 800 862 8621

14

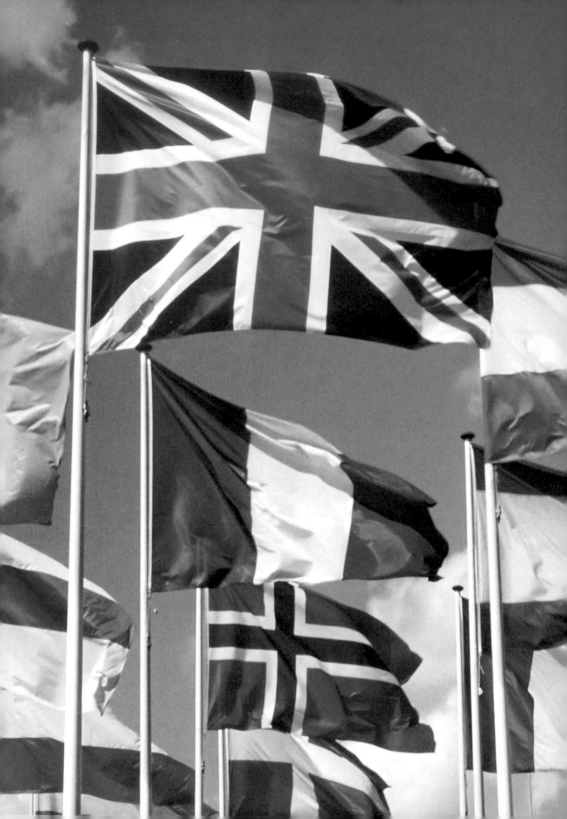

A journey of a thousand miles
begins with a single step.
—Lao Tzu

Chapter 15
Communicating Essential Multi-Lingual Phrases

Chapter Overview

These essential multi-lingual phrases represent four categories of information which you may want to communicate to health professionals and hospitality resources in restaurants, hotels, airlines, transportation, and cruise ships. Relevant phrases which may be needed while eating outside the home and traveling around the globe include:

- Food allergy phrases
- Dining phrases
- Health phrases

Each of these phrases has been translated into the following languages for your reference while traveling across the world:

- French
- German
- Italian
- Spanish

The food allergy phrases communicate:

- Allergic conditions

- 10 common food allergens

The dining phrases communicate:

- Introductions and common courtesies

- Special requests to ensure safe dining at lunch and dinner

- Clarification questions about ingredients and food preparation

The health phrases communicate:

- Types of health and store facilities

- Health professionals and symptoms

French Language Translations of Food Allergy Phrases

The following represents a partial list of phrases needed to communicate some allergy conditions and potential allergens including:

- General allergy conditions

- 10 common food allergens

English	Français
Allergy Conditions	**Conditions allergiques**
I have/am experiencing:	J'ai/je souffre:
an emergency	d'une situation de crise
anaphylactic shock	d'un choc anaphylactique
an allergic reaction	d'une réaction allergique
food allergies	d'allergies alimentaires
celiac/coeliac disease	d'une entéropathie au gluten
lactose intolerance	d'une intolérance au lactose
10 Common Allergens	**10 allergènes répandus**
I am allergic/ intolerant/hypersensitive to:	Je suis allergique/je ne tolère pas/je suis hypersensible:
corn	au maïs
dairy	aux laitages
eggs	aux œufs

English	Français
fish	au poisson
gluten	au gluten
milk	au lait
nuts	aux noix
peanuts	aux cacahuètes
shellfish	aux coquillages
soy	au soja
wheat	au blé

French Language Translations of Dining Phrases

The following represent relevant phrases needed to communicate special dietary considerations to chefs and servers in restaurants around the globe and include:

- Introductions and common courtesies

- Special requests to ensure safe dining

- Clarification questions to ensure against cross contamination

English	Français
Introductions	**Introductions**
Hello. I'm sorry, but I do not speak French.	Bonjour, je suis désolé(e), mais je ne parle pas français.
I need to special order my meal due to my food allergies	J'ai besoin d'une commande spéciale pour mon repas car j'ai des allergies alimentaires
I am on a medically prescribed allergy-free diet.	Je suis un régime médical évitant les aliments allergènes.
I need your assistance.	J'ai besoin de votre aide
Thank you for your help.	Merci pour votre aide.
I cannot eat these foods because I will become ill.	Je ne peux pas manger ces aliments parce que ça me rendrait malade.
I have a condition called celiac/coeliac ease.	Je souffre d'une maladie appelée disentéropathie au gluten.

15

English	**Français**
I cannot eat the smallest amount of gluten which is wheat, rye or barley.	Je ne peux pas absorber la moindre quantité de gluten, qu'il provienne du blé, du seigle ou de l'orge.

Foods that I can eat	**Les aliments que je peux consommer**
I can eat:	Je peux manger :
all kinds of fruit	toutes sortes de fruits
meat	de la viande
potatoes	des pommes de terre
rice	du riz
fresh stocks and broths	des bouillons frais et des consommés
all kinds of vegetables	toutes sortes de légumes
wine based vinegars	des vinaigres de vin
distilled vinegar	de vinaigre distill
rice flour or gluten-free noodles	de la farine de riz ou des pâtes sans gluten
sauce with butter, eggs, vegetables, olive oil, tomatoes, herbs	de la sauce avec du beurre, des œufs, des légumes, de l'huile, des tomates, des herbes

15

I prefer food that is:	Je préfère les plats qui sont :
broiled	grillés
grilled	grillés
pan fried	sautés à la poêle
roasted	rôtis
steamed	cuits à la vapeur

Could you suggest a few menu items that are safe for me to eat with my allergies?	Pouvez-vous me suggérer quelques plats du menu qui soient sans danger pour moi compte tenu de mes allergies ?

English	**Français**
Special Food Requests	**Demandes alimentaires spéciales**
Please:	S'il vous plait je voudrais:
salad dressing on the side	de la sauce de salade servie à part
sauce on the side	la sauce servie à part
plain	nature
No:	Non merci je ne prends pas:
bread	de pain
breading	de chapelure
bread crumbs	de miettes de pain
butter	de beurre
chocolate	de chocolat
corn starch	d'amidon
cream	de crème
croutons	de croûtons
ketchup	de ketchup
mayonnaise	de mayonnaise
pasta	de pâtes
peanut oil	d'huile d'arachide
salad dressing	de sauce pour salade
soy sauce	de sauce au soja
vegetable oil	d'huile végétale
corn tortilla	de tortilla au maïs
wheat flour tortilla	de tortilla à la farine de blé
No dish with wheat flour in the:	Pas de plat avec de la farine de blé, comme:
batter	de la pâte à frire
bouillon	du bouillon
meat/fish dusting	un farinage de viande/poisson
sauce	de la sauce
Do you have wheat free soy sauce?	Avez-vous de la sauce au soja sans blé ?

15

Clarification Points	**Points de clarification**
If you are uncertain about what the food contains, please tell me.	Si vous n'êtes pas sûr de ce que contiennent les plats, soyez gentil de me le dire.
Is this food dusted with wheat flour prior to cooking?	Est-ce que cet aliment est fariné à la farine de blé avant d'être cuit?

English	Français
Is this food cooked on the same grill as fish/meat cooked with breading?	Est-ce que cet aliment est cuit sur le même grill que d'autres poissons/ viandes préalablement enduits de chapelure?
Is this food fried in peanut oil?	Cet aliment est-il frit dans de l'huile d'arachide?
What type of garnishes are included in this dish?	Quels types de garnitures accompagnent ce plat?
What type of oil is used in the kitchen?	Quel est le type d'huile utilisé en cuisine?
Is this food fried in the same fryer as items fried with breading?	Cet aliment est-il cuit dans la même friteuse que des aliments enrobés de chapelure?
Please ask the chef whether the meal I have ordered is safe for me	Veuillez demander au chef de cuisine si le plat que j'ai commandé est sans danger pour moi.

French Language Translations of Health Phrases

The following represent relevant phrases needed to communicate special health considerations to medical professionals and hospitality staff while traveling around the globe. The health phrases include:

- Listing of health facilities
- Listing of health professionals
- Symptoms that may need to be communicated to medical professionals

English	Français
Health and Store Facilities	**Magasins de santé et paramédicaux**
I'm looking for/ need a:	Je cherche/j'ai besoin de trouver:
drug store	une parapharmacie
health food store	un magasin de produits diététiques
grocery store	une épicerie
hospital	l'hôpital
pharmacy	une pharmacie

15

English	Français
Health Professionals	**Professionnels de la santé**
I need to see/speak with a:	J'ai besoin de consulter/de parler à :
doctor	un docteur
dietician	un diététicien
nutritionist	un nutritionniste
pediatrician	un pédiatre
pharmacist	un pharmacien

Symptoms	**Symptômes**
I have severe/moderate:	Je souffre de façon sévère/modérée :
abdominal bloating	de ballonnements
abdominal cramping	de crampes abdominales
acid reflux	de reflux acide
asthma	d'asthme
bone/ joint pain	de douleur osseuse/articulaire
constipation	de constipation
diarrhea	de diarrhée
eczema	d'eczéma
fatigue	de fatigue
flatulence (gas)	de flatulence (gaz)
headaches	de maux de tête
hives	d'urticaire
migraines	de migraines
mouth ulcers	d'aphtes buccaux
nausea	de nausées
rash	d'éruption cutanée soudaine
seizures	de crises épileptiques
sinus infection	de sinusite
vomiting	de vomissements
wheezing	des troubles respiratoires

15

German Language Translations of Food Allergy Phrases

The following represents a partial list of phrases needed to communicate some allergy conditions and potential allergens and include:

- General allergy conditions

- 10 common food allergens

English **Allergy Conditions**	**Deutsch** **Allergische Reaktionen**
I have/am experiencing:	Ich habe/bin:
an emergency	einen Notfall
anaphylactic shock	anaphylaktischen Schock
an allergic reaction	eine allergische Reaktion
food allergies	Lebensmittelallergien
celiac/coeliac disease	Bauch-/Intestinalerkrankung
lactose intolerance	Laktoseintoleranz

10 Common Allergens	**10 häufige Allergene**
I am allergic/intolerant/hypersensitive to:	Ich bin allergisch/unverträglich/ überempfindlich gegen:
corn	Mais
dairy	Milchprodukte
eggs	Eier
fish	Fisch
gluten	Gluten
milk	Milch
nuts	Nüsse
peanuts	Erdnüsse
shellfish	Schalentiere
soy	Soja
wheat	Weizen

15

German Language Translations of Dining Phrases

The following represent relevant phrases needed to communicate special dietary considerations to chefs and servers in restaurants around the globe and include:

- Introductions and common courtesies

- Special requests to ensure safe dining

- Clarification questions to ensure against cross contamination

English	Deutsch

Introductions

Einleitungen

Hello. I'm sorry, but I do not speak German.

Hallo. Ich spreche leider kein Deutsch.

I need to special order my meal due to my food allergies

Ich muss wegen meiner Lebensmittelallergie eine Sonderbestellung aufgeben

I am on a medically prescribed allergy-free diet.

Mir wurde vom Arzt eine allergenfreie Diät vorgeschrieben.

I need your assistance.

Ich brauche Ihre Hilfe.

Thank you for your help.

Danke für Ihre Hilfe.

I cannot eat these foods because I will become ill.

Ich darf diese Lebensmittel nicht essen, weil ich davon krank werde.

I have a condition called celiac/coeliac disease.

Ich leide unter Verdauungsstörungen.

I cannot eat the smallest amount of gluten which is wheat, rye or barley.

Ich darf keinerlei Gluten zu mir nehmen. Gluten sind im Weizen, Roggen und Gerste enthalten.

Foods that I can eat

Lebensmittel, die ich essen darf

I can eat:

Ich darf essen:

all kinds of fruit — jedes Obst

meat — Fleisch

potatoes — Kartoffeln

rice — Reis

fresh stocks and broths — frische Brühe und Bouillon

all kinds of vegetables — jedes Gemüse

wine based vinegars — Weinessige

15

English	Deutsch
distilled vinegar	Branntweinessig
rice flour or gluten-free noodles	Reismehl oder glutenfreie Nudeln
sauce with butter, eggs, vegetables, olive oil, tomatoes, herbs	Soße aus Butter, Eiern, Gemüse, Olivenöl, Tomaten, Kräutern

I prefer food that is:

Ich möchte mein Essen:

broiled	gebraten
grilled	gegrillt
pan fried	kurzgebraten
roasted	geschmort
steamed	gedämpft

Could you suggest a few menu items that are safe for me to eat with my allergies?

Können Sie mir einige Gerichte empfehlen, die trotz meiner Allergie für mich geeignet sind?

Special Food Requests

Please:

Sonderwünsche bei der Bestellung im Restaurant

Bitte:

sauce on the side	Soße auf einem Extrateller
plain	keine Soße

No:

Kein/e:

bread	Brot
breading	Panade
bread crumbs	Semmelbrösel
butter	Butter
chocolate	Schokolade
corn starch	Maisstärke
cream	Sahne
croutons	Croutons
ketchup	Ketchup
mayonnaise	Mayonnaise
pasta	Pasta
peanut oil	Erdnussöl
salad dressing	Salatsoße
soy sauce	Sojasoße
vegetable oil	Pflanzenöl
corn tortilla	Maistortilla
wheat flour tortilla	Weizenmehltortilla

15

English	**Deutsch**
No dish with wheat flour in the:	Kein Gericht mit Weizenmehl in/an der/dem:
batter	Teig
bouillon	Bouillon
meat/fish dusting	Fleisch/Fisch
sauce	Soße

Do you have wheat free soy sauce? — Haben Sie weizenfreie Sojasoße?

Clarification Points / Klarstellungspunkte

English	**Deutsch**
If you are uncertain about what the food contains, please tell me.	Wenn Sie nicht sicher sind, was das jeweilige Lebensmittel enthält, sagen Sie es mir bitte.
Is this food dusted with wheat flour prior to cooking?	Wird dieses Lebensmittel vor dem Kochen mit Weizenmehl bepudert?
Is this food cooked on the same grill as fish/meat cooked with breading?	Wird dieses Lebensmittel auf dem gleichen Grill wie panierter/s Fisch/Fleisch gegrillt?
Is this food fried in peanut oil?	Wird dieses Lebensmittel in Erdnussöl gebraten?
What type of garnishes are included in this dish?	Welche Beilagen sind in diesem Gericht enthalten?
What type of oil is used in the kitchen?	Welches Öl wird in Ihrer Küche verwendet?
Is this food fried in the same fryer as items fried with breading?	Wird dieses Lebensmittel im gleichen Fritiergerät wie panierte Lebensmittel frittiert?
Please ask the chef whether the meal I have ordered is safe for me	Bitte fragen Sie Ihren Koch, ob ich dieses Gericht trotz meiner Allergie bestellen kann.

15

German Language Translations of Health Phrases

The following represent relevant phrases needed to communicate special health considerations to medical professionals and hospitality staff while traveling around the globe. The health phrases include:

- Listing of health facilities

- Listing of health professionals

- Symptoms that may need to be communicated to medical professionals

English
Health and Store Facilities
I'm looking for/ need a:
    drug store
    health food store
    grocery store
    hospital
    pharmacy

Health Professionals
I need to see/speak with a:
    doctor
    dietician

    nutritionist
    pediatrician
    pharmacist

Symptoms
I have severe/moderate:
    abdominal bloating
    abdominal cramping
    acid reflux
    asthma
    bone/ joint pain
    constipation
    diarrhea
    eczema
    fatigue
    flatulence (gas)
    headaches
    hives

Deutsch
Medizinische Einrichtung und Läden
Ich suche nach einer/einem:
    Drogerie
    Reformhaus
    Lebensmittelgeschäft
    Krankenhaus
    Apotheke

Auf medizinischem Gebiet tätige Personen
Ich brauche/möchte zu einem:
    Arzt
    Diätassistenten/Ernährungs wissen
      schaftler
    Diätetiker/Ernährungsberater
    Kinderarzt
    Apotheker

Symptome
Ich habe starke/n/s - mittlere/n/s:
    Blähungen
    Bauchkrämpfe
    Sodbrennen
    Asthma
    Knochen-/Gelenkschmerzen
    Verstopfung
    Durchfall
    Ekzeme
    Ermüdungserscheinungen
    Flatulenz (Darmgasbildung)
    Kopfschmerzen
    Nesselsucht

15

English	**Deutsch**
migraines	Migräne
mouth ulcers	Mundgeschwüre
nausea	Übelkeit
rash	Hautausschlag
seizures	Anfälle
sinus infection	Stirnhöhleninfektion
vomiting	Erbrechen
wheezing	keuchende Atmung

Italian Language Translations of Food Allergy Phrases

The following represents a partial list of phrases needed to communicate some allergy conditions and potential allergens and include:

- General allergy conditions

- 10 common food allergens

English	**Italiano**
Allergy Conditions	**Stato allergico**
I have/am experiencing:	Soffro di/mi trovo in:
an emergency	un'emergenza
anaphylactic shock	shock anafilattico
an allergic reaction	reazione allergica
food allergies	allergie alimentari
celiac/coeliac disease	celiachia
lactose intolerance	intolleranza al lattosio
10 Common Allergens	**10 più comuni allergeni**
I am allergic/intolerant/hypersensitive to:	Ho un'allergia/intolleranza/ipersensibilità a:
corn	granturco
dairy	latticini
eggs	uova
fish	pesce
gluten	glutine
milk	latte
nuts	noci
peanuts	arachidi
shellfish	crostacei
soy	soia
wheat	frumento

15

Italian Language Translations of Dining Phrases

The following represent relevant phrases needed to communicate special dietary considerations to chefs and servers in restaurants around the globe and include:

- Introductions and common courtesies
- Special requests to ensure safe dining
- Clarification questions to ensure against cross contamination

English	Italiano
Introductions	**Frasi di circostanza**
Hello. I'm sorry, but I do not speak Italian	Salve. Mi dispiace, non parlo italiano.
I need to special order my meal due to my food allergies	Soffro di allergie alimentari, quindi devo ordinare cibi particolari.
I am on a medically prescribed allergy-free diet.	Il mio medico mi ha prescritto una dieta priva di allergeni.
I need your assistance.	Ho bisogno del suo aiuto.
Thank you for your help.	Grazie per la cortesia.
I cannot eat these foods because I will become ill.	Non posso mangiare questi cibi, perché potrebbero farmi stare male.
I have a condition called celiac/coeliac disease.	Soffro di un disturbo chiamato celiachia
I cannot eat the smallest amount of gluten which is wheat, rye or barley.	Non posso mangiare glutine, che è contenuto nel frumento, nella segale, e nell'orzo neppure in minime quantità.
Foods that I can eat	**Cibi permessi**
I can eat:	Posso mangiare:
all kinds of fruit	tutti i tipi di frutta
meat	carne
potatoes	patate

English	Italiano
rice	riso
fresh stocks and broths	consommè e brodo fresco
all kinds of vegetables	tutti i tipi di verdure
wine based vinegars	aceti a base di vino
distilled vinegar	aceto distillato
rice flour or gluten-free noodles	spaghetti di farina di riso o senza glutine
sauce with butter, eggs, vegetables, olive oil, tomatoes, herbs	salsa a base di burro, uova, verdure, olio d'oliva, pomodori, erbe

I prefer food that is:	Preferisco i cibi:
broiled	ai ferri
grilled	grigliati
pan fried	fritti in padella
roasted	arrostiti
steamed	al vapore

Could you suggest a few menu items that are safe for me to eat with my allergies?	Potrebbe consigliarmi dei piatti del menu adatti nonostante le mie allergie?

Special Food Requests — Richieste speciali

Please:	Per favore:
salad dressing on the side	condimento per l'insalata a parte
sauce on the side	salsa a parte
plain	senza condimenti

15

No:	Niente:
bread	pane
breading	pan grattato
bread crumbs	molliche di pane
butter	burro
chocolate	cioccolato
corn starch	amido di granturco
cream	panna
croutons	crostini
ketchup	ketchup

English	Italiano
mayonnaise	maionese
pasta	pasta
peanut oil	olio di arachidi
salad dressing	condimento per l'insalata
soy sauce	salsa di soia
vegetable oil	olio vegetale
corn tortilla	tortilla di granturco
wheat flour tortilla	tortilla di farina di frumento

No dish with wheat flour in the:	Nessun piatto con farina di frumento nella/nel:
batter	pastella
bouillon	brodo
meat/fish dusting	insaporitore per carne/pesce
sauce	salsa

Do you have wheat free soy sauce?	Avete salsa di soia senza frumento?

Clarification Points

Chiarimenti

If you are uncertain about what the food contains, please tell me.	Se non sa con certezza cosa contengono i cibi, la prego di dirmelo.
Is this food dusted with wheat flour prior to cooking?	Prima della cottura questo cibo viene infarinato con farina di frumento?
Is this food cooked on the same grill as fish/meat cooked with breading?	Questo cibo viene cotto sulla stessa griglia su cui vengono cotti pesce/carni impanate?
Is this food fried in peanut oil?	Questo cibo viene cotto con olio di arachidi?
What type of garnishes are included in this dish?	Che contorni vengono serviti con questo piatto?
What type of oil is used in the kitchen?	Che tipo di olio usate in cucina?
Is this food fried in the same fryer as items fried with breading?	Questo cibo viene cotto nella stessa friggitrice usata per i cibi?
Please ask the chef whether the meal I have ordered is safe for me	Può chiedere allo chef se il cibo che ho ordinato è sicuro per me?

15

Italian Language Translations of Health Phrases

The following represent relevant phrases needed to communicate special health considerations to medical professionals and hospitality staff while traveling around the globe. The health phrases include:

- Listing of health facilities
- Listing of health professionals
- Symptoms that may need to be communicated to medical professionals

English	Italiano
Health and Store Facilities	**Strutture sanitarie e negozi**
I'm looking for/ need a:	Sto cercando/mi serve un/una:
drug store	negozio di generi vari (parafarmaceutici)
health food store	negozio di prodotti biologici
grocery store	drogheria
hospital	ospedale
pharmacy	farmacia
Health Professionals	**Personale sanitario**
I need to see/speak with a:	Devo vedere/parlare con un:
doctor	medico
dietician	dietologo
nutritionist	nutrizionista
pediatrician	pediatra
pharmacist	farmacista
Symptoms	**Sintomi**
I have severe/moderate:	Soffro in modo grave/leggero di:
abdominal bloating	gonfiore addominale
abdominal cramping	crampi addominali
acid reflux	riflusso acido
asthma	asma
bone/ joint pain	dolori alle ossa/giunture
constipation	stipsi
diarrhea	diarrea
eczema	eczema
fatigue	affaticamento
flatulence (gas)	flatulenza (gas)
headaches	mal di testa
hives	orticaria

15

English	Italiano
migraines	emicranie
mouth ulcers	ulcere della bocca
nausea	nausea
rash	rash cutaneo
seizures	attacchi
sinus infection	sinusite
vomiting	vomito
wheezing	affanno

Spanish Language Translations of Food Allergy Phrases

The following represents a partial list of phrases needed to communicate some allergy conditions and potential allergens and include:

- General allergy conditions

- 10 common food allergens

English	Español
Allergy Conditions	**Problemas alérgicos**
I have/am experiencing:	Estoy experimentando:
an emergency	una emergencia
anaphylactic shock	un choque anafiláctico
an allergic reaction	una reacción alérgica
food allergies	alergia a los alimentos
celiac/coeliac disease	una enfermedad celíaca
lactose intolerance	intolerancia a la lactosa

English	Español
10 Common Allergens	**10 alérgenos comunes**
I am allergic/ intolerant/hypersensitive to:	Soy alérgico o hipersensible:
corn	al maíz
dairy	a los productos lácteos
eggs	a los huevos
fish	al pescado
gluten	al gluten
milk	a la leche
nuts	a las nueces
peanuts	al cacahuates
shellfish	a los mariscos
soy	a la soya
wheat	al trigo

15

Spanish Translations of Dining Phrases

The following represent relevant phrases needed to communicate special dietary considerations to chefs and servers in restaurants around the globe and include:

- Introductions and common courtesies
- Special requests to ensure safe dining
- Clarification questions to ensure against cross contamination

English	Español
Introductions	**Introducciones**
Hello. I'm sorry, but I do not speak Spanish.	¡Hola! Lo siento, pero no hablo español.
I need to special order my meal due to my food allergies	Necesito pedir una comida especial, debido a mis alergias a los alimentos
I am on a medically prescribed allergy-free diet.	El médico me ha puesto a un régimen que no me cause alergias.
I need your assistance.	Necesito que me ayude.
Thank you for your help.	Gracias por su ayuda.
I cannot eat these foods because I will become ill.	No puedo comer estos alimentos, porque me enfermaré
I have a condition called celiac/cocliac disease.	Tengo un a problema, llamado "la enfermedad celíaca".
I cannot eat the smallest amount of gluten which is wheat, rye or barley.	No puedo comer ni la más mínima cantidad de gluten que provenga del trigo, el centeno o la cebada.

15

Foods that I can eat	**Alimentos que puedo comer**
I can eat:	Puedo comer:
all kinds of fruit	toda clase de frutas
meat	carne
potatoes	patatas
rice	arroz

English	**Español**
fresh stocks and broths	extractos y caldos frescos
all kinds of vegetables	toda clase de verduras
wine based vinegars	vinagres de vino
distilled vinegar	vinagre destilado
rice flour or gluten-free noodles	fideos de harina de arroz o sin gluten
sauce with butter, eggs, vegetables, olive oil, tomatoes, herbs	salsas con mantequilla, huevos, verduras, aceite de oliva, tomates y yerbas

I prefer food that is:
  broiled
  grilled
  pan fried
  roasted
  steamed

Prefiero alimentos:
  asados al fuego
  asados a la parrilla
  fritos en sartén
  asados al horno
  al vapor

Could you suggest a few menu items that are safe for me to eat with my allergies?

¿Podría recomendarme algunos platos de su menú, que pueda comer sin peligro, con mis alergias?

Special Food Requests

Please:
  salad dressing on the side
  sauce on the side
  plain

Solicitudes especiales

Por favor:
  el aliño de la ensalada aparte
  la salsa aparte
  puro, sin mezcla

No:
  bread
  breading
  bread crumbs
  butter
  chocolate.
  corn starch
  cream
  croutons
  ketchup
  mayonnaise

Nada de:
  pan
  empanizado
  miga de pan
  mantequilla
  chocolate
  fécula de maíz
  crema
  trocitos de pan frito
  salsa de tomate
  mayonesa

15

English	**Español**
pasta	pasta
peanut oil	aceite de cacahuate
salad dressing	aliño para la ensalada
soy sauce	salsa de soya
vegetable oil	aceite vegetal
corn tortilla	tortilla de maíz
wheat flour tortilla	tortilla de harina de trigo

No dish with wheat flour in the:	Ningún ingrediente con harina de trigo:
batter	en la pasta culinaria
bouillon	en el caldo
meat/fish dusting	para espolvorear la carne o el pescado
sauce	en la salsa

Do you have wheat free soy sauce?	¿Tiene salsa de soya sin trigo?

Clarification Points / Aclaraciones

Clarification Points	**Aclaraciones**
If you are uncertain about what the food contains, please tell me.	Si tiene cualquier duda acera de lo que contienen los alimentos, por favor dígamelo.
Is this food dusted with wheat flour prior to cooking?	¿Se espolvorean estos alimentos con harina de trigo, antes de cocinarlos?
Is this food cooked on the same grill as fish/meat cooked with breading?	¿Se cocina esta comida en la misma parrilla que la carne empanizada?
Is this food fried in peanut oil?	¿Se fríe esta comida en aceite de cacahuate?
What type of garnishes are included in this dish?	¿Qué tipo de aderezos trae este plato?
What type of oil is used in the kitchen?	¿Qué tipo de aceite se utiliza en la cocina?
Is this food fried in the same fryer as items fried with breading?	¿Se fríe esta comida en la misma sartén que los platos apanados fritos?
Please ask the chef whether the meal I have ordered is safe for me	Por favor, pregúntele al cocinero si la comida que he pedido es peligrosa para mí.

15

Spanish Language Translations of Health Phrases

The following represent relevant phrases needed to communicate special health considerations to medical professionals and hospitality staff while traveling around the globe. The health phrases include:

- Listing of health facilities
- Listing of health professionals
- Symptoms that may need to be communicated to medical professionals

English
Health and Store Facilities
I'm looking for/ need a:
   drug store
   health food store
   grocery store
   hospital
   pharmacy

Español
Centros médicos y tiendas de productos médicos
Busco o "necesito":
   una droguería
   una tienda de alimentos dietéticos
   una tienda de víveres
   un hospital
   una farmacia

Health Professionals
I need to see/speak with a:
   doctor
   dietician
   nutritionist
   pediatrician
   pharmacist

Profesionales de la salud
Necesito consultar a: (o "hablar con":)
   un médico
   un dietista
   un especialista en nutrición
   un pediatra
   un farmaceuta

Symptoms
I have severe/moderate:
   abdominal bloating
   abdominal cramping
   acid reflux
   asthma
   bone/ joint pain
   constipation
   diarrhea
   eczema
   fatigue
   flatulence (gas)
   headaches
   hives
   migraines

Síntomas
Tengo:...intensa(o) o moderada(o)
   distensión abdominal
   contracciones dolorosas abdominales
   reflujo ácido
   asma intensa
   dolor en los huesos o articulaciones
   estreñimiento
   diarrea
   eczema
   fatiga
   flatulencia (gases)
   dolores de cabeza
   urticaria
   migrañas

15

English	**Español**
mouth ulcers	úlceras en la boca
nausea	náusea
rash	erupción cutánea
seizures	convulsiones
sinus infection	infección de los senos nasales
vomiting	vómito
wheezing	sibilancia

15

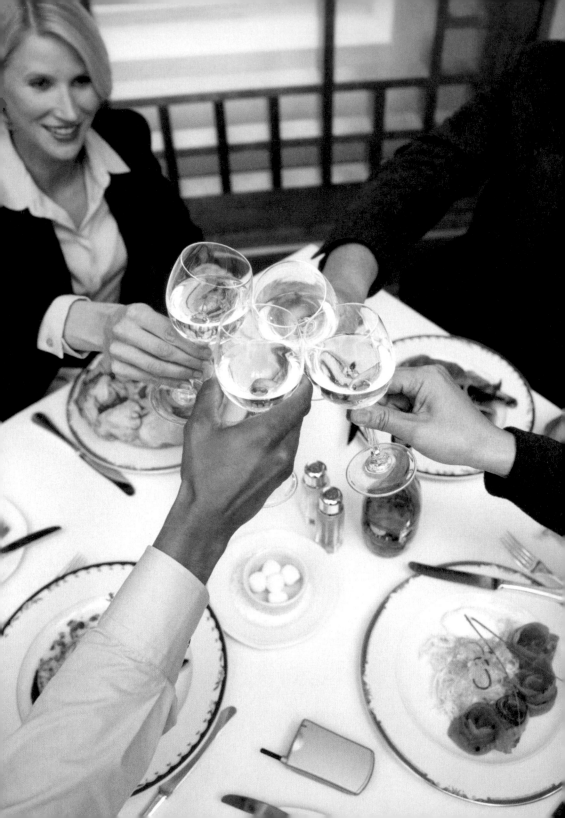

*Life is a succession of lessons
which must be lived to be understood.*
—Helen Keller

Chapter 16

Embracing the Gluten and Allergy Free Life: Our Personal Perspectives

Chapter Overview

This chapter provides our first hand insights and experiences reflecting:

- Journey to living the gluten and allergy free life—Kim's perspective

- Dealing with specialized diets: The other side of the table—Robert's perspective

16

Journey to Living the Gluten and Allergy Free Life—Kim's Perspective

I view life as a series of journeys which lead to new adventures. Every journey has its ups and downs from positive moments that you always want to savor to those so painful that you want to forget. Journeys and adventures typically take unexpected twists and turns,

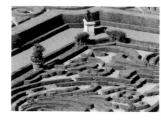

giving us the opportunity to learn something about ourselves, others and even life in general. The only failures in life, from my perspective, are when we do not learn from these opportunities.

I've definitely had my fair share of twists and turns with their accompanying lessons along the way. These range from dozens of food and environmental allergies, millions of miles of global travel, 12 orthopedic surgeries, years of misdiagnosis and finally celiac/coeliac disease. Writing this book has forced me to summarize my experiences and make sense of them. It's amazing how much I had forgotten or blocked out of my mind until now.

Although many of my lessons have been extremely challenging, I think of them as gifts, something to be appreciated. Looking back, I am now very thankful for each of these experiences, which have led to my current path in life. I'd like to share some of these with you in the hope that my experiences may help you through your unique journeys of health, adventure and travel in some way.

I have organized my journeys over the years into the following five areas:

- Early evidence of allergies and intolerances

- Journeys in traveling

- My soap opera in sports

- Discovery and diagnosis

- Living the gluten and allergy free life

Early Evidence of Allergies and Intolerances

Ever since I was a young girl, I've been allergic to cats, fish and seafood. My throat starts to close, my eyes water and breathing is difficult. Sometimes, I feel nauseous, start sneezing and wheezing. In my teenage years, after experiencing skin reactions, it was determined through the process of elimination that I was allergic to goose feathers as well as some additives in detergents, soaps, creams and make-up.

In my mid 20's, I had swollen and blood shot eyes. Again, through the process of elimination, my optometrist determined that this was an allergic reaction to thimersol, a chemical in some saline solutions for contact lenses. It still makes me laugh thinking about the questions I received from friends concerning my appearance during that time!

In my late 20's, I experienced bladder issues which were extremely rare for my age. After visiting numerous specialists and extensive testing, I consulted with my general physician. Based on her recommendation, I removed caffeine as the first part of my elimination diet. My condition improved slightly; however, the symptoms were still occurring. Next, she identified another potential culprit—aspartame. After eliminating all foods with aspartame from my diet, the issues were immediately resolved. I was so relieved that we had finally figured it out. I am eternally grateful to this physician for identifying the causes of these symptoms.

A few months later, I realized that I had the tendency to get sick within 30 to 60 minutes after eating Chinese food. Once again, through the process of elimination and investigation, we determined that Monosodium Glutamate (MSG) was the cause of my reactions.

Another situation occurred within a few minutes of receiving anesthesia for one of my surgeries. My throat started to close up and my breathing became extremely labored. Realizing that I was having an allergic reaction, I found out that they had given me penicillin. Luckily, I remembered that my great aunt had died from a shot of penicillin, so I was grateful for the injection that they gave me which immediately counteracted my reaction. Looking back, these may have been early warning signs of things to come. I just wasn't aware of my level of sensitivities at the time. In hindsight, there was a definite pattern emerging which unfortunately took over 15 years to fully decipher.

16

Journeys in Traveling

I've always been very fascinated by new places, people and cultures. The first time I realized my love for traveling was when I was five years old and my family drove to my Aunt Greta's farm in Ohio from Chicago. Throughout my childhood, for two weeks every summer, my family and I trekked throughout the United

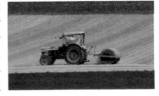

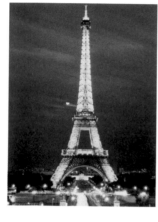

States and Canada in a camper trailer, exploring different destinations and experiencing new adventures. I loved it. For my 8th grade graduation present, my parents gave me the choice of flying to New York to visit relatives or a new bicycle. I chose the trip, of course, and still remember where I was sitting on the plane to this day!

Hearing my grandparents occasionally recite phrases in French and German always intrigued me. I started taking French lessons at the age of 13 and adored learning languages. One of my teachers in high school even taught me Spanish in her spare time after class. My first trip to Europe was at the age of 16 with my French class as an early high school graduation present. After falling in love with Paris, my new criteria for choosing a university focused on two areas: a study abroad program and a Big 10 sports program.

During my third year of college, I lived in Strasbourg, France and studied all of my courses in French. My diet primarily consisted of baguettes (French bread), petit pains au chocolat (chocolate croissants), yogurt and cheese. I backpacked through Europe, played tour guide when friends and family came to visit and felt great physically. To this day, I still meet friends in Paris one or two times a year to enjoy the culture and, of course, the outdoor cafés.

After graduating from Purdue University with a Bachelor of Arts Degree in French and a minor in Management, I worked in the world of business with domestic clients for six years. Upon earning my Masters in Business Administration with a specialization in International Management from Thunderbird, the Garvin School of International Management, I started my career at Accenture in contact center consulting. Leveraging my US-based expertise in technology, I worked with clients all over the world on a regular basis.

Discovering life and cultures in South America, Europe and Australia was extremely rewarding, both personally and professionally. I lived in Sao Paulo for seven months, Sydney for five months, Turin for three months and numerous European locations such as Geneva, London, Munich and Prague for one to two months. While living in these countries, I learned con-

16

versational skills in German, Italian and Portuguese. Throughout this time, I continued to avoid foods that I knew didn't agree with me and managed my knee-related problems.

Working in North America, my travel typically involved flying two to eight times a week. I consulted with clients all over the country from New York to San Francisco, Dallas to Toronto, Los Angeles to Washington DC and everywhere in between. I also played tour guide in the US and across the globe on numerous occasions for friends and family. I loved every minute of it. Over the past 20-plus years, I have flown over 1.5 million air miles to more than 25 countries and have eaten at least 80% of my meals in restaurants.

As glamorous as this may sound, it required a lot of energy, especially during my recuperation from four knee surgeries. While traveling from continent to continent, I was in more planes and taxis with crutches and pushed in more wheelchairs through airports than I ever care to remember. It still makes me laugh when I think of the look on some of our clients' faces as they tried to understand why I walked into strategic business meetings wearing a business suit and tennis shoes.

My Soap Opera in Sports

Since childhood, the two things that I've been most passionate about are traveling and sports. From a sports perspective, I was a healthy athletic child, teenager and young adult who loved volleyball, tennis, cheerleading, softball, basketball, swimming, diving, surfing and yes, even baton twirling. I experienced my fair share of broken bones including elbow, collarbone, fingers and wrist. These were all typical injuries due to athletics and I took them in stride.

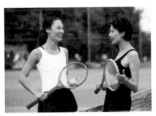

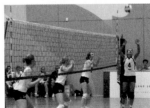

16

In celebration of our 30th birthdays, my friends and I completed our first team relay triathlon. Swimming in Lake Michigan for a mile was a challenge for me since I already had overcome two knee surgeries due to skiing and volleyball as well as four forearm reconstructive surgeries as a result of a severe car accident. Over the next few years, our teams of family and friends accomplished a total of three relay triathlons and had lots of fun in the process!

By my mid 30's, due to continuous pain and instability, I was required to have three more knee surgeries within three and a half years, just to walk. My first was arthroscopic to repair my cartilage. The second was an Anterior Cruciate Ligament (ACL) reconstruction requiring 6 ½ hours of surgery and 10 months of physical therapy to walk again. I gained weight and felt continuous abdominal bloating. I never regained the energy level that I had before this surgery.

During this time, I began experiencing acid reflux, cramping, diarrhea, flatulence, vomiting, heartburn, and indigestion. On top of all this, my third knee surgery was an ACL on the other knee, requiring three hours of surgery and five months of physical therapy. In hindsight, these traumas may have potentially triggered my gluten conditions, which were yet to be diagnosed.

Based upon my surgeries and injuries, I began an in-depth exploration of Eastern and alternative practices. These included acupuncture, Chinese medicine, herbs, reiki, reflexology and massage therapy. The combination of Eastern and Western practices with health professionals helped me recover from these injuries. However, no matter what we tried, I couldn't regain my energy level or lose the excess weight. My only "exercise" was physical therapy, restricted swimming and minimal walking. If that wasn't enough, I had to have one more knee surgery to remove the screws from my previous reconstruction requiring more anesthesia and more physical therapy.

By this time, I had grown weary of recuperating from surgeries and physical therapy. I chose boxing as my new sport to challenge myself and jumpstart my metabolism. With the patience and support of Eriks, my boxing coach, my endurance increased with semi-private boxing lessons. Finally, my first new sport in years and a great change of pace from all the injuries! Hoorah!

My excitement was short-lived as a year and a half later I lost the range of motion in my arm and could only lift it a few inches from my body. After a month of testing, the doctors determined that I needed two rotator cuff surgeries in a matter of 4 ½ months caused

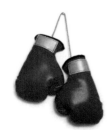

by bone spurs. I was also still experiencing stiffness, muscle cramps and inflamed joints. So back to physical therapy, walking and swimming once again.

A few years later, I was diagnosed with celiac/coeliac disease and dozens of allergies described in the next section. Finally, after following a strict gluten and allergy-free diet for two years, I started feeling as though my body was repairing itself and getting stronger. Being the athlete, I wanted to test myself from a health perspective. Could I complete another mile swim in Lake Michigan as part of a relay triathlon team after all of my surgeries, physical therapy and most recent diagnoses?

My friends and I decided to go for it. In 2004, I finished the mile swim in the largest triathlon in the US. I wish that I could say that my finishing time was stellar—unfortunately that was not the case. I was one of the last people out of Lake Michigan that day. Nevertheless, the sense of accomplishment was incredible and I achieved my goal. My journey to health had finally come full circle after 15 years of challenges, pain and great struggle. My soap opera in sports was now over. Since this time, I have continued to enjoy boxing, swimming, weight training, scuba diving and more team triathlons!

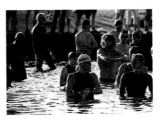

As my Dad always said, "You can accomplish anything you set your mind to as long as you're willing to work for it. It's just a matter of attitude and how determined you are to succeed to the best of your ability."

Discovery and Diagnosis

Throughout my surgeries and recuperation, my digestion, respiratory and skin related issues continued to escalate. After constant abdominal pain and diarrhea, I was so weak that I had to be driven to the doctor who immediately scheduled me for a colonoscopy. The doctor found polyps in my colon and diagnosed me with ulcerative colitis, leaky gut and Crohn's disease.

After careful analysis, I found health professionals that specialized in digestive disorders. Based upon more testing, a strict regimen of a bland diet, protein drinks, sulphasalazine, herbs and various supplements

16

was recommended. My insides were finally starting to repair themselves and my energy level was improving slightly. I still felt as though my food was not being processed appropriately, but at least my body was getting somewhat better with my symptoms occurring less frequently.

My acupuncturist, who was also an MD, began assessing the cause of my joint pain and bone spurs. She asked about my consumption of dairy which I ate on a daily basis. Needless to say, I loved milk, yogurt, cheese and cottage cheese. Upon her recommendation, I eliminated dairy from my diet and immediately began to feel a difference in my joints and my throat. I felt better and decided to avoid dairy since I never wanted to endure another surgery again!

While traveling, I was also getting sick within 30 to 60 minutes after eating airplane meals and snacks due to preservatives. I started to eliminate various foods from my diet and focus on listening to how my body responded to different foods. I followed some rotation diet recommendations including vegetables, fruits, pastas and meats. Unfortunately, at this point, I was totally unaware of any hidden allergens in foods. Although I thought I had eliminated specific potential allergens from my diet, in reality, I had not.

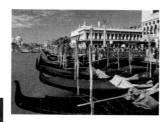

During this time, I lived in Italy. I ate incredible pasta, Italian bread, salamis and salads. My favorite meals were Veal Milanese, Chicken Parmiagana and Beef Medallions with sauce. While home in the States for a week at a time, I would avoid these foods because I enjoyed them so much more in Italy. By the end of each week in the States, I realized that I felt a bit better. Back in Italy, I continued eating my favorite foods and experienced bloating, cramping, flatulence and indigestion again. I remember thinking that my reactions were a bit unusual and maybe I just needed to reduce my amount of pasta, which I did.

I also found myself eating Mylanta, ginger, turmeric and other digestive aids on a daily basis. I was still experiencing very low energy, fatigue and lethargy. All of a sudden, extremely dark circles appeared under my eyes, my skin turned a pale grey and my nails became brittle. More things started to happen. My

16

level of headaches escalated to migraines. My nausea escalated into vomiting. My gums started bleeding and a couple of my teeth were loose. I started having palpitations and sensitivity to cold. I was unable to sleep for longer than two hours at a time and keeping foods in my body was a challenge.

What was going on with me? I attributed all of these reactions to my stress level since I had been working on various high-profile client projects requiring extremely long hours of effort and commitment. I just couldn't believe how bad I felt physically. Luckily, my two friends, Kelly and Allison, approached me in "the bunkroom" and insisted I investigate these symptoms with a doctor. I can still hear their words, "Kim, something is definitely not right and you have to do it now."

As you can imagine, after 12 surgeries coupled with a high tolerance for pain, I tried to avoid doctors at all costs (nothing personal to those of you who are doctors!). I contacted numerous professionals in the medical field for referrals and suggested that maybe, just maybe, this had to do with allergies. A multitude of allergy tests were conducted by multiple health professionals. Although there were discrepancies between the various test results, they confirmed my reactions to dairy, fish, shellfish and chemicals. I was told that I had celiac/coeliac disease as well as allergies to other food and environmental allergens. These included pork, sodium nitrates, fluoride, yeast, food dyes to name a few. I am forever thankful to my friends for their encouragement and persistence in convincing me to seek assistance.

Living the Gluten and Allergy Free Life

I categorize the timeframe immediately following my diagnosis in stages—I guess that's the consultant in me. The 1st stage in my mind is awareness—what exactly have I been diagnosed with? The 2nd stage is the information- what can I eat and what do I need to avoid? The 3rd stage is knowledge—okay now that I have this information how do I apply it to real life? The last and most important stage is power—now I can live and enjoy myself while being diligent with

16

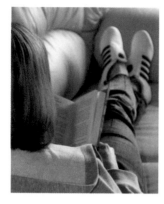

foods—feeling empowered to eat outside the home and travel where and when I want.

Going through these stages and eliminating all the allergens from my diet was difficult to say the least. As described at the beginning of this book, I spent all of my free time researching what I could and could not eat inside and outside the home, in the US and across the globe. Based on information obtained from scouring websites, reading every book I could find on the topic and contacting 100-plus associations, I studied, took notes, memorized and felt like I was back at school again. There was a lot of trial and error, an enormous learning curve and huge adjustments.

It was all worth it though. Upon understanding what needed to be eliminated from my diet including obvious as well as hidden allergens and committing to strict adherence, I began to feel a difference within one week. It was truly amazing! After over 10 years of chronic pain and 8.5 years to be diagnosed, my team of specialists figured out what I needed to do to feel better and I finally started to repair my body.

Following a gluten and allergy-free diet coupled with exercise, herbs and detoxification, my quality of life began to increase significantly. The majority of my recovery took place during the next two years. I just kept feeling better and better, younger and younger. My energy level continued to increase as my body focused on processing the proper nutrients rather than trying to protect me from the intolerable foods. Today, I'm healthier, more energetic and happier than I have been in years!!! I feel so much better than I ever did in my 30's and continue to be amazed at what our minds, bodies and spirits are capable of accomplishing.

I am also very grateful that I had traveled extensively prior to my final diagnosis and that traveling was integral to living my life. If someone tells you that they never get sick from eating outside the home, either they are very lucky, carry all their own food, eat only plain foods or cook for themselves in the kitchenette. Regardless of my experience and knowledge, I unfortunately do still get sick occasionally. During those times, while doubled over in pain and recuperating for days, I sometimes wonder to myself, why exactly am I

16

doing this? It would be so much safer for me to cook my own meals and accept the situation.

Then I remind myself of those incredible moments in time that would not have been experienced if I had stayed in my home. I would suggest that you remind yourself of your own moments in time too. Favorites of mine that inspire me to explore new restaurants with friends and family around the world are the Melnie Muki restaurant in Riga, Rothschild Chateau outside of Nice, the Enoteca in Montalcino and Wärdshuset Ulla Winbladh in Stockholm. I also remember those travel adventures that are among the top of my list includ-ing the Ocean Spirit catamaran at the Great Barrier Reef, Oktoberfest in Munich, Talsi and the Baltic Sea, Carnival in Venice, and scuba diving in Cozumel. I am just not willing to accept staying at home or remaining in my hotel room to cook all my meals while traveling. Experiencing the local culture and cuisine is key, that's all part of the fun!

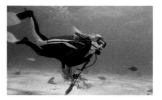

I am grateful for the support I received from family, friends and business colleagues once they understood my situation. Thank you all for helping me. Eating outside the home is a collaborative effort between the person impacted with food allergies, their dining companions and restaurant professionals. Sometimes it gets a little tiresome explaining special dietary needs on a constant basis and your help is appreciated. I've only mentioned a few of you below as examples of ways that those of you supporting friends and family with food allergies can help while in restaurants, company gatherings or at your home.

Katinka, changing plans from the comedy club to an allergy friendly restaurant in Amsterdam once you found out that they couldn't accommodate special dietary requests meant the world to me. Todd, I still laugh thinking about the restaurant in Reston that said that they couldn't serve me and you politely asked, "Can't you just make her a salad? Now that would be safe!" Camille and Eva—I appreciate your concern and diligence when ordering allergy-free take-out for me on those long nights of work in New York.

Paul, thanks for remembering my food allergies and taking me to Marks & Spencers in London based

16

upon their wide selection of "safe" foods for lunch —little did you know that I had gotten sick earlier and could only keep down hard boiled eggs that day! Ivanka, I appreciate you checking with the chef about the buffet line on New Year's Eve in Paris when I thought I was going to have to go back to the hotel to eat something safe. Faris, thanks for your patience and support after I had been so sick and of course, eating my portions at the cooking school.

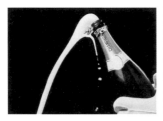

Brad—taking over the ordering process for me when I was just tired of explanations was a tremendous help. Mike—thanks for offering to eat gluten-free with me. I'm glad I declined so you could enjoy the baguettes and profiteroles for both of us. University of Chicago Celiac Program—I'll always remember the welcome package that opened my eyes to the world of gluten-free foods.

Bev—thanks for your pep talk after my diagnosis, while sitting on the floor at a closed O'Hare airport with my raw carrots and a bottle of water. Mom—I'll remember my angel food birthday cake every year going forward. Club Girls—thanks for thinking of what I could eat when each of you prepared food over the years.

Randy—your gluten and allergy-free snicker doodles, brownies and chocolate cake will go down in history for me. Bob, when I think about how my food choices have expanded from plain salad, chicken or broccoli to new things such as red wine reduction sauce and how my world opened back up again due to your diligence and knowledge, thank you. Stan, I still laugh when I think about you remembering my "food issues" as you put it, enjoying an incredible meal at the Metropolitan Grill in Seattle and then recommending that I write a book about eating out with allergies!

Highlights of my restaurant experiences after my diagnosis are thanks to the respective waiters, waitresses, managers, room service staff, owners and chefs from all over the world. You may never realize just how much you may have impacted someone's life and memories while you were working! I hope that you, the reader, will also experience similar benefits and gifts on your journey to health, adventure and

16

travel. A small sampling of my memorable gluten and allergy-free meals include:

- Café Marley in Paris for my first entrée served with an amazing allergy-free sauce

- In N Out Burger in San Francisco for the first burger I could eat with my hands (wrapped in lettuce)

- Lumi in New York City for my first gluten-free minestrone soup and Osso Bucco

- La Piazza in Chicago for my first gluten-free pasta dish

- Il Fornello in Toronto for my first gluten-free pizza

- Il Bistro in Seattle for the first time I had three allergy-free dessert choices

- W Hotel in Times Square for the first time room service reiterated my dietary requirements from a previous order captured in the computer system

- Prêt á Manger in London for my first "sandwich without the bread"

- Risotteria in New York City for my first beer (Bard's Tale) in years

- Sal e Carvão in Chicago for the amazing Brazilian churrascaria

- Bistro 990 in Toronto for an incredible gastronomic experience

- Lots of American steak and seafood restaurants including: The Palm in New York City, Keefers in Chicago, Capital Grille in Minneapolis, Old Ebbitt Grill in DC and Jackson's in Fort Lauderdale

16

In closing, I wanted to share some of my thoughts learned throughout this process: ˙

- The days of experiencing painful symptoms on a constant basis are a dim memory

- Recovery is definitely possible and doable—it just takes work

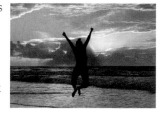

- You're in charge of your health and recovery

- The amount of hard work, adjustments and frustrations are worth it

- Learn something new every day

- Every education has its tuition

- What goes around, comes around

- Sometimes you just need to remind yourself of those moments when you've had an absolutely delicious meal and thought, "Life doesn't get any better than this!"

- Live each day to the fullest: work hard, play hard and most importantly, have fun!

Dealing with Specialized Diets: The Other Side of the Table— Robert's Perspective

How did I get here? I mean here, in front of my computer finalizing what is the culmination of years of research and writing. I have spent the majority of my adult life in front of people, either in front of guests as a restaurant service industry professional or on stage as an actor. Never in a million years did I think I would co-write a book on eating outside the home and travel for people with special dieatry requirements. In the end, it turns out that my life experiences were the perfect compliment to Kim's; one side knows the realities of living life while managing special dietary requirements and the other side knows the restaurant position on how to effectively serve those who must adhere to specialized diets. Without those two perspectives working in collaboration, this work could never have been accomplished.

Understanding guest requirements was a priority for me in my restaurant career. Looking back, I tried to determine what events in my life caused me to take this part of my job so seriously. After all, the restaurant business is transient to say the least. Many restaurants have a constantly revolving door of employees coming and going. Why was I one of those employees that stayed? The answer, I have come to believe, is that most

16

of the establishments I worked in focused on making the guest happy. I found that aspect of the job particularly rewarding, especially when it came to guests who had special dietary needs.

To further describe my perspective, I have organized my experiences into the three following sections:

- An introduction to food allergies

- In the trenches: The restaurant perspective

- Supporting friends and family with specialized diets

An Introduction to Food Allergies

I vaguely remember the first time I heard the term "food allergy." I was very young, probably in about first or second grade. Those were the days when we had snack time as part of our daily routine. When snack time came around, we usually had cookies or nuts and always a pint of whole milk. At the time, we were all taught about the "food pyramid" through government materials and films, which had catchy tunes that entertained us and provided valuable information about a well balanced diet. Although it was many years ago, I can still remember those songs and some of their lyrics! "Milk group...meat group....fruit and vegetable group....bread and cereal group."

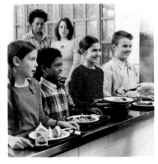

There was a classmate of mine who was shorter in stature and looked frail compared to the other kids. His complexion seemed a bit pale and he was always very quiet and reserved. When he first joined our class, the teacher announced to everyone that this boy had "food allergies" and explained that he could not drink milk, eat chocolate or peanuts. I can still remember the look of sadness on his face as we were told this information.

16

All of the children looked forward to the mid-afternoon snack, as it was a break from the arduous tasks of coloring inside the lines and reading the advanced texts from the "Dick and Jane" books, as well as a chance to boost our blood sugar levels which were depleted from the post lunch recess. We received our pints of milk and snacks, which were devoured with the utmost ferocity. This one boy, however, was set apart from the group and ate raw vegetables, special snack chips and drank fruit juice. I thought it was kind of neat that he got to eat something different than the rest of us, yet it was clear to me that he just wanted to be like the other kids and eat what we were eating.

He was only in my class a year. I believe his family moved to another town. His presence certainly impacted me though, so much so that I can remember it to this day. Half the time I can't remember what I did last week, so reminiscing about something that happened so long ago indicates to me that the experience opened my eyes to something new.

At the time, the general awareness of food allergies in the US was in its infancy. I only had a few friends diagnosed with food allergies. I did have family and friends who were very particular about what types of food they would eat. My father detested mushrooms, my sister Robbie hated peas and I would rather starve than eat fried liver and onions. It wasn't until I started working in restaurants in high school that I really got a sense of how many people had special dietary concerns or were living with food allergies.

In the Trenches: The Restaurant Perspective

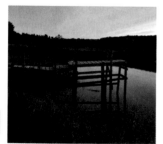

Working in the restaurant service industry is truly an adventure. Nowhere else can one come into contact with so many people on a personal level every day. One summer, I was working at a family resort in Maine on one of the most beautiful lakes in America (as rated by National Geographic Magazine). *Quisisana*, which is Italian for "a place where one heals one's self," was aptly named. It was a place where people could escape from the big cities of the East coast and enjoy a family "summer camp." Many of the guests were regular visitors, some returning to Lake Kezar and the woods of Maine every summer for 50 years.

At the time I was working as a front waiter, which is a glorified term for a busboy. We served three meals a day and it was my responsibility to fill water glasses, pour coffee and deliver bread and butter to every table. There was an elderly couple who had been coming to the resort for many years, probably decades, who sat in

16

my section for two weeks. I learned very quickly that Mrs. Shapiro did not like butter. The look on her face, when I brought her a dish of individually wrapped pats of butter, was frightening. She exclaimed, "No butter at our table!" The panic stricken look on her face was enough to make me nervous for the rest of the meal. "What did I do wrong?" I thought. "It's just butter! It's not the end of the world." Some mistakes in life you make only once and this was certainly one of them. It was none of my business why she had such a dramatic response. It was my job to make her happy, so I was very conscious about only bringing margarine to their table after that.

Looking back, I wonder if she was lactose intolerant or maybe she was on a medically prescribed diet. I never asked them about her vehement response and they never offered an explanation. She certainly was a very picky eater. The choices she made for her meals were simple and basic, if not bland. My best friend Mike and I worked as a team for the Shapiros and we still have conversations about them from time to time. "How's your tuna sandwich, Mrs. Shapiro?" we would ask. Her daily apathetic response, "Eh....it's tuna." She was clearly frustrated with her food limitations. They were very nice people though and my experience with them taught me a valuable lesson as a person working in the restaurant industry: regardless of what I thought of a special request, even if I didn't understand it, my job was to make the guest happy during their dining experience. If you make the effort to accommodate people, they leave happy and want to return because they have had an enjoyable experience with someone who cared about their needs. By the middle of the first week, Mrs. Shapiro had us well trained. We knew exactly what she wanted and didn't want, which provided her with a certain sense of comfort. She was happy to see us and felt safe at the table knowing that we were fully aware of her special needs.

Most chefs and waiters I know truly care about their patrons and take individual dietary considerations very seriously. Unfortunately, accidents do happen. During the mid-1990's, a good friend of mine was working at a popular chain restaurant at Times

16

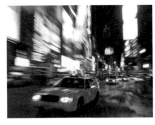

Square in New York City. A married couple came in to eat with their young son who clearly stated to my waiter friend, "No onions, please." "No problem," he thought, as he had dealt with hundreds of special requests in the past. The boy wanted a simple pasta dish with marinara sauce. My friend submitted this order with the stipulation "no onions." Somewhere between placing the order in the computer and delivering the food to the table, this important detail was lost. Nevertheless, the family seemed to enjoy the meal and left satisfied.

Unfortunately, the parents never mentioned to my friend that the boy had a serious food allergy. The next day when he came back to work, the manager asked him about the table with the special request of no onions. Apparently, the sauce contained onions and the child was sick. My friend felt horrible. He did what he was trained to do, by listing the request on the order. Should he have known the sauce had onions in it? If he didn't, shouldn't the cooks in the kitchen have known? That day, my friend realized the difference between a special order and serving a customer with a food allergy. Had he known that the child had a serious food allergy, rather than a special request, he would have been far more diligent in ensuring the proper meal was delivered. As a rule, it is extremely important to use the word "allergy" in restaurants. Failing to satisfy a simple special request has certain consequences. However, failing to deliver on an allergy request can have severe consequences. Today, restaurants know this and take it very seriously.

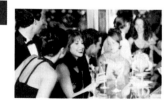

16

I witnessed a similar situation working at a popular upscale Chinese restaurant in Scottsdale, Arizona. We were very well trained on the menu and all the ingredients used in the restaurant. In fact, every server was given a mandatory test that required detailed knowledge of each dish that was served. This was not a minor hurdle or a joke—it was an absolute necessity to work on the floor of the restaurant. The tests were scrutinized so vigorously that to pass, one had to score above 85% just to work there! We were also instructed to inform the manager and chef of any guest that stated that they had a food allergy. This structure proved to be very efficient, as we had few complaints. The only flaw in this procedure was if a guest failed to declare that they had a food allergy.

One evening, a couple sat down in the section next to mine. Their food was delivered and they seemed to be enjoying the meal. Then it happened. The woman at the table turned red and was obviously going into some type of shock. The gentleman didn't know what to do; quite frankly, we didn't know what to do. Luckily, the manager did and called for an ambulance, which arrived almost immediately. After taking her vitals, they gave her a shot and she was stabilized in a short time. We were never told exactly what she had a reaction to, but we figured it was either the peanuts or the dried chili peppers that were in her meal. The event scared me. I knew that I never wanted to be responsible for someone having a severe reaction like that. From that night on, taking care of guests with food allergies and special requests became the most important part of my job.

In a very short time, regular guests with food allergies began to request seating in my section. They experienced a level of comfort when dining under my supervision and knew that I made every effort to ensure an allergy-free meal. I worked closely with each guest to determine what they could have on the menu. I would also be creative with them, "You can have this sauce, with that dish." or "Have you tried this dish? We can add this or omit that." It was actually fun and challenging for me. The kitchen didn't mind because every dish was made to order and we were encouraged to do everything possible to make the guests happy. My patrons really enjoyed it too, because they didn't have to eat the same thing every time they came to the restaurant, which can be a frustrating part of living with food allergies.

Mickey, a local helicopter pilot, was continually relieved to see me when she walked into the restaurant. If she came in on a night that I wasn't working, the next time she saw me, she would let me know about it. She was allergic to many things, including soy, poultry and wheat, which made it difficult to maneuver around a Chinese restaurant menu. She was very diligent in reminding me of exactly what she couldn't eat and how

16

all the utensils needed to be cleaned before preparing her meal. This is so important, because no matter how often you think you've repeated yourself, it is best to remind the restaurant staff of your special dietary needs.

At first, Mickey only ordered steamed vegetables and rice. Her major concern was cross-contamination. So, as soon as I saw her, I would walk right back to the kitchen and tell the chef that our special guest had arrived and it was time to clean a wok and utensils in hot soapy water. It got to be such a regular occurrence that no one in the kitchen questioned the request. As Mickey's level of comfort with me and the restaurant increased, she became more adventurous with her orders. When we would come up with something new and delicious for her that was safe, the look of excitement on her face was like a kid opening presents on Christmas!

Restaurants in New York City are wonderful in so many ways. As a city, New York is considered one of the best places in the world for dining. The pace of life in the Big Apple is so fast that the phrase "a New York minute" is not only a reality, it's a regular demand. People who live in the city just expect things to happen faster than people in most parts of the world. This includes restaurant owners, who want their tables "turned" or "served" as fast as possible, so they can afford to pay their ever-increasing rent. I worked for a few years at a popular Thai restaurant, where the staff was constantly pressured to turn their tables as fast as possible, and we did. Like most progressive establishments, we were also required to take a test on our menu knowledge so the staff was well educated on the cuisine. Much to the chagrin of the owners, the speed of my service always slowed down when I had a guest with food allergies. I felt it was more important to ensure an allergy-free dining experience for these guests than to hurry them through their meal. I always took the extra time and the regulars took notice. Once again, people requested seating in my section. They knew that if I didn't have the answer, I would take all the necessary time to discuss things with the chef.

It may seem like a basic service, but it really gave me a sense of satisfaction to help people have an enjoyable dining experience. The look of excitement on a guest's face when you introduce a new dish to them that is safe to eat is extraordinary. Communication is the key to success. When you have food allergies, dining out is a collaborative effort between you and the restaurant staff. There isn't any way around it. It may not be the case with every restaurant, but there is a growing trend in the industry to accommodate guests with special dietary requirements. This is not just for financial gain, but also for the satisfaction that any guest can dine at their establishment and have a healthy, wholesome meal. From a restaurant perspective, this pursuit is extremely rewarding.

Supporting Friends and Family with Specialized Diets

In fall 2002, my dear friend Kim was diagnosed with celiac/coeliac disease. She was in town a few days a week over a seven month period working on an enormous project for the City of New York. We were enjoying a cocktail at my favorite neighborhood haunt when she told me she had celiac/coeliac disease. Celiac disease? I had never heard of it and probably couldn't have spelled it if you asked. As we talked about it, I learned another new term I had no knowledge of...gluten. I was very aware of wheat allergies, as I came across them often in the business and was used to modifying orders for people on low carbohydrate diets. Gluten, however, was a detail that I never received the memo on. In fact, after hearing about it, I asked many of my friends in the restaurant business if they knew what gluten was. Most of them had never heard of it.

Kim was at a loss. She discovered she had a permanent intolerance to gluten, which is hidden in so many foods. I saw the frustration on her face, as she looked at the menu when we went out to dinner. "It has a sauce, I can't have that." "I don't know what's in that and I don't want to get sick." Soon I realized that she was living an extremely cautious life, which was completely out of character for her, because she didn't want to get sick. Who could blame her? I began to take a more active role in the ordering process with her and our collaboration yielded more choices for her to eat on a regular basis. After all, I'd worked in restaurants for

16

a long time, cooking was a passion for me and I wasn't shy about asking questions.

As a team, we got very good at dining out together. Our meals were great, she had more options and she rarely got sick when we ate out. We developed an interesting approach to ordering by analyzing the menu and figuring out which questions to ask like, "Is there soy sauce in that marinade?" and "Do you have a designated fryer for the fries or do you use one fryer for everything?" It was a learning process for us as well as the servers who took our orders. They would say things like, "Wow, I would have never thought about that" or "Soy sauce has wheat in it?" It was a fun challenge and it allowed us to enjoy our dining experiences more often without the fear of her getting sick.

About a year later, my brother discovered that he was allergic to wheat. He had struggled, like most people, for some time trying to figure out what he was eating that was making him sick. He went through the process of the elimination diet and cut out various food allergens for periods of time to see if there was any improvement to his overall health. When he finally got to wheat, the results were dramatic. He lost over twenty pounds and had more energy on a daily basis than he had had in years. His frequency of having hives decreased considerably and his skin looked so healthy that people often thought that he was younger than me! I don't know what that says about me, but he's my elder by a few years, so the visual change was amazing.

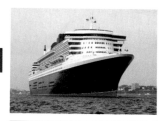

Rick and I are great friends. We have so much in common and are amazed that we are related. One of our shared passions is travel. We have had the oppor-tunity to explore the Caribbean, Mexico and Central America together on a number of occasions. I was very excited to take him on a cruise through the Panama Canal, which is an experience I have been fortunate to enjoy a few times in my life. One of my traditions is to get up at 5 a.m., have breakfast and be out on the deck to view the ship's passing through the first lock. Once through the first set of locks, the afternoon is spent drinking Bloody Marys or Bloody Caesars, depending on whether I was with Canadians or Americans. Rick and I stuck to tradition and had a wonderful afternoon,

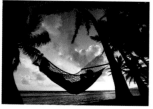

16

until he started to feel sick and his hives began to surface. Throughout the entire vacation we had been very diligent about ordering wheat-free meals, but we obviously missed something. Through the process of elimination, we determined there was only one possible culprit...the Bloody Mary mix. I went back to the bartender and asked to see the bottle of the mix and sure enough, printed in big letters, the label stated wheat as an ingredient. The next few days Rick felt terrible. He was sick to his stomach, often doubled over in pain and especially uncomfortable because of those huge itchy hives. His eyes and lips were also swollen. He ended up staying in his cabin for the next three days until he felt better and his symptoms went away. Twenty percent of our vacation was ruined because of that drink. We had no idea wheat could be a hidden allergen in Bloody Mary mix, but we certainly learned our lesson during that trip.

I consistently make an extra effort when I dine or travel with anyone with food allergies. I have found that having an extra watchful eye is both helpful and comforting to everyone at the table. Whether I am dining with my family or friends, I try to assist as much as I can by leveraging my knowledge of food and asking the right questions when appropriate.

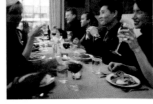

It is important to take a proactive role in the dining experience when you are out with people you care about, because the frustrations and fears associated with having food allergies can be a lot for one person to handle. That is why I feel this book is important for those individuals living with specialized diets. It is also for their loved ones, health professionals and people in the restaurant industry. At the end of the day, the more one knows about food preparation and the more the restaurant knows about your situation, the less likely you are to get sick. It's that simple!

16

Santé!   **Chin Chin!**

¡Salud!   **Cheers!**

Chok-dee!

歡呼!   चीयर्श

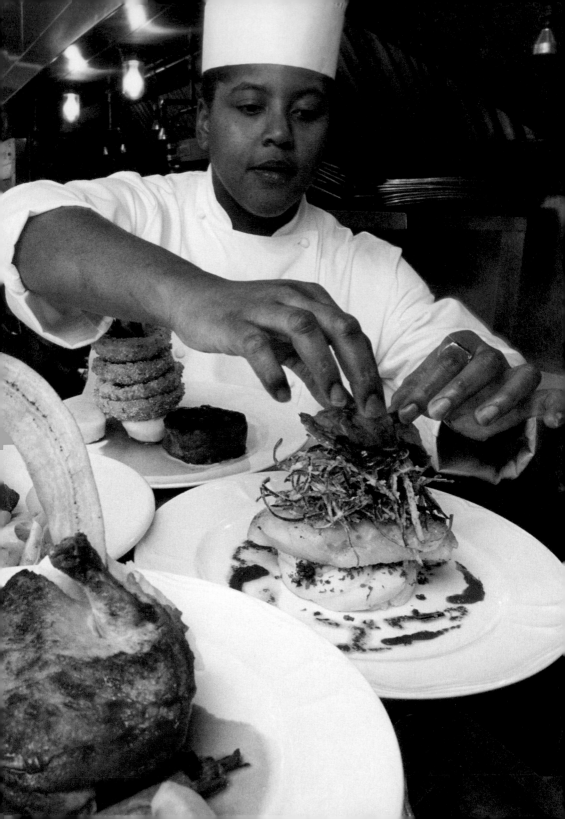

*Friends are angels who lift us
to our feet when our wings have trouble
remembering how to fly.*
—Unknown

Appendix I
Contributors to Let's Eat Out

Appendix Overview

The following describes the backgrounds and qualifications for the contributors who reviewed the contents of this book from a culinary and health perspective. We appreciate the recommendations, information and advice provided to us for:

- International cuisine reviews
- Other content reviews
- Product reference materials

Contributors for International Cuisine Reviews

The following contributors have reviewed the respective seven international cuisines detailed in this book and have provided their knowledge and expertise to help ensure that this information is as accurate as possible for:

- American Steak and Seafood
- Chinese

- French

- Indian

- Italian

- Mexican

- Thai

American Steak and Seafood Cuisine
The contributors for American Steak and Seafood cuisine include:

- Tim Gannon—Founder and Executive Chef: Outback Steakhouse® headquartered in Tampa, FL US

- domenica catelli—Chef: domenica's way in Houston, TX US

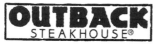

Outback Steakhouse®
In 1988, three fun-loving entrepreneurs who believed in serving consistent high-quality food at reasonable prices in a casual, relaxed atmosphere founded *Outback Steakhouse®* in Tampa, Florida. With the free-spirited attitude of the Australian lifestyle in mind, they created generous portions of steaks, chicken, ribs, seafood and pasta with big, bold flavors, hand-made seasonings and sauces, served with a unique, "no worries" hospitality.

Today, *Outback Steakhouse®* owns and operates nearly 800 Outback units across the United States and internationally through joint venture partnerships and existing franchise agreements. Its growing family of restaurants has expanded to include Carrabba's Italian Grill, Fleming's Prime Steakhouse and Wine Bar, Roy's Restaurants, Lee Roy Selmon's, Bonefish Grill, Cheeseburger in Paradise and Paul Lee's Chinese Kitchen.

Outback Steakhouse® introduced a gluten-free menu in an effort to accommodate the special dietary needs of its customers. Remember to involve a manager when you dine at *Outback Steakhouse®*, as they are well trained in food allergies and will help to ensure a gluten-free dining experience for you. A copy of the gluten-free menu as of June 2005 is provided. Visit the company website for a listing of specific locations and the most up-to-date gluten-free menu.

Outback Steakhouse®
2202 N. West Shore Boulevard Suite 500
Tampa, FL 33607, United States
Phone: 813-282-1225, Facsimile: 813-286-2247
http://www.outbacksteakhouse.com

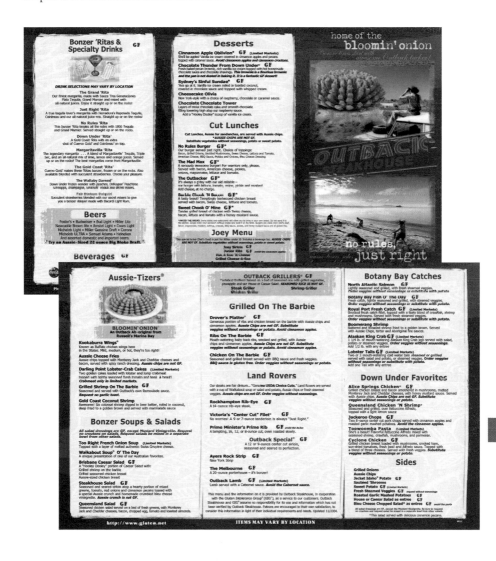

domenica's way

domenica's way

Chef domenica catelli believes that preparing delicious healthy food is a way to restore a disappearing family ritual and further bond our deepest friendships. Through her website, domenica's way, and teaching, she strives to replace bad eating habits, reconnect individuals to their body's nutritional wants and needs, and provides a creative, fun and intimate avenue to re-connect family relationships. An alchemist in the kitchen, she has enjoyed the role of celebrity chef. When teaching her popular cooking classes, she demonstrates how busy moms and dads need to make a successful life change. domenica has the recipes children respond to and has carved a way of cultivating food that is as close to nature as possible. Her expertise is preparing food so fresh and delicious that the preservatives and dyes found in processed food begin to taste foreign—as they should—and we no longer crave them.

Previously, domenica was the executive chef at the Stanford Inn in Mendocino, California. She has worked on food segments for the Oprah Winfrey show. She is a recipe developer for the James Beard Award Winning cookbook, *Back to the Table,* by Art Smith, Oprah Winfrey's chef. Along with chefs such as Jamie Oliver, Tyler Florence and Sarah Moulton, domenica is a member of the chef's advisory board for *Common Threads,* a non-profit organization dedicated to improving children's lives by embracing diversity through food and other artistic expression as a vehicle for positive change. She is the Women Chefs and Restaurateurs scholarship recipient and was trained in organic farming while in Italy. domenica resides in Houston, Texas with her husband Michael and daughter Chiara. She contributes to the Houston Farmers' Market and collaborates with Monica Pope, a premier chef with national acclaim.

domenica's way
Phone: 713-269-4619
domenicacatelli@houston.rr.com
http://www.domenicasway.com

Chinese Cuisine

The contributors for Chinese cuisine include:

- P. F. Chang's China Bistro®: headquartered in Scottsdale, AZ US

- Sueson Vess—Founder and President: Special Eats™ in Chicago, IL US

P. F. Chang's China Bistro®

Founded in 1993, *P.F. Chang's* is a US-based restaurant chain that has been embraced by diners across the country. The goal of a P.F. Chang's meal is to attain harmony of taste, texture, color and aroma by balancing the Chinese principles of *fan* and *t'sai*. *Fan* foods include rice, noodles, grains and dumplings, while vegetables, meat, poultry, and seafood are *t'sai* foods.

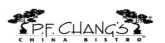

P.F. *Chang's* cuisine is reflective of China's evolving culinary landscape. The menu features traditional Chinese offerings and innovative dishes that illustrate the emerging influence of Southeast Asia on modern Chinese cuisine. *P.F. Chang's* chefs are respectful of the culture and traditions that are behind the dishes they prepare. Working in a dramatic exhibition kitchen, they use Mandarin style wok cooking to prepare the dynamic menu. Using only the freshest, highest quality ingredients, their chefs create lightly sauced dishes that allow natural flavors to emerge and stimulate the senses.

The recommendations for gluten intolerant diets at *P.F. Chang's China Bistro* were developed because they were receiving an increasingly large volume of requests via their website for information on dishes that were or could be made gluten-free.

Because every dish at *P.F. Chang's* is made to order, *P.F. Chang's* has always been able to accommodate their guests' dietary needs and preferences. When *P.F. Chang's* started researching the issues regarding gluten-free diets, they felt it would be best to design a menu that their guests with intolerance to gluten could specifically ask for and order from. The menu has been available since March 2003 and the feedback *P.F. Chang's* has received from their guests in over 100 locations has been extremely positive.

Remember to involve a manager when you dine at

RECOMMENDATIONS FOR GLUTEN INTOLERANT DIETS

ASK YOUR SERVER FOR THESE SUBSTITUTIONS

CHANG'S CHICKEN IN SOOTHING LETTUCE WRAPS
With our Gluten Free Sauce.

SHANGHAI CUCUMBERS 素
With wheat free soy sauce.

ORIENTAL CHICKEN SALAD
Without wonton strips.

GINGER CHICKEN AND BROCCOLI - STEAMED
With our Gluten Free Sauce.

CANTONESE SHRIMP OR SCALLOPS

PHILIP'S BETTER LEMON CHICKEN

火CHANG'S SPICY CHICKEN OR SHRIMP

CHANG'S LEMON SCALLOPS

MOO GOO GAI PAN

SHRIMP WITH LOBSTER SAUCE

火MANGO CHICKEN

STEAMED FISH OF THE DAY
With wheat free soy sauce.

CANTONESE CHOW FUN*
Substitute in rice "stick" noodles and our Gluten Free Sauce.

火SINGAPORE STREET NOODLES*
Substitute our Gluten Free Sauce for the Singapore sauce.

SPINACH STIR-FRIED WITH GARLIC*素

GARLIC SNAP PEAS*素

BUDDHA'S FEAST - STEAMED*素

P.F. Chang's Gluten Free Sauce contains garlic, ginger, rice wine, chicken stock, Sichuan pepper, salt, sugar and wheat free soy sauce.

---

*Marinated chicken, shrimp, scallops or calamari can be added to these dishes. These marinades contain cornstarch.

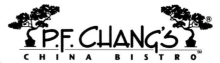

火 Spicy　素 Vegetarian

Products containing gluten are prepared in our kitchens.

P.F. Chang's, as they are well trained in food allergies and will help to ensure a gluten-free dining experience for you. A copy of the gluten-free menu, as of June 2005, is provided. For a listing of specific locations and the most up-to-date gluten-free menu, visit the company website.

P.F. Chang's China Bistro®
15210 N. Scottsdale Rd. Suite 300
Scottsdale, AZ 85254, United States
Phone: 602-957-8986, Facsimile: 602-957-8998
http://www.pfchangs.com

Special Eats™

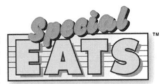

Sueson Vess is president and founder of *Special Eats™,* a company created solely to assist others on the healthy path to embracing gluten and dairy-free living. She is also the author of *Special Eats Simple, Delicious Solutions for Gluten-Free & Dairy-Free Cooking.*

When Sueson was diagnosed as gluten intolerant she resolved to be the best possible gluten-free cook so no one would realize they were eating "special food". As a past restaurateur and chef with 25 years experience in marketing and training, teaching others to embrace gluten-free living is the fulfillment of her dream. Additionally, Sueson leads a support group and provides consulting/training services to restaurants, grocery retailers and corporations.

Sueson helps those with food allergies, celiac/coeliac disease and/or parents of children on the autism spectrum by teaching gluten-free/casein-free (GFCF) cooking classes, developing delicious recipes and providing instructions for meal planning. The learning process addresses understanding and accepting the changes associated with the new lifestyle, as well as:

- Increased awareness of new or unfamiliar products and ingredients

- How to shop with confidence and improve label reading skills

- Where to locate products and ingredients

- Healthy product substitutions

- Creating a safe kitchen, free from cross-contamination

- Tips for traveling and eating in restaurants

Special Eats™
2100 Manchester Road, Suite 1640
Wheaton, IL 60187, United States
Phone: 630-846-4605, Facsimile: 630-510-8250
http://www.specialeats.com

French Cuisine

The contributors for French cuisine include:

- Nicolas Bergerault – Founder and President: L'atelier des Chefs in Paris, France

- Stephane Tremolani – Former Executive Chef: French Embassy in Rome, Italy

L'atelier des Chefs

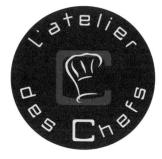

L'atelier des Chefs is headquartered in the 8th arrondissement of Paris, within walking distance of the Champs Elysées. Founded by Nicolas Bergerault and his brother François, it is a new style of cooking school targeted at younger generations (aged 25-45). Classes are for those who enjoy the art of cooking, as well as those who have never learned. The goal of *L'atelier des Chefs* is to bring people back to the kitchen, while re-discovering the pleasure of cooking.

L'atelier des Chefs offers five classes a day, ranging from 1/2-hour to 2-hour courses, six days a week in an open garden setting complete with sky lights, racks of wine and fine grocery products. This "à la carte" program allows students to have a "hands-on" approach to cooking; thereby engaging students in the creative world of the culinary arts. *L'atelier des Chefs* partners with major specialty food manufacturers and takes pride in building its classes around these high quality ingredients, along with common items found in your kitchen, to make the learning experience as accessible as possible.

Courses are taught in French; however, most of

I

the chef-instructors also speak English or Italian. Since cooking classes are a collaborative effort, *L'atelier des Chefs* is the perfect environment for corporate team-building exercises for up to 100 people. *L'atelier des Chefs* has also been featured in many periodicals including *Le Figaro, The Christian Science Monitor, The Beautiful Life* and *Periscope*. Visit the company website for class descriptions, course schedules and specialized corporate events.

L'atelier des Chefs
10 Rue de Penthiévre, 75008 Paris, France
Phone: 33 01 53 30 05 82
http://www.atelierdeschefs.com

Stepane Tremolani

Stephane Tremolani received his degree from the famed *Le Lycée Hôtelier de Nice* and traveled the world perfecting his culinary knowledge as a private chef to an international businessman. While in New York City, Stephane had the opportunity to create gastronomic adventures for many major celebrities and socialites. Most recently, he served as Executive Chef at the French Embassy in Rome, also known as the "Palazzo Farnese." Stephane was raised in Grasse, which is located in the south of France. He is a dual citizen of both France and Italy, through his mother's family from Provence and his father's wine-making family from Perugia.

Before he began his life in the kitchen, he worked in the perfume industry. Having a highly developed sense of smell, he skillfully mixed new fragrances in both Grasse, the birthplace of perfume, and in Paris. In recognition of his talent as an artist, he was selected by the Cultural Council of Southeast France to create hand-painted religious frescos in ceramic to adorn the walls of the "Chapelle Sainte Croix," a 15th century church in Guillaumes, during its restoration. His ceramics studio is currently located in Grasse, outside Nice.

Indian Cuisine

The contributors for Indian cuisine include:

- Samir Majmudar—Owner: Rani Indian Bistro in Brookline, MA US

- Tariq Zaman—Owner: The Spice Company in Moseley, Birmingham, UK

Rani Indian Bistro

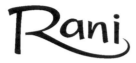

Located in the Coolidge Corner area of Brookline, Massachusetts and easily accessible from downtown Boston, *Rani Indian Bistro* specializes in Hyderabadi cuisine from the Andhra Pradash State of India. Restaurateur Samir Majmudar worked for years in the hotelier industry in India before moving to the States to continue his career. He has owned and operated a number of restaurants in the Boston area prior to focusing all of his energy on *Rani*.

Along with his wife, Prakruti, a strict vegetarian who specializes in the preparation of vegetarian items, and Head Chef Paul Gomes, Samir brings a great enthusiasm for food from his native land, as well as a passion for wine. Hyderabadi cuisine combines Hindu and Muslim influences, offering many vegetarian items, as well as a host of savory chicken and lamb dishes. Chilies and nuts play a large part in the preparation of their dishes; however, each is carefully marked on the menu as a courtesy for those adhering to specialized diets. There are many options that do not contain nuts or are mild in flavor for those who are not fond of spicy food.

The chefs at *Rani Indian Bistro* make an effort to carefully combine ingredients in each dish, so you can capture the essence of every herb or spice in a way that makes you truly appreciate the dedication and pride that goes into their food. *Rani* is open daily for lunch from 11: 30 a.m. to 3 p.m. and dinner from 5 p.m. to 10:30 p.m.

Rani Indian Bistro
1353 Beacon Street, Brookline, MA 02446, United States
Phone: 617-734-0400, Facsimile: 617-566-1278
http://www.ranibistro.com

The Spice Company

The Spice Company is the latest joint venture between Tariq Zaman and Lynne Brooks. Tariq's previous experience includes *Spice Avenue* and the *Spice Exchange*, plus he has extensive knowledge of the hospitality sector. Tariq and Lynne's view of the restaurant business is good food and good company—a view that has earned them five star ratings by restaurant critics. Their approach to *The Spice Company* is a commitment to all things fresh and modern.

The Spice Company is located in the popular and eclectic village of Moseley, only 2 miles from Birmingham city centre. The restaurant features authentic Indian cuisine, highlighted by a wine list that includes "New World" wines from Chile and Argentina, as well as standard favourites from Australia, France, Italy and New Zealand. It is due to open in September 2005 and is set in a historic building, which has been transformed into an ultra-modern lounge and restaurant. *The Spice Company* will be open Monday through Saturday from 11 a.m. to 2:30 p.m. for lunch and 5:30 p.m. to 11 p.m. for dinner.

The Spice Company
23 A, St. Mary's Row
Moseley, Birmingham B13 8HW, United Kingdom

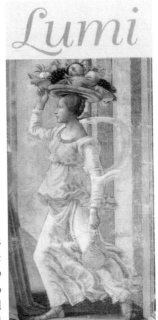

Italian Cuisine

The contributors for Italian cuisine include:

- Arber Murici—General Manager: Lumi in New York, NY US

- Stephane Tremolani—Former Executive Chef: French Embassy in Rome, Italy

Lumi

With a focus on regional Italian cuisine, *Lumi* is located in the heart of New York City's Upper East Side and was featured in Patricia Cornwell's book, *Food to Die For*. Set in a charming townhouse, it features two dining rooms and an outdoor café. *Lumi* was opened to the public in April of 1995 by restaurateur Lumi

Lumi

Gluten Free Dinner Menu

~~ Gli Antipasti ~~

Stagione   7.00
Salad of Assorted Seasonal Greens

Spinaci   8.50
Salad of Baby Spinach, Apples, Parmesan and Walnuts

Frisee   8.50
Salad with Gorgonzola and Pine Nuts

Insalata di Asparagi con Latughette   9.50
Asparagus, Endive, Radicchio, Orange and Mashe Salad
with Shavings of Parmesan Cheese in a Citrus Vinaigrette

Vegetali e Funghi alla Griglia   8.50
A Variety of Grilled Vegetables and Mushrooms

Insalata Caprese   12.50
Buffalo Mozzarella with Tre Colore Salad, Tomatoes and Basil

Carpaccio d'Anatra con Melone e Verdure   9.50
Thinly Sliced Duck Carpaccio with Cantaloupe and Greens

Minestra   7.00
Soup of the Day.

Risotto   P.A
Preparation changes daily.

~~ Pesce ~~

Salmone al Vapore   23.50
Steamed Filet of Salmon, with Red Cabbage
and Marinated Cucumbers

Merluzzo alla Livornese   23.50
Codfish Filet, Cooked in a Traditional Tuscan Spicy
Tomato Sauce

Grigliata Mista di Mare   24.00
Grilled Shrimp, Squid and Scallops, Served with
Canelini Beans and Endive

Dentice al Forno con Radicchio e Indivia   27.50
Red Snapper Filet, Roasted with Herbs and White Wine,
Served with Italian Red Chicory and Endive

Branzino   Market Price
Whole Roasted Wild Striped Bass
Preparation Changes Daily

~~ Carne ~~

Tagliata di Manzo alle Erbe Aromatiche   29.50
Rib Eye Steak Grilled with Herbs, Served with
Roasted Spring Vegetables and Mashed Potatoes

Polletto al Forno con Cime di Rape   23.00
Whole Baby Chicken Split and Roasted, Served with
Broccoli Rab and Roasted Potatoes

Petto di Anatra con Melone e Vin Santo   25.00
Breast of Duck, Sautéed with a Touch of Vin Santo,
Served with Fresh Melon and Vegetables

****
American Express, Visa, and Master Card Accepted

Devine whose previous experience included *Il Cantinori*, *Sapore di Mare*, *Le Madri* and *Cocco Pazzo*. The restaurant is operated by Lumi herself, along with her management team of Chef Daniel Catana and General Manager Arber Murici.

In addition to its popular regional Italian cuisine, *Lumi* features an eclectic, ever evolving wine list representing growing regions from America, France, Italy and Spain. Your host, Arber Murici will personally guide you through the wine list or perhaps offer you a special selection from his reserve list.

Lumi is proud to be part of the Westchester Celiac Sprue Support Group's Gluten-Free Restaurant Awareness Program. A gluten-free menu is available daily and features many specialties typically avoided by people with gluten and wheat allergies such as soups, pasta, gnocchi, Osso Bucco, meat and fish entrees with sauces, lamb chops, flourless chocolate cake, gelato and sorbeto. *Lumi* is open daily from 11:30 am to 11:30 pm or later.

Lumi
963 Lexington Avenue
New York, NY 10021, United States
Phone: 212-570-2335, Facsimile: 212-288-6410
http://www.luminyc.com

Stephane Tremolani

Refer to the French cuisine description for Stephane Tremolani's culinary experience as former Executive Chef at the French Embassy in Rome, Italy.

Mexican Cuisine

The contributors for Mexican cuisine include:

- Freddy Sanchez—Owner and Chef: Adobo Grill in Chicago, IL US

- The Crawley Family: El Sombrero Patio Cafe in Las Cruces, NM US

Adobo Grill

As part of the daVINCI Group, *Adobo Grill* first opened its doors to the public in 2000. Adjacent to Piper's Alley in Chicago's Old Town district, the restaurant is set in an urban atmosphere complete with exposed red brick, Southwestern colors, bright Mexican inspired artwork and two vintage bars featuring over 90 tequilas. Specializing in authentic regional Mexican cuisine, *Adobo* serves everything from its signature table-side prepared guacamole to Oaxacan black mole with epazote-infused black beans.

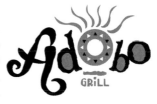

Owner and Chef Freddy Sanchez created a gluten-free menu to provide *Adobo's* gluten intolerant guests with many choices ranging from guacamole, ceviche,

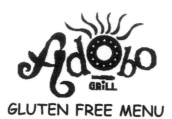

GLUTEN FREE MENU

ANTOJITOS

Guacamole con Totopos   Adobo's famous guacamole; *prepared tableside!*
Served with jicama chips $7.50

"Cevichazo"   Tuna ceviche marinated with Ají amarillo-guava salsa, papaya-watercress salad $9.50
Crab ceviche with sour orange-chile habañero salsa, avocado and pico de gallo $9.95
Shrimp with classic Mexican cocktail sauce and pico de gallo $9.50
Scallops marinated in lime & orange juice, tomatoes, chile serrano, avocado $9.50
A tasting of all ceviches $15.95

Tamales de Pollo   Chicken barbacoa tamales in a corn husk with chile chilcosle salsa,
sour cream and fresco cheese $5.95

Ensalada de Jícama y Mango   Jícama and mango salad with cucumber, mixed greens, pumpkin seed
vinaigrette, chile piquín $5.95

PLATILLOS PRINCIPALES

Enchiladas en Mole Verde   Roasted butternut squash & shiitake mushrooms enchiladas basted in
mole verde, topped with cotija cheese, red onion and sour cream $13.95

Lomito en Mole Negro Oaxaqueño   Grilled pork tenderloin in Oaxacán black mole, poblano rice,
sautéed spinach with cacahuanzitle corn $16.95

Enchiladas en Mole Rojo   Chicken enchiladas basted in mole rojo and topped with sour cream, añejo
cheese, red onion and radishes $14.95

Tilapia a la Talla   Sautéed tilapia marinated in chile guajillo and ancho, served with wild mushrooms
in escabeche and fire-roasted chile poblano machuca $16.95

Please notify your server of any food allergies
Private party rooms available for groups from 15 to 85
18% gratuity added to parties of 6 or more
Guacamole gift sets available-$25.00 each

and enchiladas to other popular Mexican specialties such as tamales, rellenos and jicama-mango salad in pumpkin vinaigrette. The "FiestAdobo" vibe caught on and a second *Adobo Grill* opened in Chicago's Wicker Park neighborhood during the summer of 2004.

The daVINCI Group's first restaurant was *VINCI*, an Italian establishment opened in 1991 by chef/owner Paul LoDuca. *VINCI* has been offering a gluten-free menu for many years, so gluten intolerant guests can still enjoy wonderful Italian dishes, such as polenta, pasta dishes and panna cotta dessert.

A copy of *Adobo's* gluten-free menu as of June 2005 is provided. Visit the company's web sites for the most up-to-date gluten-free menus.

Adobo Grill
1610 N. Wells St., Chicago, IL, United States
Phone: 312-266-7999, Facsimile: 312-266-9299
http://www.adobogrill.com
Adobo Grill
2005 W. Division St., Chicago, IL, United States
Phone: 773-252-9990, Facsimile: 773-252-1834
http://www.adobogrill.com

VINCI
1732 N. Halsted St., Chicago, IL, United States
Phone: 312-266-1199, Facsimile: 312-266-8143
http://www.vincichicago.com

El Sombrero Patio Cafe

Opened in 1956 by family matriarch Ophelia Carrillo, *El Sombrero Patio Cafe* is owned and operated by the Crawley family and specializes in Southern New Mexican cuisine. More than just a restaurant, it is widely considered an institution to the residents of the Mesilla Valley. New Mexican green and red chile from Hatch is featured on the menu, as well as traditional Southwest specialties such as burritos, churros, enchiladas, fajitas, tamales and tostadas compuestas.

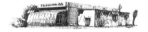

El Sombrero Patio Cafe currently does not have a menu for those following specialized diets. However, they hope to implement one by the end of 2005 for their customers with food allergies. Their hours of operation are Monday through Thursday from 11 am to 8:30 pm and Thursday through Friday from 11 am to 9 pm. The restaurant is closed on Sundays and holidays.

El Sombrero Patio Cafe
363 S. Espina, Las Cruces, NM 88001, United States
Phone: 505-524-9911, Facsimile: 505-526-4394

Thai Cuisine

The contributors for Thai cuisine include:

- Pam Panyasiri—Owner and Chef: Pam Real Thai Food in New York, NY US

Pam Real Thai Food

Located on the western fringes of midtown Manhattan, or "Hell's Kitchen" as the locals still refer to it, is the famed *Pam Real Thai Food* restaurant, which opened in 2001. Owned by Chef Pam Panyasiri and her husband Ron, *Pam Real Thai Food* is a restaurant beloved by New York food aficionados. *The New York Times'* food Critic Mark Bittman declared it, "...one of the strongest contenders for the title 'Best Thai Food in the City'." Chef Panyasiri and her restaurant have been featured in many of the city's other newspapers, restaurant guides and radio stations including *AM New York, The Daily News, The New York Post, The Village Voice* and *Zagats*.

Chef Panyasiri's recipes are inspired by her mother's cooking, which she enjoyed daily while growing up in Bangkok, Thailand. These recipes have changed very little over the years and she has learned to be pragmatic in the kitchen due to the lack of availability of traditional Thai ingredients. In fact, her father still sends 10-pound bags of dried authentic Thai chili peppers every month from Thailand. Chef Panyasiri prides herself on using only the freshest ingredients available in New York and very rarely uses canned or pre-made ingredients. As an example, she squeezes over a case of fresh limes daily for her dishes!

Since most of her dishes are made to order, Chef Panyasiri often caters to guests with food allergies. "No peanuts, no problem!" she says with a smile. Daily specialties include spicy *Larb Gai* and her famous *Ox Tail Soup*. Seafood lovers will be impressed with her *Crispy Whole Fish*, which is available with eight different sauces. *Pam Real Thai Food* is open daily from 11:30 am to 11 pm.

Pam Real Thai
404 W. 49th Street, New York, NY 10019, United States
Phone: 212-333-7500, Facsimile: 212-333-3743
http://www.pamrealthai.com

Contributors for Other Content Reviews

The following contributors have provided their health and dietary insights to the development of this book:

- University of Chicago Celiac Disease Program
- Case Nutrition Consulting
- Vital Health, Inc.

University of Chicago Celiac Disease Program

The University of Chicago Celiac Disease Program (UCCDP) serves children and adults throughout the United States. Its mission is to raise diagnosis rates for celiac disease and meet the critical needs of people with the condition, through education, research and advocacy. There are currently five primary areas of focus including: the celiac disease information line, gluten-free care package program, annual celiac blood screening, patient and professional education and celiac disease research.

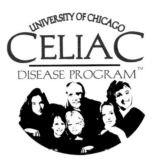

The information line provides medical information to help people receive a timely celiac diagnosis and counsels physicians with questions about celiac disease testing. The care package is a basket of food and resource materials to instruct newly diagnosed patients and dietitians on the gluten-free diet. The free blood screening draws participants throughout the United States. It helps families overcome problems with insurance and individuals by providing test results in order to encourage their doctors to diagnose them. A team of speakers works year-round to educate medical professionals, people with celiac disease and the public about diagnosing and treating this condition. The University of Chicago has one of two research teams in the world that is working to understand the nature of the immune system in the gut and the earliest response of the intestine to the presence of gluten.

Michelle Melin-Rogovin, the executive director of UCCDP, manages these programs and works with Dr. Stefano Guandalini, the section chief of gastroenterology, hepatology and nutrition at the University of Chicago's Comer Children's Hospital. As the founder and director of the UCCDP, Dr. Guandalini has studied the condition and diagnosed patients for over three decades. He is also a professor of pediatrics at the University of Chicago, Pritzker School of Medicine and the immediate past president of the Federation of International Societies for Pediatric Gastroenterology, Hepatology, and Nutrition.

University of Chicago Celiac Disease Program
5839 South Maryland Avenue, MC 4069
Chicago, IL 60637, United States
Phone: 773-702-7593
http://www.celiacdisease.net

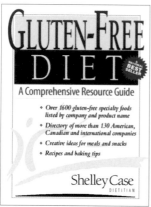

Case Nutritional Consulting

A Registered Dietitian, Shelley Case earned a Bachelor of Science degree in Nutrition and Dietetics from the University of Saskatchewan and completed her Dietetic Internship at the Health Sciences Centre in Winnipeg. For the past 25 years, Shelley has helped thousands of people change poor eating habits and manage a variety of disease conditions through good nutrition. She specializes in nutrition counseling for gastrointestinal disorders such as celiac disease, food allergies and intolerances, heart disease and diabetes.

Gluten-Free Diet: A Comprehensive Resource Guide (2005 edition) by Shelley Case, RD, includes the gluten-free (GF) diet by food groups, foods and ingredients allowed, to avoid and to question; US and Canadian labeling regulations; nutrition information; shopping and meal planning guidelines; cross contamination issues; use of alternative grains; recipes; over 1900 GF specialty products listed by company, product name and package size; directory of more than 160 American, Canadian and international companies; resources (cookbooks, books, magazines, newsletters, websites, celiac groups) and more! This national best seller is an excellent reference for every person with gluten intolerance, health professional, culinary professional and food retailer who needs comprehensive information on this complex diet.

Shelley and her work have been featured on the NBC *Today Show* and in publications such as *Gastro-*

enterology, Practical Gastroenterology, Today's Dietitian, Canadian Living Magazine and *The Toronto Star* newspaper. She is also a member of the medical advisory boards of the Celiac Disease Foundation, Gluten Intolerance Group of North America and the Canadian Celiac Association, as well as the advisory board of *Living Without* magazine.

Case Nutritional Consulting
1940 Angley Court
Regina, Saskatchewan S4V 2V2, Canada
Phone/Fax: 306-751-1000
info@glutenfreediet.ca
http://www.glutenfreediet.ca

Vital Health, Inc.

Over the past 30-plus years, Barbara Griffin, NMD, CNC has worked and lived within the framework of natural wellness. She was introduced to naturopathy and received her original training in a Naturopathic clinic in Germany. Barbara has a Naturopathic degree from Arkansas College of Natural Health and is a Certified Nutritional Consultant from the Yamuni Institute of Healing Arts, PanAmerican Institute of Bioenergetic Medicine, International College of Bionutrition. She is an active member of the World Organization of Natural Medicine Practioners, International Parliament of Safety & Peace, International Society of Electrodermologist (Fellowship–Board Certification), American Association of Nutritional Consultants, American Association of Drugless Practitioners, National Board of Examiners in Integrated/Alternative Medicine and Natural Health Science and the North Carolina Board of Naturopathic Examiners.

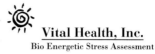

Barbara developed her own personal style of natural wellness and opened *New Vitality Health Foods,* in 1988. The store flourishes as an educational and nutritional center now run by her daughter, Diana Sourek, MS, CNC, Nutritional Consultant. *New Vitality Health Foods* provides an extremely large variety of gluten and allergy-free product selections.

Barbara currently directs her own wellness center, *Vital Health, Inc.,* that addresses a whole body approach

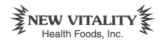

to health with the intention of facilitating well-being and optimal health amongst her 5000-plus clients. Her advanced levels of education and training in many established integrative therapies, along with her practical experience and caring ways, puts her services in high demand. Vital Health's specialties include: Electrodermal Screenings, Sensitivity Screenings, Iridology, NES, Naturopathy, Nutrition, EAV, SKASYS, Neuroemotional Therapy, Neuromodulation Technique, Cold Laser Therapy, Emotional Stress Integration and Neuro-link Technique.

Barbara has taken a non-invasive approach in identifying food intolerance in the body and has appeared on an ABC-TV special presentation of *Healthbeat* entitled, "Food for Thought".

Vital Health, Inc
9031 West 151st Street, Ste 210
Orland Park, IL 60462, United States
Phone: 708-226-1131
http://www.vitalhealth.org

New Vitality Health Foods, Inc
9177 West 151st Street
Orland Park, IL 60462, United States
Phone: 708-403-0120
http://www.newvitalityhealth.com

Product Reference Materials

As mentioned in the beverage and snack chapters, the following information provides an overview of the guides and directories detailing country specific product names and manufacturer/brand listings by organization. To purchase these guides or to obtain more information, contact each of the organizations directly:

Canada	Canadian Celiac Association – *Pocket Dictionary of Ingredients*
France	Association Française des Intolérants au Gluten – *Liste des Produits Autorisés*
Ireland	The Coeliac Society of Ireland – *A List of Gluten-Free Manufactured Products*
Italy	Associazione Italiana Celiachia – *Il Prontuario in Internet*
Netherlands	Vodeinscentrum – *Lijst van Gluten-vrije Merkatikelin*
New Zealand	*Manufactured Foods Database*
Spain	Federación de Asociaciones de Celíacos de España – *La Lista de Alimentos Sin Gluten*
United Kingdom	Coeliac UK - *Gluten Free Food and Drink Directory*
United States	Celiac Sprue Association – *The CSA Gluten-Free Product Listing*
United States	Clan Thompson™ – *Celiac Smart Lists and Celiac Pocket Guides*

I

Canada
Canadian Celiac Association
Pocket Dictionary of Ingredients—Acceptability of Foods and Food Ingredients for the Gluten-Free Diet

- Pocket-size dictionary has been developed to assist persons in selecting acceptable foods and interpreting food labels so that they may avoid foods containing gluten. It provides a brief description of each item along with an assessment of its acceptability for the gluten-free diet.

- Published in English and French

Phone: 905-507-6208
http://www.celiac.ca

France
Association Française des Intolérants au Gluten
Liste des Produits Autorisés

- 60-plus page booklet listing products by category with brand names and specific items. Also contains a list of brands to be avoided regardless of product and contact numbers for various companies

- Published in French and updated annually

Phone: 33-1-56-08-08-22
http://www.afdiag.com

Ireland
The Coeliac Society of Ireland
A List of Gluten-Free Manufactured Products

- 200-plus page pocket-sized book listing products by category with brand names and specific items. Also contains a list of stores and respective gluten-free items as well as definitions of foods and basic ingredients

- Published in English and updated annually

Phone: 353-1-872-1471
http://www.coeliac.ie

Italy
Associazione Italiana Celichia
Il Prontuario in Internet

- Online food and drink database providing gluten-free manufacturers and products available thoughout Italy.

- Published in English and Italian

Phone: 39-50-580-939
http://www.celiachia.it

Netherlands
Vodeinscentrum
Lijst van Glutenvrije Merkatikeln

- 200-plus page book listing products by category with brand names and specific items. Also contains background information, contact information for celiac/coeliac associations and manufacturers

- Published in Dutch and updated regularly

Phone: 31-33-247-1040
http://www.coeliakievereniging.nl

New Zealand
Manufactured Foods Database

- 30-plus page electronic internet listing of products by category with brand names and specific items

- Available in English

http://mfd.co.nz

I

Spain
Federación de Asociaciones de Celíacos de España
La Lista de Alimentos Sin Gluten

- 300-plus page pocket-sized book listing products by category with brand names and specific items, color coded, with an index

- Published in Spanish and updated annually

Phone: 34-91-713-01-47
http://www.celiacos.org

United Kingdom
Coeliac UK
Gluten Free Food and Drink Directory

- 400-plus page pocket-sized book or online guide listing over 11,000 products by category, brand names and specific items. Also contains a list of stores, respective gluten free items, appendices and index

- Available in English and updated regularly

Phone: 44-1494-437-278
http://www.coeliac.co.uk

United States
Celiac Sprue Association
The CSA Gluten-Free Product Listing

- 375-plus page listing of products by category with brand names and specific items. Contains detailed notes, contact information for 125-plus vendors and products both alphabetically, and by state. Also contains a glossary of common terms associated with celiac/coeliac disease, restaurant cards and guidelines for managing this condition.

- Published in English and updated annually

Phone: 1-402-558-0660
http://www.csaceliacs.org

Clan Thompson™

Clan Thompson™ Celiac SmartLists and Pocket Guides

- Celiac SmartLists are a series of database software programs which make it easy to find gluten information on thousands of items using Windows PCs or Palm handheld devices. The SmartList databases also contains information on regional items, mail order, online and health food store items.

- Celiac Pocket Guides contain hundreds of products from the Celiac SmartList databases. These paper Pocket Guides include foods, over the counter drugs, prescription drugs and everything else fitting right inside your pocket or purse for easy reference during shopping.

- Available in English and updated regularly

http://www.clanthompson.com

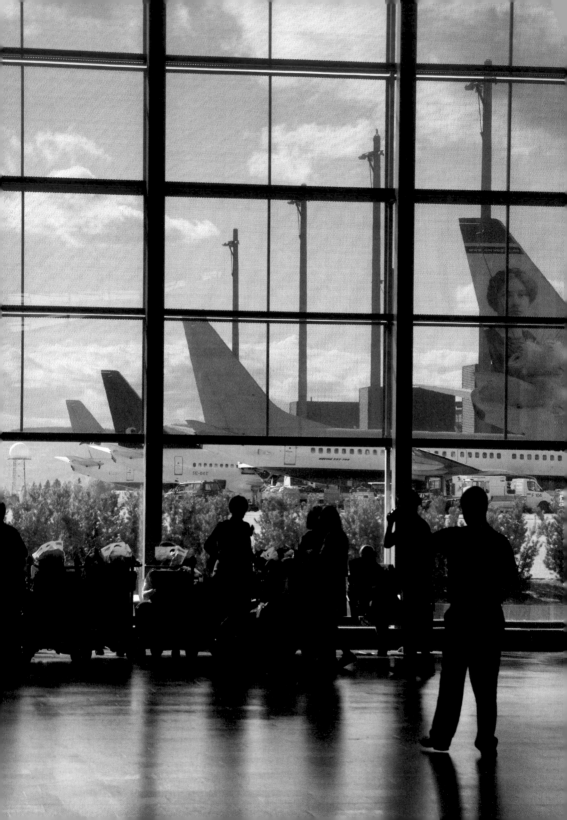

You'll be bothered from time to time by
storms, fog, and snow. When you are, think of
those who went through it before you,
and say to yourself, "What they could do, I can do."
—Antoine de Saint-Exupéry

Appendix II
Global Association and Organization Listings

Appendix Overview

The following global listings provide you with points of reference for supplemental information about eating outside the home and traveling around the world. These listings represent three categories of organizations which may be useful to you while at home or on the road and include:

- 80-plus food allergy associations and related organizations

- 60-plus celiac/coeliac associations

- 55-plus autoimmune associations and related organizations

Contacting these associations and organizations may benefit you in a number of ways. You may be able to obtain additional educational materials concerning medical considerations, relevant research, newsletters and allowable foods or products. Additional eating and travel related information specific to each association's

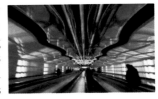

II

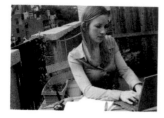

geographic region may also be available. Some of these reference materials are free of charge and others need to be ordered from the respective organization.

You may also be interested in becoming a member of these associations in order to participate in educational conferences, receive regular communications in your areas of interest and access timely medical research findings. We recommend that you contact these organizations directly if you have any questions about their materials, memberships and overall benefits.

These materials have been compiled based upon research and information provided by association professionals as of June 2005. Contact information changes from time to time, so it is recommended that you use this as a guide and refer to the respective website for the most up-to-date information.

Each of the global listings outlines the following contact information when available:

- Respective country

- Organization name

- Telephone number

- Website or email address

Food Allergy Association and Organization Listings by Country

Australia

Allergy Unit: Royal Prince Alfred Hospital
Phone: 61-2-9565-1464
http://www.cs.nsw.gov.au/rpa/allergy

Anaphylaxis Australia Inc.
Phone: 1300-728-000
http://www.allergyfacts.org.au

Australian Society of Clinical Immunology and Allergy (ASCIA)
Phone: 0425-216-402
http://www.allergy.org.au

Belgium

Allergie Preventie
Phone: 32-56-25-89-16
http://www.astma-en-allergiekoepel.be

Astmastichting België vzw
Phone: 32-1-625-31-11
http://www.astma-en-allergiekoepel.be

Fondation pour la Prévention des Allergies
Phone: 32-2-511-67-61
efa.belgium@skynet.be

Bulgaria

Association of Bulgarians with Bronchial Asthma (ABBA)
Phone: 359-2-980-4546
asthma@mail.gb

Association of Patients with Bronchial Asthma
Phone: 359-2-986-2493
simona_ralcheva@abv.gb

Canada

Allergy Asthma Information Association
Phone: 1-416-679-9521
http://www.calgaryallergy.ca/aaia/.ca

Anaphylaxis Canada
Phone: 1-416-785-5666
http://www.anaphylaxis.ca

Association Quebecoise des Allergies Alimentaires Canada
Phone: 1-514-990-2575
http://www.aqaa.qc.ca

Asthma Society of Canada
Phone: 1-416-787-4050
http://www.asthma.ca

Canadian Lung Association
Phone: 1-613-569-6411
http://www.lung.ca

Canadian Society of Allergy and Clinical Immunology (CSACI)
Phone: 1-613-730-6272
http://www.csaci.medical.org

Health Canada
Phone: 1-613-957-2991
   or 1-866-225-0709
info@hc-sc.gc.ca

Osteoporosis Society of Canada
Phone: 1-416-696-2663
http://www.osteoporosis.ca

II

Czech Republic
Czech Initiative for Asthma
Phone: 42-0-22-42-66-229
http://www.cipa.cz

Denmark
Astma-Allergi Forbundet
Phone: 45-4-343-59-11
http://www.astma-allergi.dk

Europe
European Academy of Allergology and Clinical Immunology (EAACI)
Phone: 32-2-640-77-80
http://www.eaaci.org

European Federation of Allergy and Airways Diseases Patients' Association (EFA)
Phone: 32-2-646-99-45
http://www.efanet.org

European Public Health Alliance (EPHA)
Phone: 32-2-230-3056
http://www.epha.org

Finland
Allergia-ja Astmaliitto
Phone: 358-9-473-351
http://www.allergia.com

France
Association Française pour la Prévention des Allergies (AFPRAL)
Phone: 33-1-4818-0584
http://www.prevention-allergies.asso.fr

Fédération Française des Associations et Amicales d'Insuffisants Respiratoires (FFAAIR)
Phone: 33-565-621-371
http://www.ffaair.org

Germany
Deutscher Allergie-und Asthmabund e.V. DAAB
Phone: 49-2161-8149-40
http://www.daab.de

Greece
ANIKSI
Phone: 30-10-6564110
http://www.allergyped.gr

Hungary
MAKIT Hungarian Society Of Allergology and Clinical Immunology
Phone: 36-1-335-0915
http://www.makit.hu

National Society of Asthmatic and Allergic Patients in Hungary (ABOSZ)
Phone: 36-2-63-89-774

Ireland
Asthma Society of Ireland
Phone: 353-1-878-8511
http://www.asthmasociety.ie

Italy
Federasma
Phone: 39-0-574-541353
http://www.federasma.org

Food Allergy Italia
Phone: 3402391230
http://www.foodallergyitalia.org

Lithuania
Association of Allergic Children Clubs
Phone: 370-37-327092

Netherlands
Astma Patiënten Vereninging VbbA/LCP
Phone: 31-26-325-4483
wana@home.nl

Nederlands Astma Fonds AF
Phone: 31-33-343-1212
http://www.astmafonds.nl

Nederlands Anafylaxis Netwerk
Phone: 31-78-639-0356
http://www.anafylaxis.net

Stichting VoedselAllergie
Phone: 31-33-46550
http://www.stichtingvoedselallergie.nl

Vereniging voor Mensen met Constitutioneel
Eczeem (VMCE)
Phone: 31-33-2471044
http://www.vmce.nl

New Zealand
Allergy New Zealand
Phone: 09-303-2024 or 0800-34-0800
http://www.allergy.org.nz

Norway
Norges Astma- og Allergiforbund (NAAF)
Phone: 47-23-35-35-35
http://www.naaf.no

Portugal
Associacão Portuguese de Asmaticos (APA)
Phone: 351-2-2332-6212
http://www.apa.org.pt

Slovenia
Pulmonary and Allergic Patients' Association of
Slovenia DPBS
Phone: 386-1-5616320
http://www.astma-info.com

South Africa
Allergy Society of South Africa
Phone: 27 21-4479019
http://www.allergysa.org

Spain
Asociación Gallega de Asmáticos y Alérgicos
Phone: 34-981-228008
http://www.accesible.org/asga

Sweden
Astma och Allergi Förbundet
Swedish Asthma and Allergy Association
Phone: 46-8-506-282-00
http://www.astmaoallergiforbundet.se

Switzerland
aha! Schweizerisches Zentrum für Allergie,
Haut und Asthma
Phone: 41-31-359-90 00
http://www.ahaswiss.ch

United Kingdom
Action Against Allergy
Phone: 44-20-8892-4950
http://www.actionagainstallergy.co.uk

Allergy UK
Phone: 44-1322-619864
http://www.allergyfoundation.com

Anaphylaxis Campaign
Phone: 44-1252-373793
http://www.anaphylaxis.org.uk

Arthritic Association
Phone: 44-1323-416550
http://www.arthriticassociation.org.uk

II

British Allergy Foundation BAF - Allergy UK
Phone: 44-20-83038525
http://www.allergyuk.org

British Dietetic Association
Phone: 44-121-200-8080
http://www.bda.uk.com

British Nutrition Foundation
Phone: 44-20-7404-6504
http://www.nutrition.org.uk

Food Standards Agency
Phone: 44-20-7276-8000
http://www.food.gov.uk/

IBS Network
Phone: 44-114-272-32-53
http://www.ibsnetwork.org.uk

Medic-alert Foundation
Phone: 44-20-7833-3034 or 0800-581420

National Asthma Campaign
Phone: 44-207-226-22-60
http://www.asthma.org.uk

National Eczema Society
Phone: 44-20-7281-3553
http://www.eczema.org

National Osteoporosis Society
Phone: 44-1761-471771
http://www.nos.org.uk

UK Department of Health
Phone: 44-207-210-4850
http://www.dh.gov.uk

United States
Allergy and Asthma Network-Mothers of Asthmatics, Inc.
Phone: 1-800-878-4403
http://www.aanma.org

American Academy of Allergy, Asthma & Immunology
Phone: 1-414-272-6071
http://www.aaaai.org

American Academy of Dermatology
Phone: 1-847-330-0230
http://www.aad.org

American Board of Allergy and Immunology
Phone: 1-215-592-9466
http://www.abai.org

American College of Allergy, Asthma & Immunology
Phone: 1-847-427-1200
http://www.acaai.org

American Dietetic Association
Phone: 1-800-877-1600
http://www.eatright.org

American Medical Association
Phone: 1-800-621-8335
http://www.ama-assn.org

American Society for Nutritional Sciences
Phone: 1-301-634-7050
http://www.asns.org

Asthma and Allergy Foundation of America (AAFA)
Phone: 1-202-466-7643
http://www.aafa.org

II

Autism Research Institute
Phone: 1-619-563-6840
http://www.autismresearchinstitute.com

Cure Autism Now (CAN)
Phone: 1-323-549-0500
   or 1-888-8-AUTISM
http://www.canfoundation.org

Food Allergy Anaphylaxis Network (FAAN)
Phone: 1-800-929-4040
http://www.foodallergy.org

Food Allergy Initiative
Phone: 1-212-527-5835
http://www.foodallergyinitiative.org

Food and Drug Administration
Phone: 1-888-463-6332
http://www.fda.gov

La Leche League International
Phone: 1-847-519-7730
http://www.lalecheleague.org

Medic Alert Foundation
Phone: 1-888-633-4298
http://www.medicalert.org

National Arthritis, Musculoskeletal and Skin Diseases Information Clearinghouse
Phone: 1-301-495-4484
   or 1-877-22-NIAMS
http://www.nih.gov/niams

National Center for Complementary and Alternative Medicine
Phone: 1-888-644-6226
http://www.nccam.nih.gov

National Heart, Lung & Blood Institute (NLHBI)
Phone: 1-301-592-8573
http://www.nhlbi.nih.gov

National Institutes of Health
Phone: 1-301-496-4000
http://www.nih.gov

Pathways Medical Advocates
Phone: 1-262-740-3000
http://www.pathwaysmedicaladvocates.com

Talk About Curing Autism (TACA)
Phone: 1-949-640-4401
http://tacanow.com

World Allergy Organization (WAO-IAACI)
Phone: 1-414-276-1791
http://www.worldallergy.org

II

Celiac/Coeliac Association and Organization Listings by Country

Algeria
La Maladie Coeliaque, ou Intolerance au Gluten
http://www.ifrance.com/gluten

Argentina
Asistencia al Celiaco de la Argentina
Phone: 54-4292-6373
http://www.acela.org.ar

Asociacion Celiaca Argentina
Phone: 54-221-483-8371
http://www.celiaco.org.ar/uk.asp

Asociacion Pro Ayuda Al Celacio
Phone: 54-351-423-9217

Australia
Coeliac Society of NSW
Phone: 61-2-9411-4100
http://www.nsw.coeliac.org.au

Coeliac Society of South Australia Inc
Phone: 61-8-8365-1488
http://www.coeliac.org.au

Coeliac Society of Tasmania Inc
Phone: 61-3-6344-4279
http://www.coeliac.org.au

Coeliac Society of Victoria Inc
Phone: 61-3-9808-5566
http://www.coeliac.org.au

Coeliac Society of Western Australia
Phone: 61-8-9444-9200
http://www.wa.coeliac.org.au

Queensland Coeliac Society Inc
Phone: 61-7-3854-0123
http://www.qld.coeliac.org.au

Austria
Osterreichische Arbeitsgeminschaft Zoliakie
Phone: 43-1-667-1887
  or 43-1-982-4005
http://www.go.to.zoeliakie

Belgium
B.C.V.- S.M.B.C.
Phone: 32-2-216-83-47

Viaamse Coeliakie Verenigingg
Phone: 32-1623-8964
http://www.vcv.coeliakie.be

Bermuda
Coeliac Support Group of Bermuda
Phone: 1-441-232-0264

Brazil
ACELBRA
Phone: 55-51-333-3000
http://www.acelbra.org.br/2004/index.php

Bulgaria
Bulgarian Coeliac Society
Ms Isadora Zaidner
Pl Slavieikov 9, Sofia 1000, Bulgaria

Canada
Canadian Celiac Association
Phone: 1-905-507-6208
http://www.celiac.ca

Association Quebecoise des Allergies Alimentaires
Phone: 1-514-990-2575
http://www.aqaa.qc.ca

Fondation Quebecoise de la Maladie Coeliaque
Phone: 1-514-529-8806
http://www.fqmc.org

Hamilton Chapter of the Canadian Celiac
Association
Phone: 1-905-572-6775
http://www.penny.ca/Hamilton.htm

Edmonton Chapter of the Canadian Celiac
Association
Phone: 1-780-482-8967
http://www.celiac.edmonton.ab.ca

Chile
COACEL
Phone: 56-2 44-2828
http://www.coacel.prenssam.cl

Croatia
Hrvatsko Drustvo za Celijakiju
Phone: 385-1-664-514
http://www.celiac.inet.hr

Cuba
Grupo de Celiacos de Cuba
Phone: 53-7-91-41-28

Czech Republic
Czech Coeliac Society
Phone: 420-2-8659-0654
http://www.coeliac.cz

Denmark
Danish Coeliac Society
Phone: 45-70-10-10-03
http://www.coeliaki.dk

Estonia
Estonian Coeliac Society
Phone: 372-48-96-824

Farof Islands
Coeliakifclag Foroya
coliaki@post.olivant.fo

Finland
The Finnish Coeliac Society
Phone: 358-3-2541-321
http://www.keliakia.org

France
Association Française Des Intolérants Au Gluten
(A.F.D.I.A.G.)
Phone: 33-1-56-08-08-22
http://www.afdiag.org

Germany
Deutschz Zoliakie-Gesellschaft e.V.
Phone: 49-711-454514
http://www.dzg-online.de

Gran Canaria
ASOCEPA Asociacion de Celiacos
Phone: 34-9-28-859-044

Hungary
Liszterzekenyek Erdekkepviseletenek
Phone: 36-1-438 0233
coeliac@matavnet.hu

Iceland
Samtok Folks meo Glutenopol
Phone: 354-860-3328
magnus@esso.is

Ireland
The Coeliac Society of Ireland
Phone: 353-1-872-1471
http://www.coeliac.ie

Israel
The Celiac Association of Israel
Phone: 972-3-678-1481
http://www.celiac.org.il

II

Italy
A.I.C. Associazione Italiana Celiachia
Phone: 39-50-580-939
http://www.celiachia.it

Associazione Ciliaci Emilia Romagna
Phone: 39-51-391980
http://www.ceserobo.bo.it/celiaci

Latvia
AML Children's Hospital
Phone: 371-7-621330
amlbs@lanet.lv

Lithuania
Lithuanian Coeliac Society
Phone: 370-2-720-270
uvaidas@altavista.net

Luxembourg
Association Luxembourgeoise des Intolerants au Gluten (A.L.M.C.)
Phone: 352-52-02-79
theism@gmx.net

Malta
Coeliac Assocation Malta
Phone: 356-21-370-778
edros@global.net.mt

Mexico
Celiacos Asociacion en Mexico
http://www.celiacosdemexico.com

Netherlands
Nederlandse Coeliakie Vereniging
Phone: 31-33-247-1040
http://www.coeliakievereniging.nl

New Zealand
Coeliac Society of New Zealand (Inc)
Phone: 64-9-820-5157
http://www.mfd.co.nz

Norway
Norsk Coliakiforening
Phone: 47-22-799170
http://www.ncf.no

Paraguay
FUPACEL, Fundacion Paraguaya de Celiacos
Phone: 595-21-61-18-80
http://www.fupacel.org

Poland
Fundacja "Przekreslony Klos"
Phone: 48-22-631-59-14
http://bezgluten.pologne.pl/oferta.php

Portugal
Clube dos Celiacos
Phone: 351-96-32-30-165
eurotema@mail.telepac.pt

Romania
Aglutena Romania
Phone: 40-69-21-76-22

Russia
Saint-Petersburg Coeliac Society
Phone: 7-7-095 -248-1800
http://www.celiac.spb.ru

Slovenia
Slovensko Drustvo za Celiakijo
Phone: 386-2-300-63-50
http://www.drustvo-celiakija.si

South Africa
Coeliac Society of South Africa
Phone: 27-11-440-3431
coeliac@netactive.co.za

Spain
Federación de Asociaciones de Celíacos de España (F.A.C.E.)
Phone: 34-91-713-01-47

II

http://www.celiacos.org
S.M.A.P. Celiacs de Catalunya
Phone: 34-93-412-17-89
http://www.celiacscatalunya.org

Sweden
Svenska Celiakiforbundet
Phone: 46-8-730-05-01
http://www.celiaki.se

Switzerland
Association Suisse Romande de la Coeliakie
Phone: 41-21-796-33-00
http://www.coeliakie.ch

Gruppo Celiachia della Svizzera Italiana
Phone: 41-79-614-0779
http://www.celiachia.ch

Schweizerische Interessengemeinschaft fur Zoliakie
Phone: 41-61-271-6217
http://www.zoeliake.ch

United Kingdom
Coeliac UK
Phone: 44-1494-437278
http://www/coeliac.co.uk

United States
Celiac Disease Foundation
Phone: 1-818-990-2354
http://www.celiac.org

Celiac Sprue Association/United States of America
Phone: 1-402-558-0660
http://www.csaceliacs.org

Gluten Intolerance Group
Phone: 1-206-246-6652
http://www.gluten.net

The American Celiac Society
Phone: 1-973-325-8837
amerceliacsoc@netscape.net

Uruguay
Asociacion Celiaca del Uraguay (ACELU)
Phone: 598-2-902-2362
http://www.acelu.org

II

Autoimmune Association and Organization Listings by Country

Australia

Lupus Australia Foundation
Phone: 03-9650-5348
http://www.lupusvic.org.au

Lupus Association of NSW
Phone: 02-9878-6055
  or 1-800-802-088
http://www.lupusnsw.org.au

Lupus Association of Tasmania
http://www.users.bigpond.net.au/
  lupustas

Multiple Sclerosis Australia
Phone: 02-9646-0600
http://www.msaustralia.org.au

Scleroderma Association of NSW
Phone: 9798-7351 or 1-800-068-061
http://www.sclerodermansw.org

Scleroderma/Lupus Support Society
Phone: 61-2-4294-6146
rossiter@mail.newcastle.edu.au

Scleroderma Assoc of Queensland
Phone: 61-7-5527-0490
info@scleroderma.org.au

Scleroderma Foundation of Victoria
Phone: 61-3-9288-3651
Sclerofv@alphalink.com.au

Australian Crohn's and Colitis Association
Phone: 61-3-9726-9008
http://www.acca.net.au

Belgium

F.A.R.E.S.
Phone: 32-2-51-22-936
http://www.fares.be

Canada

Lupus Canada
Phone: 1-800-661-1468
  or 1-905-513-0004
http://www.lupuscanada.org

Lupus Foundation of Ontario
Phone: 1-905-894-4611
  or 1-800-368-8377
http://www.vaxxine.com/lupus

Lupus Society of Alberta
Phone: 1-888-242-9182
  or 1-403-228-7956
http://www.lupus.ab.ca

Multiple Sclerosis Society of Canada
Phone: 1-416-922-6065
  or 1-800-268-7582
http://www.mssociety.ca

Europe

European Lupus Erythematosus Federation
http://www.elef.rheumanet.org

Hungary

Hungarian Respiratory Society
Phone: 36-1-355-8682
http://www.resphun.com

Norway

Landsforeningen for Hjerte -og Lungesyke LHL (Norwegian Heart and Lung Association)
Phone: 47-22799300
http://www.lhl.no

II

Singapore
Lupus Assocation Singapore
http://www.home1.pacific.net.sg/~lupusas

Switzerland
Lungenliga Schweiz (Swiss Lung Association)
Phone: 41-31-378-20-50
http://www.lung.ch

United Kingdom
Arthritis Research Campaign
Phone: 44-1246 558033
http://www.arc.org.uk

British Lung Foundation (BLF)
Phone: 44-20-7831-5831
http://www.lunguk.org

Diabetes UK
Phone: 44-20-7424-1000
https://www.diabetes.org.uk

Insulin Dependent Diabetes Trust
Phone: 44-1604-622837
http://www.iddtinternational.org

Lupus UK
Phone: 44-708-731251
http://www.lupusuk.com

Multiple Sclerosis International Federation
Phone: 44-20-7620-1922
http://www.msif.org

Multiple Sclerosis Society of UK
Phone: 44-20-8438-0700
http://www.mssociety.org.uk

National Association for Crohn's & Colitis (NACC)
Phone: 44-845-130-2233
http://www.nacc.org.uk

St. Thomas' Lupus Trust
Phone: 44-20-7188-3562
http://www.lupus.org.uk

United States
American Association of Diabetes Educators
Phone: 1-800-338-3633
http://www.diabeteseducator.org

American Autoimmune Related Diseases Association
Phone: 1-586-776-3900
http://www.aarda.org

American College of Rheumatology
Phone: 1-404-633-3777
http://www.rheumatology.org

American Diabetes Association
Phone: 1-800-342-2383
http://www.diabetes.org

American Foundation of Thyroid Patients
Phone: 1-281-855-6608
http://www.thyroidfoundation.org

American Thyroid Association
Phone: 1-703-998-8890
http://www.thyroid.org

Arthritis Foundation
Phone: 1-404-872-7100
   or 1-800-568-4045
http://www.arthritis.org

Barbara Volcker Center for Women & Rheumatic Diseases
Phone: 1-212-606-1000
http://www.hss.edu/departments

II

Center for Arthritis and Autoimmunity
Phone: 1-212-598-6516
http://www.med.nyu.edu/hjd/
rheumatology/arthritis

Chronic Fatigue Syndrome CFIDS Association of America
Phone: 1-704-365-2343
http://www.cfids.org

Crohn's & Colitis Foundation of America
Phone: 1-800-932-2423
http://www.ccfa.org

Diabetes Action Research and Education Foundation
Phone: 1-202-333-4520
http://www.diabetesaction.org

Fibromyalgia Alliance of America
Phone: 1-614-457-4222
http://www.stanford.edu/~dement/
fibromyalgia.html

Indian Health Service National Diabetes Program
Phone: 1-505-248-4182
diabetesprogram@mail.ihs.gov

International Foundation for Functional Gastrointestinal Disorders
Phone: 1-414-964-1799
    or 1-888-964-2001
http://www.iffgd.org

Intestinal Disease Foundation
Phone: 1-412-261-5888
http://www.intestinalfoundation.org

Juvenile Diabetes Research Foundation International
Phone: 1-800-533-CURE
http://www.jdf.org

Lupus Foundation of America
Phone: 1-202-349-1155
http://www.lupus.org

Multiple Sclerosis Foundation
Phone: 1-954-776-6805
    or 1-800-225-6495
http://www.msfacts.org

Myasthenia Gravis Foundation of America
Phone: 1-651-917-6256
    or 1-800-541-5454
http://www.myasthenia.org

National Fibromyalgia Research Association, Inc.
Phone: 1-503-588-1411
http://www.nfra.net

National Institute of Arthritis and Musculoskeletal and Skin Diseases
Phone: 1-301-495-4484
    or 1-877-22-NIAMS
http://www.niams.nih.gov

National Institutes of Health—Office of Rare Diseases
Phone: 1-301-402-4336
    or 1-800-999-6673
http://rarediseases.info.nih.gov

National Multiple Sclerosis Society
Phone: 1-800-344-4867
http://www.nmss.org

National Organization for Rare Disorders
Phone: 1-203-744-0100
    or 1-800-999-6673
http://www.rarediseases.org

National Psoriasis Foundation
Phone: 1-503-244-7404
    or 1-800-723-9166
http://www.psoriasis.org

II

Pediatric Crohn's & Colitis Association
Phone: 1-617-489-5854
http://www.pcca.hypermart.net

Scleroderma Foundation
Phone: 1-978-463-5843
  or 1-800-722-4673
http://www.scleroderma.org

Scleroderma Research Foundation
Phone: 1-415-834-9444
  or 1-800-441-CURE (2873)
http://www.srfcure.org

Sjogren's Syndrome Foundation
Phone: 1-301-718-0300
  or 1-800-475-6473
http://www.sjogrens.org

S.L.E Foundation
Phone: 1-212-685-4118
  or 1-800-74-LUPUS
http://www.lupusny.org

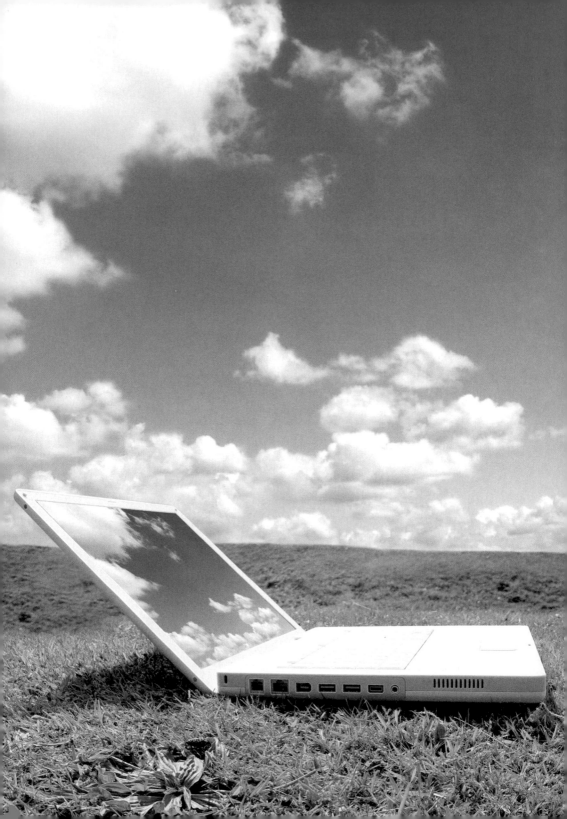

No problem is insurmountable.
With a little courage, teamwork and determination,
a person can overcome anything.
—B. Dodge

Appendix III
Additional Global Resource and Reference Listings

Appendix Overview

The following provide you with additional resources and points of reference for supplemental information about eating outside the home and traveling around the world from food allergy, celiac/coeliac and autoimmune disease perspectives. These include:

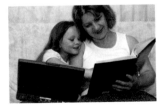

- Helpful websites

- Helpful reading materials

- Contact listings for stores and online websites carrying allergy-free products by country

Helpful Websites

These websites are additional sources of information and are categorized by:

- Food allergies and specialized diets

- Gluten-free lifestyles: chefs, cooking schools, restaurants, and travel information

III

- Gluten-free lifestyles: education and awareness

- Autoimmune disease

These website listings have been compiled based upon research and confirmed as of June 2005. Website links and the associated information may change from time to time.

Food Allergy and Specialized Diet Related Websites

Allallergy.net
http://www.allallergy.net

Allergic Child
http://www.allergicchild.com

Allergic Living Magazine
http://www.allergicliving.com

Allergy Action
http://www.allergyaction.org

Allergy Alerts
http://www.inspection.gc.ca

Allergy/Asthma Information Association
http://www.calgaryallergy.ca/aaia

Allergy Directory
http://www.allergy-network.com/allergyuk

Allergy Induced Autism
http://www.autismmedical.com

The Allergy Site
http://www.theallergysite.co.uk

Asthma and Allergy Information and Research
http://www.users.globalnet.co.uk/~aair/anaphylaxis.htm

Auckland Allergy Clinic Site
http://www.allergyclinic.co.nz

Autism File
http://www.autismfile.com

Center for Food Safety and Applied Nutrition
http://www.cfsan.fda.gov

Certified Allergen Control
http://www.certification-allergies.com

Dietary Intervention for Autistic Spectrum Disorder
http://www.gfcfdiet.com

European Federation of the Associations of Dietitians
http://www.efad.org

Food Allergy & Anaphylaxis Alliance
http://www.foodallergyalliance.org

Food Allergy & Intolerance Center
http://www.allergyhealthonline.com

Food Allergy Center
http://www.nutramed.com/foodallergy/
index.htm

Food Allergy Directory
http://www.food-allergy-info.com

Food Allergy/ Intolerance Site
http://www.foodcanmakeyouill.co.uk

Food Allergy News for Kids
http://www.fankids.org

Food Allergy News for Teens
http://www.fankids.org/FANTeen

Food Allergy Survivors Together
http://www.angelfire.com/mi/FAST

Foods Matter Publication
http://www.foodsmatter.com

Food Standards Agency-UK
http://www.food.gov.uk

Food Standards Australia New Zealand (FSANZ)
http://www.foodstandards.gov.au

Health Canada—Santé Canada
http://www.hc-sc.gc.ca

Lactose Intolerance Site
http://www.lactose.co.uk

Living Without Magazine
http://www.livingwithout.com

Milk Free Kids
http://www.milkfree.org.uk

National Institute of Allergy and Infectious Diseases (NIAID)
http://www.niaid.nih.gov

No Cow's Milk for Me Thanks
http://www.lactoseintolerance.co.uk

Parents of Food Allergic Kids (POFAK)
http://www.kidswithfoodallergies.org/
eve

Peanut Aware
http://www.peanutaware.com

Resource for Autism
http://www.autism-resources.com

Talk Asthma
http://www.talkasthma.com

Talk Eczema
http://www.talkeczema.com

**Trusted Advisor—
Book Recommendations Program**
http://www.chapters.indigo.ca

York Nutritional Laboratories
http://www.yorktest.com
http://www.yorkallergyusa.com

III

Gluten-Free Lifestyle Websites For Chefs, Cooking Schools, Restaurants and Travel

Ballymaloe Cookery School—Cork, Ireland
http://www.cookingisfun.ie

Bel Cibo—Gluten-Free Cooking
http://www.belcibo.com

Bob and Ruth's Gluten-Free Dining & Travel Club
http://www.bobandruths.com

Buona Forchetta—Villa Holidays and Cooking School in Italy
http://www.buonaforchetta.co.uk

Celiac Chicks Web Log
http://www.celiacchicks.com

Celiac Travel Information Site
http://www.celiactravel.com

Gluten Evolution Workshops
http://www.glutenevolution.com

Gluten-Free Cooking School—Arizona, US
http://www.glutenfreecookingclub.com

Glutenfreeda On-Line Cooking Magazine
http://www.glutenfreeda.com

Glutenfreeda Travel Vacations
http://www.glutenfreedavacations.com

Gluten-Free Meal Delivery
http://www.glutenfreemeals.com

Gluten-Free On the Go – UK/Europe
http://www.gluten-free-onthego.com

Gluten-Free Restaurant Awareness Program
http://www.glutenfreerestaurants.org

Gluten-Free Toronto Restaurant Pages
http://www.geocities.com/
glutenfreetoronto

My Chef Megan
http://www.mychefmegan.com

Natural Gourmet Cookery School—New York, US
http://www.naturalgourmetschool.com

Pam's Celiac Kitchen
http://www.celiackitchen.com

The Ruby Range Gluten and Casein-Free Cooking and Lifestyle School—Colorado, US
http://www.therubyrange.com

The Seasonal Kitchen
http://www.theseasonalkitchen.com

Special Eats
http://www.specialeats.com

Travel Professionals International— for Celiac Vacations
http://www.tpiworldwide.com

III

Gluten-Free Lifestyle Websites For Education and Awareness

Association of European Coeliac Societies (AOECS)
http://www.aoecs.org

AOECS Youth-Association of European Coeliac Societies
http://www.aoecs.de.vu

Celiac.com—Celiac Disease & Gluten-Free Resource
http://www.celiac.com

Celiac Disease Center at Columbia University
http://www.celiacdiseasecenter.columbia.edu

Celiac Disease Meetup Groups
http://www.celiacdisease.meetup.com

Celiac Disease Webring
http://www.webring.com/cgi-bin/webring?ring=celiac

Celiac/Coeliac Message Board
http://www.coeliacs.proboards3.com

Clan Thompson's Celiac Site
http://www.clanthompson.com

Club Celiac for Children with Celiac Sprue
http://www.clubceliac.com

Coeliac Awareness
http://www.coeliacawareness.org.uk

Delphi Forums Archive/Listserv
http://www.forums.delphiforums.com/celiac

Dermatitis Herpetiformis Online Community
http://www.dermatitisherpetiformis.org.uk

Gluten-Free Canada
http://www.glutenfreecanada.com

Gluten-Free Diet Resource Guide
http://www.glutenfreediet.ca

GlutenFreedom
http://www.glutenfreedom.net

Gluten-Free Living Publication
http://www.glutenfreeliving.com

The Gluten-Free Page
http://www.gflinks.com

Mayo Clinic GI Center
http://www.mayoclinic.org

National Foundation for Celiac Awareness
http://www.celiacawareness.org

National Institutes of Health (NIH) Consensus
http://www.consensus.nih.gov

NRG Solutions – Allergy Testing
http://www.nrgsolutions.net

Online Magazine for Wheat-Free Diets
http://www.wheat-free.org

Raising our Celiac Kids (R.O.C.K.)
http://www.celiackids.com

III

Savory Palate Press
http://www.savorypalate.com

Stanford University Celiac Support
http://www.celiacsupport.stanford.edu

St. John's Celiac Listerv
http://www.maelstrom.stjohns.edu/
archives/celiac.html

University of Chicago Celiac Disease Program
http://www.uchospitals.edu/specialties/
celiac/index.php

University of Maryland Center for Celiac Research
http://www.celiaccenter.org

Autoimmune Related Websites

American Association for Chronic Fatigue Syndrome
http://www.aacfs.org

Autoimmune Technologies
http://www.autoimmune.com

Best Diet for Multiple Sclerosis
http://www.ms-diet.org

Celiac and Sjögren's Syndrome
http://www.dry.org

Fibromyalgia Network
http://www.fmnetnews.com

Inova Diagnostics Inc.
http://www.inovadx.com

International Scleroderma Network
http://www.sclero.org/isn/a-to-z.html

Juvenile Diabetes Foundation- Local Chapter
http://www.jdf.org/chapters/
homepage.php

National Institute of Diabetes & Digestive & Kidney Diseases
http://www.niddk.nih.gov

National Multiple Sclerosis Society
http://www.nmss.org

Prometheus Laboratories
http://www.prometheus-labs.com

Scleroderma Family & DNA Registry
http://www.uth.tmc.edu

The Thyroid Society
http://www.the-thyroid-society.org

Helpful Reading Materials

Since the focus of this book is on eating outside the home and traveling, related cookbooks have been excluded from the listing below. The following reading materials have been published between 2000 and 2005. These books and magazines are categorized by: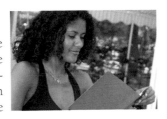

- Food allergies

- Celiac/coeliac disease and gluten-free lifestyles

- Autoimmune disease

Food Allergy Reading Materials

Allergic Living Magazine
Peter M. Wilmshurst, Publisher

The Allergy and Asthma Cure
Fred Pescatore
John Wiley & Sons Inc., 2003

The Allergy Bible: The Definitive Guide to Understanding, Diagnosing and Treating Allergies and Intolerances
Linda Gamlin and
Jonathan Brostoff MD
Quadrille Publishing, 2001

The Allergy Exclusion Diet: The 28-Day Plan to Solve Your Food Intolerances
Alison Edwards
Hay House, 2003

Allergy-free Diet Plan for Babies and Children
Carolyn Humphries
Foulsham, 2004

Allergy Free Naturally
Rick Ansorge
Rodale Press, 2001

Allergy Magazine—UK
Magazine Marketing Company

The Allergy Sourcebook: Everything You Need To Know
Merla Zellerbach
McGraw-Hill, 2000

American Academy of Pediatrics Guide to Your Child's Allergies and Asthma: Breathing Easy And Bringing Up Healthy Active Children
Michael J. Welch MD, American Academy of Pediatrics
Villard, 2000

The Asthma and Allergy Action Plan for Kids
Allen Dozor and Kate Kelly
Simon and Schuster, 2004

Asthma Survival: The Holistic Treatment Program for Asthma
Robert S. Ivker DO and
Todd Nelson ND
Penguin Putnam, 2001

III

Atlas of Allergy
P. Ewan
Parthenon Publishing, 2005

The Bible Cure For Allergies
Dr. Don Colbert
Creation House Press, 2003

Complete Idiots Guide to Food Allergies
Lee H. Freund
Alpha Books, 2003

The Complete Kid's Allergy and Asthma Guide
Milton Gold
Robert Rose Inc, 2003

Cure Your Allergies ... Live Your Life
Martin F. Healy
C.W. Daniel Company, 2004

Dealing With Food Allergies
Janice Vickerstaff Joneja
Bull Publishing, 2003

Earl Mindell's Allergy Bible
Earl Mindell R.Ph., Ph.D
Warner Books, 2003

Food Allergies and Food Intolerance: The Complete Guide to Their Identification and Treatment
Jonathan Brostoff MD and
Linda Gamlin
Healing Arts Press, 2000

Food Allergies: The Complete Guide to Understanding and Relieving Your Food Allergies
William E. Walsh
Wiley Trade Publishing, 2000

Food Allergy: Adverse Reactions to Food and Food Allergies
D. D. Metcalfe
Blackwell Publishing, 2003

The Food Allergy Cure: A New Solution to Food Cravings, Obesity, Depression Headaches, Arthritis, and Fatigue
Dr. Ellen Cutler
Three Rivers Press, 2003

Food Allergy Field Guide: A Lifestyle Manual for Families
Theresa Willingham
Savory Palate, 2000

Food Allergy Relief
James Braly MD and Jim Thompson
McGraw-Hill, 2000

Food Allergy Survival Guide: Surviving and Thriving With Food Allergies and Sensitivities
Vesanto Melina MS, RD, Dina Aronson MS, RD, and Jo Stepaniak MSEd
Healthy Living Institutes, 2004

Food and Nutritional Toxicology
Stanley T. Omaye
CRC Press LLC, 2004

Food Intolerance Bible: A Nutritionist's Plan to Beat Food Cravings, Fatigue, Mood Swings, Bloating, Headaches & IBS
Antoinette Savill
Thorsons, 2005

Get to Know Your Gut: "Everything You Wanted to Know About Burping, Bloating, Candida, Constipation, Food Allergies, and Farting but Were Afraid to Ask"
John Sauers
Marlowe & Company, 2005

Good Gut Guide: Help for IBS, Ulcerative Colitis, Crohn's Disease, Food Allergies and Other Gut Problems
Stephanie Zinser
Harpercollins (UK), 2003

How To Live With A Nut Allergy: Everything You Need to Know if You are Allergic to Peanuts or Tree Nuts
Chad Oh and Carol Kennedy
McGraw-Hill, 2004

Las Alergias
Andrea Wallrafen
Alfaomega Grupo Editor, 2003

Living Without Magazine
Peggy A. Wagener, Publisher

The Parent's Guide to Food Allergies: Clear and Complete Advice from the Experts on Raising Your Food-Allergic Child
Marianne S. Barber
Owl Books, 2001

The Peanut Allergy Answer Book
Michael C. Young
Fair Winds Press, 2001

Sinus Survival: The Holistic Medical Treatment for Sinusitis
Robert S. Ivker
Jeremy P. Tarcher, 2000

Year in Allergy 2004
S.T. Holgate, A. Edwards, S.H. Arshad, C. Venter, and K.S. Babu
Clinical Publishing Services, 2004

Your Hidden Food Allergies Are Making You Fat
Roger Deutsch and Rudy Rivera MD
Prima Lifestyles, 2002

III

Celiac/Coeliac Disease and Gluten-Free Lifestyles Reading Materials

Dangerous Grains: Why Gluten Cereal Grains May Be Hazardous to Your Health
James Braly MD and Ron Hoggan MA
Avery Publishing Group, 2002

Diet Intervention and Autism: Implementing a Gluten Free and Casein Free Diet for Autistic Children and Adults: A Guide for Parents
Rosemary Kessick and
Marilyn Le Breton
Jessica Kingsley Publishers, 2001

Eating Gluten-Free with Emily, A Story for Children with Celiac Disease
Bonnie Kruszka
Woodbine House Inc., 2004

The Gluten-Free Bible: The Thoroughly Indispensable Guide to Negotiating Life without Wheat
Jax Peters Lowell
Owl Books, 2005

Gluten-Free Diet: A Comprehensive Resource Guide
Shelley Case, BSc, RD
Case Nutrition Consulting, 2005

Gluten-Free for a Healthy Life: Nutritional Advice and Recipes for Those Suffering from Celiac Disease and Other Gluten-Related Disorders
Kimberly A. Tessmer
New Page Books, 2003

Gluten-Free Friends: An Activity Book for Kids
Nancy Patin Falini, MA, RD, LDN
Savory Palate Press, 2005

Gluten-Free Living Magazine
Ann Whelan, Editor/Publisher

Going Against the Grain: How Reducing and Avoiding Grains Can Revitalize Your Health
Melissa Diane Smith
McGraw-Hill, 2002

Kids with Celiac Disease: A Family Guide to Raising Happy, Healthy, Gluten-Free Children
Danna Korn
Woodbine House Inc., 2001

Living Well With Celiac Disease: Abundance Beyond Wheat or Gluten
Claudine Crangle
Trafford Publishing, 2002

Lose Wheat, Lose Weight
Antoinette Savill, Dawn Hamilton
Thorsons, 2001

No Grain No Pain: How to Thrive Not Just Survive Living Gluten-Free
Shirley Hartung
Shirley Hartung, 2000

No More Cupcakes and Tummy Aches
Jax Peters Lowell
Xlibris, 2004

A Personal Touch On... Celiac Disease (The #1 Misdiagnosed Intestinal Disorder)
Berlin
Personal Touch Publishing, 2004

III

The No-Grain Diet- Conquer Carbohydrate Addiction and Stay Slim for Life
Joseph Mercola MD with Alison Rose Levy
Penguin Group, 2003

The Ultimate Gluten-Free Diet: The Complete Guide to Coeliac Disease
Pete Rawcliffe
Vermillion, 2004

Waiter, Is There Wheat in My Soup? The Official Guide on Dining Out, Shopping, and Traveling Gluten-Free and Allergen-Free
LynnRae Ries
What No Wheat Publishing, 2005

Wheat-Free, Worry-Free: The Art of Happy, Healthy Gluten-Free Living
Danna Korn
Hay House, 2002

Your Wheat Free, Gluten Free Diet Plan
Carolyn Humphries
Foulsham, 2000

Autoimmune Disease Reading Materials

American Diabetes Association Complete Guide to Diabetes
American Diabetes Association
McGraw-Hill, 2002

Arthritis Survival: The Holistic Treatment Program for Asthma
Robert S. Ivker DO, Todd Nelson ND
Penguin Putnam, 2001

The Autoimmune Connection: Essential Information for Women on Diagnosis, Treatment and Getting on With Your Life
Rita Baron-Faust and Jill P. Buyon
McGraw-Hill, 2004

Autoimmune Diseases and Their Environmental Triggers
Elaine A. Moore
McFarland & Company, 2002

Autoimmune Diseases "The Enemy from Within"
Yehuda Shoenfeld MD and Gisele Zandman-Goddard MD
Bio-Rad Laboratories, 2004

The Bible Cure For Autoimmune Diseases
Donald Colbert
Creation House, 2004

Cfids, Fibromyalgia, and The Virus-Allergy Link: Hidden Viruses and Uncommon Fatigue/Pain Disorders
R. Bruce Duncan
Longman Publishing Group, 2000

Diabetes for Dummies
Alan L. Rubin
For Dummies, 2004

How to Eat Away Arthritis
Laurie Aesoph
Prentice-Hall Press, 2003

III

The Inflammation Syndrome
Jack Challem
John Wiley & Sons Canada, 2003

*Living Well with Autoimmune Disease:
What Your Doctor Doesn't Tell You...That
You Need to Know*
Mary J. Shomon
HarperCollins Canada, 2002

Living with Lupus, The Complete Guide
Sheldon Paul Blau MD and Dodi Schultz
 Da Capo Press Lifelong Books, 2004

Lupus Underground
Anthony De Bartolo
Hyde Park Media, 2004

*Mind-Body Harmony: How to Resist and
Recover From Auto-Immune Diseases*
Dr. Terry Willard
Key Porter, 2003

The Sjogren's Syndrome Survival Guide
Teri P. Rumpf
New Harbinger Publications, 2003

Textbook of Autoimmune Diseases
Robert G. Lahita
Lippincott Williams & Wilkins
Publishers, 2000

*Thriving With Your Autoimmune Disorder:
A Woman's Mind-Body Guide*
Simone Ravicz PhD, MBA
New Harbinger Publications, 2000

*What Your Doctor May Not Tell You About
Autoimmune Disorders: The Revolutionary,
Drug-Free Treatments for Thyroid Disease,
Lupus, MS, IBD, Chronic Fatigue; Rheu-
matoid Arthritis, and Other Diseases*
Deborah Mitchell and Stephen B. Edelson
Warner Books, 2003

*Women and Autoimmune Disease: The
Mysterious Ways Your Body Betrays Itself*
Robert G. Lahita and Ina Yalof
Regan Books, 2005

III

Contact Listings for Stores and Online Websites Carrying Allergy-Free Products by Country

The following listings, by country, reflect a sampling of stores that carry allergy-free products across the globe. These stores encompass both physical brick and mortar buildings as well as on-line websites. The selection of products varies significantly from country to country, store to store and website to website.

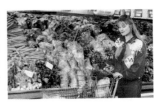

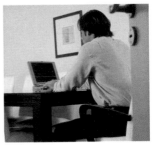

Some are dedicated to allergy and specifically gluten-free products and may have hundreds to thousands of allergy-free foods for purchase. Other stores have dedicated sections with aisles and aisles of allergy-free products, while others provide gluten and allergy-free listings of their products. Many general supermarkets are starting to provide allergy-free products for their customers based upon geographic region. It is acknowledged that this represents a partial listing of available stores worldwide. Depending upon your location, more stores may be available.

This listing gives you a starting point on where to purchase gluten and allergy-free products anywhere in the world while away from home and on the road. Each of the 100-plus store listings outlines the following contact information when available:

- Respective country
- Store name
- Telephone number
- Toll-free telephone number
- Website

These materials have been compiled based upon research conducted as of June 2005. Contact information may change so it is recommended that you use this as a guide and contact the specific brick and mortar or on-line store for the most up-to-date information.

III

Australia
Coles Myer Ltd.
Phone: 61-3-9829-3111
http://www.colesmyer.com

Orgran/Roma Foods Products
Phone: 613-9776-9044
http://www.orgran.com

Woolworths Ltd.
Phone: 61-2-9323-1555
http://www.woolworths.com.au

Belgium
Delhaize
Phone: 32-2-412-21-11
http://www.delhaize.be

Canada
The Big Carrot Natural Food Market
Phone: 1-416-466-2129
http://www.thebigcarrot.ca

El Peto Products Ltd.
Phone: 1-519-650-4614
Toll-free: 800-387-4064
http://www.elpeto.com

Envirokidz Organic Cereals
Phone: 1-604-248-8777
http://www.envirokidz.com

Glutino
Phone: 1-450-629-7689
Toll-free: 800-363-3438
http://www.glutino.com

Kingsmill Foods Company Limited
Phone: 1-416-755-7124
http://www.kingsmillfoods.com

Kinnikinnick
Phone: 1-780-424-2900
Toll-free: 877-503-4466
http://www.kinnikinnick.ca

Kokimo Kitchen
Phone: 1-905-344-7960
Toll-free: 888-344-7977
http://www.kokimokitchen.com

Loblaw Companies Limited
Phone: 1-416-922- 8500
http://www.loblaw.com

Natural Food Mill Bakery
Phone: 1-705-721-0919
Toll-free: 800-353-3178
http://www.naturalfoodmill.com

Northern Quinoa Corp.
Phone: 1-306-542-3949
Toll-free: 866-368-9304
http://www.quinoa.com

Panne Rizo
Phone: 1-604-736-0885
http://www.pannerizo.com

Provigo Inc.
Phone: 1-514-383-8800
http://www.loblaw.com

Specialty Food Shop,
The Hospital for Sick Children
Phone: 1-416-813-5294
Toll-free: 1-800-737-7976
http://www.specialtyfoodshop.com

Whole Foods Market, Inc.
Phone: 1-416-944-0500
http://www.wholefoodsmarket.com

III

Czech Republic
Albert
Phone: 420-323-613-111
http://www.ialbert.cz

Delvita A.S.
Phone: 42-0311609111
http://www.delvita.cz

Denmark
SuperBrugsen
Irma A/S &
Kvickly
Phone: 45-43-86-43-86
http://www.coop.dk
http://www.superbrugsen.dk
http://www.irma.dk
http://www.kvickly.dk

France
Auchan
Phone: 33-3-28-37-67-00
http://www.auchan.com

La Vie Claire
Phone: 33-1-472-67-80 00
http://www.lavieclaire.com

Maison Poetto
Phone: 33-4-91-49-03-77
http://www.maisonpoetto.com

Monoprix
Phone: 33-1-42-82-34-56
http://www.galerieslafayette.com

Naturalia
Phone: 33-1-55-80-77-81
http://www.naturalia.fr

Germany
ALDI Group
Phone: 49-201-85-93-0
http://www.aldi.com

Ireland
Dunnes Stores
Phone: 353-1-475-1111
http://www.dunnesstores.com

Heron Quality Foods Ltd.
Phone: 353-0-233-9006
http://www.glutenfreedirect.com

Superquinn
Phone: 353-1-630-2000
http://www.superquinn.ie

SuperValu (Musgrave Group PLC)
Phone: 353-21-452-2222
http://www.musgrave.ie

Italy
Esselunga
Phone: 39-02-923-671
http://www.esselunga.it

Naturalia
Phone: 39-047-3221012
http://www.naturalia.it

Schär
Phone: 39-047-3293300
http://www.schaer.com

Luxembourg
Cactus
Phone: 39-71-21 - 597
http://www.cactus.lu

III

The Netherlands
Albert Heijn B.V.
Phone: 31-75659-9111
http://www.ah.nl

Laurus N.V.
Phone: 31-73-622-3622
http://www.laurus.nl

Le Poole
Phone: 31-57-127-1702
http://www.glutenvrij-lepoole.nl

Natuurwinkel B.V., De
Phone: 31-0341-565150
http://www.denatuurwinkel.com

PureFood QoLp
Phone: 31-70-317-9065
http://www.purefood.nl

Super de Boer
Phone: 31-52-822-2222
http://www.superdeboer.nl

Slovenia
Interspar
http://www.interspar.at

Spain
El Cortés Ingles
Phone: 34-91-402-8112
http://www.elcortesingles.es

Switzerland
gfShop
Phone: 41-55-442-05-26
http://www.gfShop.ch

United Kingdom
Allergyfree Direct
Phone: 44-128-835-6396
http://www.allergyfreedirect.com

ASDA Group Limited
Phone: 44-113-243-5435
http://www.asda.co.uk

Boots Group PLC
Phone: 44-115-950-6111
http://www.boots-plc.com

Buy Allergy Free
Phone: 44-1803-782956
http://www.buyallergyfree.com

Co-operative Group (CWS) Limited
Phone: 44-161-834-1212
http://www.co-op.co.uk

Dietary Needs Direct
Phone: 44-152-757-9086
http://www.dietaryneedsdirect.co.uk

Glutafin
Phone: 44-122-571-1801
http://www.glutafin.co.uk

Gluten Free Foods Ltd.
Phone: 44-208-953-4444
http://www.glutenfree-foods.co.uk

Gluten Free Foods Direct
Phone: 44-175-763-0725
http://www.glutenfreefoodsdirect.co.uk

Goodness Direct
Phone: 44-871-871-6611
http://www.goodnessdirect.co.uk

Harrods
Phone: 44-207-730-1234
http://www.harrods.com

III

Holland and Barrett Retail Ltd.
Phone: 44-247-624-4400
http://www.hollandandbarrett.com

Iceland Foods PLC
Phone: 44-124-483-0100
http://www.iceland.co.uk

Juvela
Phone: 44-151-228-1992
http://www.juvela.co.uk

Lifestyle Healthcare Ltd.
Phone: 44-149-157-0000
http://www.gfdiet.com

Marks and Spencer Group PLC
Phone: 44-207-935-4422
http://www.marksandspencer.com

Nutrition Point Ltd.
Phone: 44-70-41-544-044
http://www.nutritionpoint.co.uk

Sainsbury PLC
Phone: 44-207-695-6000
http://www.j-sainsbury.co.uk

Somerfield PLC
Phone: 44-117-935-9359
http://www.somerfield.co.uk

Tesco PLC
Phone: 44-1992-632-222
http://www.tesco.com

Waitrose Limited
Phone: 44-1344-424-680
http://www.waitrose.com

Wheat and Dairy Free Supermarket Limited
http://www.wheatanddairyfree.com

Wm Morrison Supermarkets PLC
Phone: 44-1274-494-166
http://www.morereasons.co.uk

United States
Acme Markets
Phone: 1-610-889-4000
http://www.acmemarkets.com

Albertson's Inc.
Phone: 1-208-395-6200
Toll-free: 1-888-746-7252
http://www.albertsons.com

Atkin's Natural Foods Market
Phone: 1-918-663-4137
Toll-free: 1-800-800-3133
http://www.atkins.com

Basha's
Phone: 1-480-895-5396
http://www.bashas.com

Celiac Specialties
Phone: 1-586-598-8180
http://www.celiacspecialties.com

Dietary Shoppe Inc.
Phone: 1-215-242-5302
http://www.dietaryshoppe.com

Dietary Specialties
Toll-free: 1-888-640-2800
http://www.dietspec.com

Ener-G Foods Inc.
Phone: 1-206-767-6660
Toll-free: 1-800-331-5222
http://www.ener-g.com

III

Enjoy Life Foods
Phone: 1-773-884-5070
Toll-free: 1-888-503-6569
http://www.enjoylifefoods.com

Fred Meyer Stores, Inc.
Phone: 1-503-232-8844
Toll-free: 1-800-858-9202
http://www.fredmeyerstores.com

Fresh Fields
Phone: 1-512-477-4455
http://www.wholefoodsmarket.com

Fruitful Yield
Toll-free: 1-800-469-5552
http://www.fruitfulyield.com

Gelsons
Phone: 1-310-638-2842
http://www.gelsons.com

Genuardi's Family Markets, Inc.
Phone: 1-610-277-6000
http://www.genuardis.com

Gluten-Free Mall
Phone: 1-707-537-3011
http://www.glutenfreemall.com

Gluten-Free Market, Inc.
Phone: 1-847-419-9610
http://www.glutenfreemarket.com

Gluten-Free Pantry
Phone: 1-860-633-3826
Toll-free: 1-800-291-8386
http://www.glutenfreepantry.com

Gluten-Free Trading Company
Phone: 1-414-747-8700
Toll-free: 1-888-993-9933
http://www.food4celiacs.com

Gluten Solutions Inc.
Phone: 1-858-292-4564
Toll-free: 1-888-845-8836
http://www.glutensolutions.com

Hy-Vee, Inc.
Phone: 1-515-267-2800
Toll-free: 1-800-289-8343
http://www.hy-vee.com

Jewel-Osco
Phone: 1-708-531-6000
http://www.jewelosco.com

Kroger Company
Phone: 1-513-762-4000
http://www.kroger.com

Miss Robens—Your Allergy Grocer
Phone: 1-301-665-9580
Toll-free: 1-800-891-0083
http://www.allergygrocer.com

Ralph's Grocery Company
Phone: 1-310-884-9000
http://www.ralphs.com

Safeway, Inc.
Phone: 1-925-467-3000
http://www.safeway.com

Shaws Supermarkets, Inc.
Phone: 1-508-313-4000
http://www.shaws.com

Shop by Diet—Natural Health Foods
Phone: 1-630-355-4840
http://www.shopbydiet.com

Special Order Market & Bakery
Phone: 1-630-264-7128
http://www.specialordermarket.com

III

The Stop and Shop Supermarket Company
Phone: 1-781-380-8000
http://www.stopandshop.com

Trader Joe's Company, Inc.
Phone: 1-626-599-3700
http://www.traderjoes.com

Ukrop's Super Markets
Phone: 1-804-379-2233
Toll-free: 1-800-868-2270
http://www.ukrops.com

Wegmans Food Markets, Inc.
Phone: 1-585-328-2550
Toll-free: 1-800-934-6267
http://www.wegmans.com

Whole Foods Market, Inc.
Phone: 1-512-477-4455
http://www.wholefoodsmarket.com

Wild Oats Markets, Inc.
Phone: 1-303-440-5220
http://www.wildoats.com

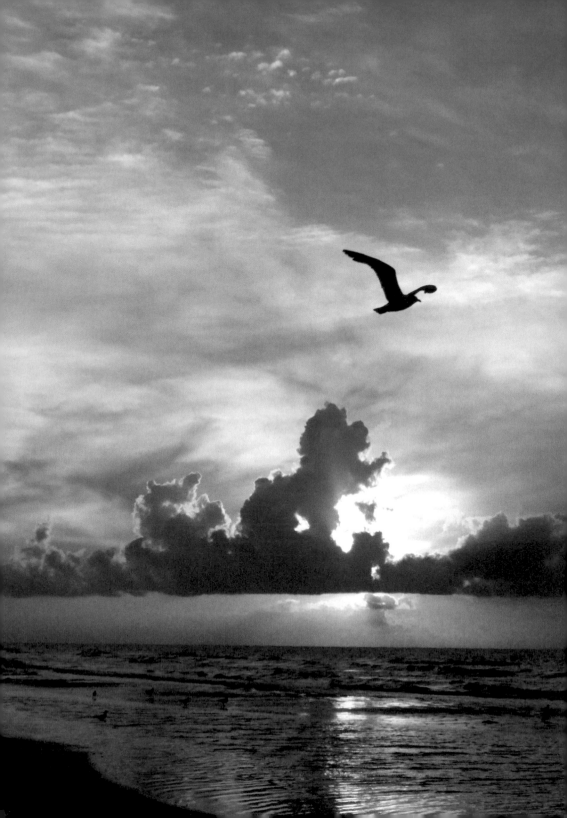

Go confidently in the direction of your dreams.
Live the life you've imagined.
—Henry David Thoreau

Appendix IV
About the Authors and Additional Products

Appendix Overview

The following materials outline additional information about:

- Background of the authors
- AllergyFree Passport™ overview
- Pocket-size cuisine passports

Background of the Authors

Kim Koeller has spent the last 23 years eating 80% of her meals in restaurants across the globe while managing over a dozen food-related allergies/sensitivities and celiac/coeliac disease. Robert La France has spent over twelve years in the restaurant industry and devotes his spare time to a passion for the culinary arts. Collectively, they have traveled over 2 million miles across the globe, dined in 30-plus countries on four continents, and have conversational skills in French, German, Italian, Portuguese and Spanish.

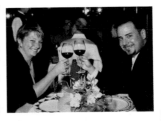

IV

Kim Koeller

Kim has been living with various food allergies and sensitivities for the past 30-plus years. Her food-related allergies include gluten, seafood, dairy, fish, pork, food colorings, food additives/preservatives such as aspartame, monosodium glutamate (MSG), and sodium nitrate. She also has chemical and environmental allergies to ammonia, penicillin, thimersol, chlorox, sodium fluoride, mold, and cat/dog hair and in 2002, was diagnosed with celiac/coeliac disease.

Prior to establishing AllergyFree Passport™, Kim was a partner with Accenture, the world's leading management consulting and technology services organization and spent 75% of her time traveling across the globe. In this role, she worked with Fortune 500 clients delivering sales and service related business solutions on a worldwide basis, has been a keynote speaker and presented at 100-plus US and international conferences to audiences of up to 1000 participants. The combination of Kim's health concerns and her extensive domestic and international travels has provided her with a practical understanding of dining out with special dietary requirements.

She holds a Masters of Business Administration (MBA) degree in International Management from Thunderbird, the Garvin School of International Management and a Bachelors of Arts degree in the French language from Purdue University.

Robert La France

Robert has spent over 12 years in the restaurant industry and has worked extensively with Asian, European and North American cuisines. The spectrum of his professional experience has ranged from small single restaurant operations to large publicly traded companies with 100-plus locations. He has interacted with restaurant guests across many areas of service including: bus boy, food runner, waiter, head waiter, bartender and trainer. Over the past 15 years, he has devoted his time to a passion for the culinary arts. Independent study and cooking sessions with professional chefs have given him a breadth and depth of understanding, as well as a practical working knowledge of most international cuisines.

The combination of restaurant operations and his culinary pursuits has afforded Robert a unique understanding of the impact of living with food allergies. He has witnessed the struggles and anxieties associated with dining out, as his brother has wheat allergies and his close friend has celiac/coeliac disease and other food sensitivities. His experience in the restaurant industry has given him deep insight to guest requirements, fears of cross contamination and hidden allergens in food preparation. From a dining perspective, supporting family and friends and having compassion for restaurant clients with specialized diets has always been an important part of his personal and professional life.

With over twenty years as a professional actor and singer, Robert has extensive media and public performance experience. He has performed for over 1 million people in live theatrical productions, starred in travel programs, films, and recorded voiceovers for radio and television. He attended Arizona State University under a full talent-based scholarship and graduated Cum Laude with a Bachelors of Music degree in Vocal Performance.

Kim and Robert now promote awareness of food allergies and celiac/coeliac disease as President and Executive Vice President respectively of AllergyFree Passport™.

AllergyFree Passport™ Overview

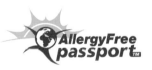

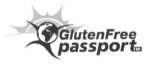

The mission of AllergyFree Passport™ and its affiliates, including GlutenFree Passport™, is to empower individuals with food allergies and specialized diets to safely dine outside the home, travel and explore the world. It is our vision to substantially impact the awareness of food allergies, autoimmune diseases and specifically celiac/coeliac disease. We intend to achieve this vision through our media products and services on a worldwide basis, as well as increase the number of:

- Individuals who safely dine out and travel with food allergies and specialized diets

IV

- Restaurants, hotels, airlines, cruise lines and railroads that offer allergy-free meals as part of their standard menus

- Hospitality, travel and transportation resources that provide allergy-free services

On a worldwide basis, we will:

- Educate the public with food allergies and specialized diets on what to eat and how to order

- Educate professionals in the hospitality and tourism industry about food allergies and special dietary requirements

- Minimize the anxiety associated with eating outside the home and traveling

Our goals for restaurant guests include being able to:

- Communicate their food requirements

- Order allergy-free menu items

- Enjoy local allergy-free meals and delicacies

- Facilitate worry free travel

- Have fun

In addition to the pocket-sized cuisine passports described on the next page, additional media products are under development dealing with specialized diets and travel. Be sure to view our websites for announcements of our new releases. If you would like to be included in our mailing list, obtain information on our consulting and educational services or have feedback, please contact us at:

27 North Wacker Drive, Suite 258
Chicago, IL 60606-2800
United States
Phone: 1-312-952-4900
Facsimile: 1-312-372-2770
info@allergyfreepassport.com
http://www.allergyfreepassport.com
http://www.glutenfreepassport.com

Pocket-Size Cuisine Passports

As part of the *Let's Eat Out!* series, R & R Publishing has also produced pocket-size cuisine passports for your convenience. These light-weight passport-size materials are designed to be carried with you anywhere and anytime. The dimensions of each passport are approximately 3-3/4" by 5-3/8" by ½".

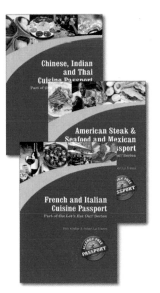

The cuisine passports contain sample menus, item descriptions and preparation requests from each cuisine chapter, as well as the associated quick reference guides. These passports are grouped by the following cuisines:

- *American Steak & Seafood and Mexican Cuisine*

- *Chinese, Indian and Thai Cuisine*

- *French and Italian Cuisine*

An additional pocket-size reference passport is available which includes essential multi-lingual phrases in French, German, Italian and Spanish. To obtain these pocket-size passports or to inquire about special printings, volume discount pricing and foreign rights, please contact us at:

R & R Publishing, LLC.
446 N. Wells Street, Suite 254
Chicago, IL 60610
United States
Phone: 1-312-371-4442
Toll Free: 1-866-564-1440
Facsimile: 1-312-276-8001
info@rnrpublishing.com
http://www.rnrpublishing.com

IV

Common Allergen and Ingredient Index

Due to the proliferation of the common 10 allergens and 65-plus ingredients/ preparation techniques identified throughout this book, only the initial descriptions are listed within this index and are not identified in the *General Index*.

General Index

Due to the proliferation of the common 10 allergens and 65-plus ingredients/ preparation techniques identified throughout this book, only the initial descriptions are listed within the *Allergen and Ingredient Index* and are not identified in this index.